Practical EHR

Electronic Record Solutions for Compliance and Quality Care

Stephen R Levinson, MD

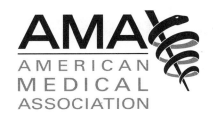

AMA
AMERICAN
MEDICAL
ASSOCIATION

Internet address: www.ama-assn.org

Additional copies of this book may be ordered by calling 800 621-8335 or from the secure AMA web site at www.amabookstore.com. Refer to product number OP 324408.

Library of Congress Cataloging-in-Publication Data

Levinson, Stephen, MD.
Practical EHR: electronic record solutions for compliance
and quality care/ by Stephen R. Levinson.
      p. ; cm.
  Includes bibliographical references and index.
  Summary: "The book focuses on the medical history and physical examination (H&P) feature of
  EHR and effective physician training for its use"—Provided by publisher.
  ISBN 978-1-57947-987-9 (alk. paper)
  1. Medical records—Data processing. 2. Medical history taking—Data processing. 3. Physical
diagnosis—Data processing. I. American Medical Association. II. Title.
  [DNLM: 1. Medical Records Systems, Computerized. 2. Forms and Records Control—methods.
3. Practice Management, Medical. WX 173 L665p 2008]

R864.L48 2008
610.285—dc22

                                                                                    2008009081

ISBN: 978-1-57947-987-9
BP08-P-034

CONTENTS

PART 4: PRACTICE TRANSFORMATION AND HEALTH INFORMATION TRANSFORMATION

Physicians, medical practice administrators, and hospital administrators are all asking critical questions about electronic health records (EHRs):

"Should I get an EHR?"

"Which one should I get?"

"How much will it cost?"

"Will it increase my income?"

"Will it take care of evaluation and management (E/M) coding issues?"

"Will it be faster than what I am using now?"

"How do I know what questions I should ask?"

As I crisscross the United States discussing quality care solutions for E/M documentation and coding, almost every organization includes a meeting with its task force on EHRs. These task forces are exploring the potential for future integration of EHRs into their medical practice or trying to untangle usability and/or compliance issues related to an existing software system.

The need to successfully address these questions requires us to focus on one of the EHR's critical components: the medical history and physical examination (H&P) record and how this component affects physicians and patients at the point of care. This medical record feature and effective physician training for its use are the primary concerns for physicians, the cornerstones for the potential success of EHRs in promoting quality patient care, and the primary focuses of this book.

As the systemic questions raised by physicians and their medical practices are confronted, how easily and comfortably physicians can integrate an electronic H&P record into patient care, a process essential for the success of the EHR, must also be considered. Despite the critical importance of the design and functionality of the medical H&P record for physicians, the medical and compliance requirements for this component of the EHR are rarely mentioned at national policy meetings on health information technology (HIT), and, in many respects, they have not been successfully addressed by software programs currently on the market. The challenge of the transition to EHRs is compounded by the fact that most physicians have lacked compliance training and sufficiently sophisticated medical record tools in their existing paper record environment to achieve the high-quality H&P performance and documentation of their early training years under the time constraints of current medical practice. This lack of an effective paper system and discomfort with current E/M standards further hinder physicians' ability to evaluate their needs for optimal design and function of these new software systems.

Most of the national HIT work groups and task forces dedicated to refining the features of EHRs have focused on interconnectivity, interoperability, Internet security, computerized physician order entry, clinical decision support, and a myriad of other items that depend on optimal use of information already entered into an EHR system. Although all of these issues are unquestionably important, they should not be considered to the exclusion of designing an effective electronic H&P record. This component of the EHR is required to aid physicians in providing high-quality medical care to patients at the point of care and to facilitate efficient and compliant documentation of the care so that the clinical data entered into the EHR system is reliable and meaningful.

Regardless of whether a physician's medical record format is paper or electronic, the H&P record must meet medical practice standards for this powerful diagnostic tool, including the following:

- A structured framework that promotes quality care
- E/M compliance
- Usability and *intuitivity* (a term that describes software designs that match the way physicians have been taught to practice medicine and document their care)
- Efficiency
- Integrity of clinical documentation
- Productivity

HEALTH SYSTEM TRANSFORMATION AND EHR STANDARDS FOR THE MEDICAL H&P RECORD

It was October 23, 2004, during the final day of the first Health Information Technology Summit ("HIT Summit"), when I first noted the discrepancy between the system-wide goals of policy makers who are developing the standards for EHRs and the EHR requirements of practicing physicians working to provide care for patients. This conference sparked my enthusiasm for HIT by highlighting its potential benefits for patient safety, interoperability, and enhancing population health. As a physician, I was also particularly interested in how these software systems address the medical H&P record. All physicians are taught that the H&P diagnostic modality is the most valuable tool for facilitating quality patient care. When I asked one of the conference's physician leaders how I could participate in a work group to develop improvements and standards for the H&P component of EHRs, he responded that there was no such work group and that there had been no consideration that this area was an important issue. In the nearly 4 years since that meeting, I have been drawing attention to the importance of this topic during work group meetings of the eHealth Initiative (eHI) and by presenting this topic at national HIT conferences.

---

eHI

The eHealth Initiative and its foundation are national, "independent, nonprofit affiliated organizations whose missions are to drive improvement in the quality, safety, and efficiency of health care through information and information technology."[1] Its membership includes an entire spectrum of organizations that are working together to promote health care evolution, such as medical organizations (including the American Medical Association); consumer groups; employers and health care purchasers; health plans; HIT suppliers; hospitals; laboratories; pharmaceutical and medical device manufacturers; pharmacies; public health agencies; quality improvement organizations; standards groups; and state, regional, and community-based organizations.[2]

---

[1]eHealth Initiative web site, http://www.ehealthinitiative.org/
[2]Ibid.

Why is it important to develop improvements and national standards for the H&P component of EHRs? A review of the standards currently used to certify EHRs underscores the need to bring attention to the design and functionality of the medical H&P portion of EHRs. The current and proposed criteria of the Certification Commission for Healthcare Information Technology (CCHIT)[3] include 51 measures of interoperability and 264 measures of functionality. Yet, of these 315 measures, none provides direct criteria to fulfill medical H&P standards of E/M compliance, adherence to standardized diagnostic methods, usability, or efficiency.[4] As a consequence, EHR systems may achieve certification without successfully addressing these concerns, even though these capabilities are of critical importance to physicians and fundamental to their ability to document high-quality patient care.

SURVEYING THE CURRENT MEDICAL RECORD LANDSCAPE

Current reports indicate that approximately 15% to 25% of physicians are using some form of an EHR.[5] However, this does not necessarily mean that they are using their systems to record and store medical H&P data, ie, the portion of a patient record that physicians use to document and review patient care. A recent study from the Robert Wood Johnson Foundation reported that "less than one in 10 are using what experts define as a 'fully operational' system that collects patient information, displays test results, allows providers to enter medical orders and prescriptions, and helps doctors make treatment decisions."[3(p1)6] Numerous practices and hospitals use only the laboratory connectivity (ie, electronically ordering studies and/or accessing results), nurses' notes, pharmacy, and/or radiology capabilities of EHRs and they have deferred implementing the medical H&P record. To move forward with this component of the EHR, physicians and administrators must find a set of quality-based *guidelines* that will assist them in achieving a successful "health information transformation." They require an approach that will facilitate the patient encounter, optimize medical outcomes, and provide a high probability of successful EHR implementation, minimal aggravation, and a reasonable and immediate positive return on their investment.

To meet these goals, it is essential to address the finding by coders and compliance experts of significant compliance failures and omissions in the E/M documentation and coding features of existing EHR systems. The severity and urgency of this concern are underscored by the recently published report that:

"The HHS Office of Inspector General (OIG) has drafted what appears to be a preliminary 'National Medicare Fraud Alert,' which alerts federal and state government and law enforcement agencies to the 'use of medical

---

[3]CCHIT was established in 2004, originally as a private sector organization to certify HIT products. The US Department of Health and Human Services awarded CCHIT a 3-year contract in 2005 to develop and evaluate certification criteria and create an inspection process for HIT. (http://www.cchit.org/about/overview.htm)
[4]CCHIT, "Proposed Functionality for 2007 Certification of Ambulatory EHRs"
[5]Robert Woods Johnson Foundation, "Electronic Health Records Still Not Part of Routine Practice," Washington D.C., October 11, 2006, page 1
[6]Ibid, page 1

documentation software programs in a manner that results in the upcoding of Office Evaluation and Management Services.' "[7]

This article also advises medical practices using EHRs to "be careful that your electronic medical records (EMR) software doesn't cause billing of E/M services at higher levels than your providers actually deliver. The potential of such upcoding has attracted the government's attention. . . . You could face recoupments, false claims allegations and civil monetary penalties—even if you inadvertently upcode without any intent to commit fraud."[8] It further cautions against documenting medical charts that appear "cloned." Finally, because many EHR systems currently incorporate E/M coding engines that have noncompliant functionality and fail to address medical necessity, compliance experts have advised practices to "turn off the coding function of EHRs."[9]

Several branches of the federal government are actively advocating the use of EHRs, while the investigative branch is issuing alerts that suggest these same EHRs may promote noncompliance and even false claims. This irony reveals a significant contradiction that has not been adequately appreciated or addressed. If this inconsistency is to be resolved with a positive outcome, software developers, medical practices, and compliance experts must work together. Their task is to supplement current successful EHR functionality for storing and processing data with additional features for physician-friendly H&P record interface designs that reliably facilitate optimal patient care and compliant, individualized medical documentation.

An Old Challenge in a New Package

The challenge creating a medical record design that is easy to use, physician-friendly, and capable of meeting all of today's requirements for efficiency, compliance, and promoting quality care is not new. It is confronted by medical students as soon as they leave the sheltered environment of the second year of medical school, where, armed with nothing more sophisticated than a pen and a blank sheet of paper, they have been allowed 1 hour or more to evaluate each patient and document their care.

Practical E/M[10] explores ways of meeting these same challenges in the world of paper records. It combines the method physicians learn and use to evaluate patients, compliance-based medical record tools, and design features that increase efficiency to optimize the patient care and documentation process. *Practical EHR* explores how to achieve similar solutions in the more complex and potentially more rewarding environment of EHRs.

GOALS

The immediate and long-term goals of this book are to help physicians, medical practices, and all those involved in HIT to:

■ Recognize the value and critical importance of the medical H&P component of EHRs.

---

[7]Vogenitz, Wendy, "EMR & E/M: Beware of Software's Potential to Upcode," Part B News, May 01, 2006 Volume 20, Issue 18.
[8]Ibid
[9]Rappoport, Bruce, MD, "Electronic Health Records, Friend or Foe," Presentation at Annual Conference of American Academy of Professional Coders, April 2006 and April 2007.
[10]Levinson, Stephen R., MD, *Practical E/M: Documentation and Coding Solutions for Quality Patient Care*, AMA Press, 2005.

- Identify individual practice requirements for success with EHRs and develop the criteria and benchmarks that EHR systems must meet to satisfy these requirements.

- Describe a logical and systematic *protocol* that provides medical practices with control over EHR selection, design customization, effective physician training, successful practice transformation, and an ongoing improvement process.

- Define a set of baseline *standards* for the design features and functionality of the medical H&P component of EHRs.

Practical EHR suggests specific, attainable measures for medical H&P record functionality, physician training and transformation experience, positive return on investment, and physician satisfaction. Success in each of these areas is mandatory to create content-rich, individualized medical documentation. Achieving this level of quality data in the electronic H&P record will provide a solid foundation for a system-wide electronic network with interconnectivity, interoperability, and development of evidence-based protocols that can enhance quality and patient safety.

There must also be a reliable transformation model to ensure that medical practices experience a successful transition to EHRs and avoid potentially costly consequences for physicians, patients, and our health care system. Physicians are currently under extreme economic constraint, with only limited time and finite resources to commit to the implementation of EHRs. Therefore, EHRs must help, not hinder, the real-time care of patients and individualized documentation that facilitates quality and continuity of care. In addition to incorporating the long-term health care improvements and efficiencies envisioned by policy makers, administrators, and payers, the progression to EHRs must place medical requirements for the quality care of individual patients first. Now is the time to invest the intellectual resources required to create a predictable, successful, and quality-based electronic H&P standard that fulfills the current, and future, needs and goals of physicians and patients.

SUGGESTIONS FOR USING THIS BOOK

This book is designed as a comprehensive reference on the principles of *Practical EHR*. It focuses on meeting physicians' medical requirements for effective electronic H&P record design and on the protocols for physicians' optimal use of such tools during patient care. The book is organized into four related but independent sections, which allow for structured reading in addition to usefulness as a reference resource. Physicians are encouraged to read the first four parts of the book in the order most appropriate for their current needs.

All readers are encouraged to first read Part 1, which introduces the issues facing medical practices that are involved in investigating or using EHRs. These four chapters highlight the diagnostic process physicians are taught for providing optimal care and they examine the role of E/M compliance as a codification of that process, which can, therefore, be used as a guide for H&P record designs to meet physicians quality care needs.

Most readers will want to read the book in its normal order, continuing directly on to Parts 2 and 3, which explore in depth the potential obstacles that various designs can create for physicians and then consider design solutions that prevent such problems. Practices that are currently beginning their investigations into EHRs may prefer to jump from Part 1 directly to Part 4, which suggests a practice transformation protocol that includes selection of an appropriate transformation team and proceeds through creation of criteria and benchmarks, system selection, physician training, and system verification before implementation. The practice leaders can then focus on Parts 2 and 3 in preparation for this process.

The appendices at the end of the book include a variety of practical tools, ranging from templates for evaluating costs of paper systems and overhead costs to sample templates and to a collection of *Practical EHR* axioms discussed throughout this book. Readers are encouraged to keep a photocopy of the templates in Appendix F on hand for quick reference when reading Parts 2 and 3. In addition, everyone who is involved in the design and use of EHRs are particularly encouraged to review Appendix E, which summarizes the importance of adhering to *Practical EHR* principles to avoid designs and practices that can create potential difficulties with compliance, patient care, and liability issues.

References

1. eHealth Initiative. http://www.ehealthinitiative.org. Accessed March 20, 2007.

2. CCHIT. Proposed Functionality for 2007 Certification of Ambulatory EHRs.

3. Robert Wood Johnson Foundation. *Electronic Health Records Still Not Part of Routine Practice.* Washington, DC: Robert Wood Johnson Foundation; October 11, 2006:1.

4. Vogenitz W. EMR and E/M: beware of software's potential to upcode. *Part B News.* 2006;20(18).

5. Rappoport B. Electronic health records, friend or foe. Presented at: Annual Conference of American Academy of Professional Coders; April 2006 and April 2007. St. Louis, MO and Seattle, WA.

6. Levinson SR. *Practical E/M: Documentation and Coding Solutions for Quality Patient Care.* Chicago, IL: AMA Press; 2005.

Preparing this book has called for investigating solutions that can integrate software's significant potential for enhanced information management with the diagnostic capabilities of the physicians' history and physical. The transition to electronic health records also encourages all of us involved in patient care to consider the future implications of this evolution for the rest of our health care system, ranging from the need to properly prepare medical students and residents to the potential for electronic information exchange among physicians, hospitals, patients, and research organizations.

I want to extend thanks to Michael Beebe of the American Medical Association, whose 2004 request that I write *Practical E/M* expanded my opportunities and created the potential to tackle the "high hanging fruit" of developing an approach capable of synthesizing software technology with the science and art of medicine. Thanks also to my editors Marsha Mildred and Lisa Chin-Johnson, whose efforts help ensure that the language and explanations are realistic and understandable by physicians, administrators, and software developers alike.

Neither this book, nor the concepts that drive it, would have been possible without my wife Barbara. Her questioning and her insights have encouraged workable solutions, and I continue to appreciate her much-needed tolerance of my involvement with health care issues. The benefits of our 1995 discussion of the complexities of the Documentation Guidelines led to the core concept that integrates compliance principles with quality care: when H&P designs incorporate compliance rules into physicians' optimal care process, physicians are able to satisfy documentation and coding requirements while practicing high-quality medical care.

Finally, this book is especially dedicated to my two physician daughters, Randi and Kimberly. In addition to contributing essential real-time insights on how medical schools and residency programs currently address the medical record, they have offered their honest criticism and their encouragement in contributing what time they could manage to help edit this work and make it as meaningful and reader-friendly as possible. Most importantly, their personal passions for providing the best care to patients, and for striving to make our health care system work better for everyone, draws my highest respect and admiration, and it inspires me to continue contributing to solutions for the medical profession.

Stephen R. Levinson, MD, completed his undergraduate and medical education at Johns Hopkins in 1971, followed by specialty training in Head and Neck Surgery at UCLA, which he completed in 1976. He was a member of a private group medical practice in Connecticut for 26 years. Since leaving active medical practice in 2002, Dr. Levinson has continued to dedicate his energies to physicians' concerns, quality patient care issues, and the challenges surrounding the health of our health care system.

Throughout his career, he has participated on numerous medical committees at the county, state, and national medical society levels, working on Medicare issues, quality guidelines, and insurer compliance and reimbursement conflicts.

Dr. Levinson's involvement in E/M coding and documentation began in 1991, when two different medical societies asked that he become one of a small number of physicians to be trained by AMA and HCFA as an E/M coding educator. During the training program, he commented that the proposed E/M training approach would likely create problems for, and resistance from, physicians. In response to this challenge, he worked to develop an E/M protocol and "Intelligent Medical Records" (IMR) paper-based chart tools that make E/M compliance part of physicians' optimal patient care process. This effort culminated in the publication of *Practical E/M: Documentation and Coding Solutions for Quality Patient Care* by the AMA Press in 2005. Since that time, in addition to continuing to provide presentations and consultations for physician organizations, he has delivered E/M presentations and webcasts for the American Health Information Management Association (AHIMA) and the American Academy of Professional Coders (AAPC).

Dr. Levinson first explored electronic health records in the mid 1990s, when several software companies requested his input concerning E/M compliance. This gave him an opportunity to examine not only the compliance issues associated with electronic H&P designs, but also the challenges the electronic format could create for usability and for recording meaningful clinical information. In 2003 he began to develop workable solutions to these compliance and quality care challenges, starting with adapting and enhancing *Practical E/M* principles and IMR designs to fit the electronic format. During the ensuing four years, he also contributed to work groups of the eHealth Initiative (www.ehealthinitiative.org), a Washington, DC-based organization whose mission is to improve the quality and safety of health care through health information technology (HIT). This effort provided the opportunity to have discussions with national leaders in HIT and to present concepts on design requirements for future EHRs at several national Health Information Technology Summits. This focus on meeting all of physicians' electronic H&P needs by combining successful EHR design with effective physician preparation has come together in *Practical EHR*.

Introduction: *The Highway to Health Care Evolution*

The goal of the public and private movement for system-wide implementation of electronic health records (EHRs) is the creation of an interconnected and interoperable national health information network (NHIN, or "highway"). Like our national Interstate highway system for interconnected transportation, system-wide implementation of EHRs is intended to provide an efficient and effective route for communication of health information. The vision for Interstate highways was the creation of an infrastructure capable of moving more people to more destinations with greater efficiency, fewer twists and turns along the route, and less risk of getting lost along the way. Similarly, the vision driving the movement to create an EHR infrastructure is to promote our population's health, increase patient safety, reduce duplication of testing and treatments, prevent medical errors, and increase cost-effective health care provision.

Lessons From the Creation of the National Interstate Highway System

One of the benefits of working with a transportation metaphor is the real-world model for successful development of such a national network and for appreciating the benefits of that accomplishment that it provides. In the 1950s, the creation of our national Interstate highway system was a centerpiece of President Eisenhower's 8-year presidency. The creation of this transportation network encountered significant development, design, financial, and political hurdles. However, as described by Cox and Love[1] in their 1998 book, *The Best Investment a Nation Ever Made,* the significant benefits of this effort continue today.

"Without a first class system of Interstate highways, life in America would be far different—it would be more risky, less prosperous, and lacking in the efficiency and comfort that Americans now enjoy and take for granted."[1(p1)]

This book concludes that "The Dwight D. Eisenhower System of Interstate and Defense Highways, in place and celebrating its 40th anniversary, must surely be the best investment a nation ever made. Consider this:

- It has enriched the quality of life for virtually every American.
- It has saved the lives of at least 187,000 people.
- It has prevented injuries to nearly 12 million people.
- It has returned more than $6 in economic productivity for each $1 it cost.
- It has positioned the nation for improved international competitiveness.

continued

- It has permitted the cherished freedom of personal mobility to flourish.
- It has enhanced international security."[1(p1)]

Clearly, physicians, software developers, health policy advocates, and politicians should be willing to invest the effort required to achieve a similar level of success for an NHIN (highway).

The report of the Institute of Medicine (IOM), *Crossing the Quality Chasm*,[2] released in 2001, described the implementation of EHRs as a critical first step on the journey to improving our medical system and preparing to get to the other side of a documented gap in health care quality. Specifically, the IOM concluded that EHRs are required to build the infrastructure for a new set of systems and tools that will promote health care advances.

The publication of this pioneering report identifying a system-wide quality chasm also, I believe, marked the first stage of the development of a previously unrecognized *electronic chasm*. This is a significant gap in the electronic highway, which physicians, administrators, and software designers must cross together when transitioning from the traditional paper-based documentation system to an electronic system, before more sophisticated systems can be successfully integrated into our health care structure as a whole.

Practical EHR is dedicated to defining and bridging this electronic chasm and ensuring that skilled physicians have optimal medical record tools that help them provide high-quality diagnostic and therapeutic medical insights for patients at the point of care. Achieving these goals will be critical for the treatment of individual patients and for ensuring that the data entered into the clinical record will be as reliable, accurate, and complete as possible. Other health care providers and the greater medical community also require high-quality individualized documentation in medical records for patient care, outcomes research, and future health advancements. To accomplish this, *Practical EHR* calls for electronic history and physical examination (H&P) record design and functionality that helps physicians to record care easily, accurately, and efficiently, including a thorough description of diagnostic considerations and management options. *Practical EHR* also emphasizes that designs for EHRs must facilitate *compliant* H&P methods as an integral component of providing optimal patient care.

Data Integrity and Data Integration

The electronic H&P record is the clinical foundation of the medical record, and there must be clinical integrity of this information *before* it is shared. Because there is currently a significant variation in the quality of H&P documentation in paper and existing EHRs, EHRs must introduce designs and guidance that meet recognized standards for *compliant* clinical documentation. This will ensure that the documented history, evaluation, and course of management can be relied on as records are shared throughout the health care system.

Medical practices find this electronic transition difficult. They need a "health information transformation" roadmap to guide them from their present paperbound H&P approach to an electronic approach. This approach will provide a logical and systematic analysis of practice needs, development of criteria for EHR selection and customization, physician training for optimal use of enhanced records, and performance trials with benchmarks to ensure success.

A FRESH FOCUS

Most current discussions, publications, and national meetings address how the various components of our health care system can use data that have already been stored electronically: the benefits of medical practices transmitting stored electronic information to various external sites (such as distant practice locations, laboratories, and pharmacies) and receiving electronic data (such as laboratory results, radiographic images, and guidelines for clinical decision support) from outside sources. However, these discussions generally presume that all data that have been entered into EHRs, including the medical H&P data, are complete and fully reliable. However, with regard to the focus on the H&P record, examination reveals that many software designs fail to ensure that this is the case, and others create barriers to thorough, individualized H&P documentation.

The H&P record is critically important to physicians who want to provide the best patient care. Not only should the medical chart reflect the care provided, it should also facilitate and guide the ability of physicians to provide care. As they explore the introduction of EHRs, medical practices need to be in control of the selection and implementation processes. They need to know not only how to evaluate the software available for the H&P record, but also how to establish standards the designs must fulfill to be acceptable.

Practical EHR, therefore, shifts the focus of EHR evaluation to addressing the core issues that practices must consider to ensure an effective H&P record:

- How physicians (or others) enter clinical data
- What information needs to be entered and by whom
- How the electronic H&P record can best be designed to facilitate entry of these data
- Which interface design is most appropriate for each component of clinical documentation
- How the design and functionality of the electronic H&P record affect patient care

Practical EHR also calls for the application of standards for clinical data entry to ensure the integrity and usability of the recorded information. The quality of this clinical data is responsible for the medical decisions physicians make concerning the subsequent care of their patients; to achieve "quality out," the health care system requires the clinical record to promote "quality in." This new attention to the design of the electronic H&P record highlights the aspect of EHRs that currently presents the most significant challenges for physicians attempting to make the transition to EHRs. It is critical for medical practices to bring these concerns to the attention of EHR system vendors to encourage and compel them to create and implement improvements that will enable successful transformation.

Spotlight on the National Health System—Identifying Systemic Problems and the Quality Chasm

On November 1, 1999, the IOM published its health care report, *To Err Is Human: Building a Safer Health System,*[3] which provided statistics revealing that *health system errors* are the cause of many patient deaths every year. After reviewing two large studies of hospital admissions, one in 1984 and one in 1992, the IOM concluded "Preventable adverse events are a leading cause of death in the United States. When extrapolated to the over 33.6 million admissions to U.S. hospitals in 1997, the results of these two studies imply that at least 44,000 and perhaps as many as 98,000 Americans die in hospitals each year as a result of medical errors."[3] Even the lower estimate exceeded the annual number of US deaths for three of our more notable medical ills: traffic accidents, breast cancer, and AIDS.[3(p26)]

The book created a national sensation. I recall hearing government representatives and news summaries reporting that medical errors were a national epidemic, the equivalent of a fully loaded 747 crashing every day. However, beneath the headlines, this report also pointed out that medical errors are multifactorial, rather than the result of individual events or individual human error. It concluded "Preventing errors and improving safety for patients require a *systems approach* [emphasis added] in order to modify the conditions that contribute to errors. People working in health care are among the most educated and dedicated workforce in any industry. The problem is not bad people; the problem is that the system needs to be made safer."[3(p49)] *To Err Is Human* emphasizes building safer systems that minimize chances for human error. Such an effort clearly requires problem identification and implementation of superior medical *processes* and *tools*.

Merely 16 months later, in March 2001, the IOM released *Crossing the Quality Chasm: A New Health System for the 21st Century.*[2] It is hard to believe that a follow-up report could achieve the stature of the landmark publication *To Err Is Human,* but this book's impact was at least the equal of its predecessor. It built on the previous depiction of medical errors and identified the need for an organized effort to increase the quality of medical care and patient safety throughout the entire health care system. Citing several studies, it reported, "The frustration levels of both patients and clinicians have probably never been higher. . . . Health care today harms too frequently and routinely fails to deliver its potential benefits."[2(p1)] To emphasize the degree of concern and the urgency of reform, it emphasized that "Between the health care we have and the care we could have lies not just a gap, but a *chasm.*"[2(p1)] Once again, an IOM report had spotlighted systemic problems and called for systemic solutions. It recommended the development of health care systems that are "designed to produce care that is safe, effective, patient-centered, timely, efficient, and equitable."[2(p1)]

Pogo

This case of a publication raising nationwide awareness of current technology being part of the current problem harkens back to the impact of Walt Kelly's cartoon "Pogo" on the ecology movement, when he published the picture that ultimately became the poster for "Earth Day" in 1970. The image captured Pogo standing in his home, Okeefenokee Swamp, which was covered with litter. Pogo's insightful summary was "We have met the enemy, and he is us."[4]

The two IOM reports have similarly brought nationwide attention to the shortcomings of a health care system that is fragmented into separate compartments. The present lack of connectivity among various compartments impedes the sharing of patient data, information about disease processes, and advances in diagnostic and therapeutic care.

The Quality Chasm

Crossing the Quality Chasm also emphasized the need to develop and implement new systems designed to *integrate* our fragmented health care system, and it further identified "the critical role of information technology (IT) in the design of those systems."[2(p1)] This summary statement clearly indicated that health information technology (HIT) is the *vehicle that will be used to design the systems* needed to cross the quality chasm. HIT, therefore, assumes the role of the master system required for gathering and sharing medical information. It creates the health information infrastructure that can foster "improvements in safety, effectiveness, patient-centeredness, timeliness, efficiency, and equity."[2(p176)]

The Electronic Chasm

The *electronic chasm* can be characterized by contrasting the critical characteristics that physicians want and need for the medical H&P record with the design features that EHR systems currently provide. This gap widens when contrasting the differences between physicians' perceptions of how their medical record should contribute to patient care with the perceptions of policy makers and payers about the desired and required features of EHRs.

During consultations with medical groups and hospital organizations on medical record compliance and quality care, I frequently ask physicians and administrators to list the reasons they want to purchase an EHR system, ie, What do they want it to do that is new or better for them and their patients than what they are doing now? At HIT meetings, respected public and private policy leaders also present a variety of lists of the goals that HIT must fulfill to help cross the health care system's quality chasm. These have culminated in two Executive Orders on HIT, articulated by President Bush on April 27, 2004, and August 22, 2006. Both sets of lists, from physicians and hospitals on the one hand and the leaders of HIT transformation on the other, demonstrate thoughtful insight and significant goals for improvement. Yet, these two sets of lists *share no common goals.*

What does this mean? At the very least, we have a *chasm* in our *electronic* perception and a pressing need to increase the communication and understanding on all sides: between our leaders—who address the essential vision of improving the process, tools, and quality of the health care system—and physicians and administrators—who must implement the vision and must have it "work" at the *point of care* (the medical environment in which the patient, physician, information system, and administrative system come together to provide patients with the best possible care).

This division in perception is a clarion call to delve more deeply into the issues, practical and theoretical, that are contributing to and widening the electronic chasm. Recognizing and addressing this gap is critical to ensure that the systems being built are themselves designed to help physicians meet standards for quality care and patient safety. Although the national vision and goals for HIT encompass the entire health care system, this evolution can only be successful if it builds on clinical systems that help physicians at the level of providing excellent care to individual patients. Our responsibility as physicians, patients, and participants in the national health transformation process is to promote a heightened sensitivity to the fact that these electronic systems themselves are subject to flaws in design and functionality, just like the health care system we are requesting them to repair. All such flaws must be identified and addressed vigorously so that they do not create a cascade of new problems and unintended consequences that could inadvertently interfere with care and endanger patient safety.

This "healing" process must begin with the creation of an easy-to-use and clinically effective electronic system for quality medical H&P documentation. The medical H&P record is an essential component of providing, and recording, quality patient care. However, creating an intuitively usable electronic system capable of integrating efficient and compliant documentation with high-quality care during patient encounters has proven a difficult challenge for physicians and software developers. With the goal of overcoming this challenge, this book will concentrate specifically on optimizing the design and functionality of the electronic H&P component and creating a transformation model for integrating EHR systems into the clinical aspects of the patient care process at the point of care.

THE BIG PICTURE: A NHIN

In his July 2004 presentation, "Framework for Strategic Action," David Brailer, MD (first national coordinator for Health Information Technology), proposed that one of the goals for overall health system transformation is "interconnecting clinicians so that clinicians can exchange health information using advanced and secure electronic communication."[5] This translates to the goal of constructing of a NHIN, which should enable effective communication among all health care stakeholders. Analysis of this project and its benefits can be facilitated by viewing this effort metaphorically, as the building of a national health information *highway system.*

■   The health information highway must have a solid infrastructure. The hardware and software for connectivity and information exchange must be standardized, safe, and secure and require no more than reasonable maintenance. It must also be designed to accommodate future improvements, technological and medical, without becoming obsolete.

■   Effective "rules of the road" are needed to ensure the safety and security of all who use this highway. Several groups are currently developing national standards for interconnectivity and interoperability, privacy, and secure transmission of data. However, recognition is lacking of the need to include compliance and data integrity *standards* for use of the electronic H&P record. *Practical EHR* advocates the immediate need to address this deficit. It is necessary to incorporate these standards to ensure that the NHIN can successfully share *clinical information* among EHRs designed by different vendors.

■   The vehicles (EHR systems) that will drive on the highway must be built to meet these same H&P record standards. They must provide safety systems (compliance, usability, efficiency, and quality tools) to ensure that the "drivers" (physicians) are able to operate safely while following the rules of the road, ultimately getting the drivers and passengers (patients) safely from their point of origin (health problems) to their destination (improved health and/or quality of life).

■   The drivers need to be educated and skilled. They must know the H&P rules of the road and how to use their new EHR vehicles safely and effectively. Their "driving" skills must be assessed (by performing compliance and quality reviews before and after EHR implementation) to ensure that drivers and their software vehicles function together effectively to meet these H&P standards.

It is critical to recognize that creating this health information highway will require a significant coordinated and cooperative effort, financial resources, knowledge, skill, and commitment. These resources must be mobilized now to avoid starting with an infrastructure that will prove inadequate to support the desired health care improvements. A thoroughfare cannot be built for a horse and buggy and then expected to permit racecars to move easily over the dirt and ruts. A quality infrastructure must be built from the outset, designed to serve all who use the system, to reap the positive benefits in the future.

PROBLEM IDENTIFICATION AND PROBLEM SOLVING

In 1930, John Dewey (the highly respected American philosopher, psychologist, and educational reformer) observed, "a problem stated is well on its way to solution."[6] The first priority, therefore, is to appreciate that the electronic chasm represents an important and multifaceted problem, a challenge that must be successfully defined in order that it can be overcome.

By defining the critical issues that medical practices encounter with transformation to EHRs and that physicians experience using an electronic H&P record at the point of care, this book intends to promote understanding, encourage readers' insights, stimulate consideration of a variety of potential solutions, and, thereby, provide medical practices with control over the process of investigating and adopting an EHR system. It provides tools that each medical practice can use to assess its own circumstances so that it has the ability to evaluate current EHR systems, define customizations needed to meet its clinical needs, properly train its physicians, and be prepared to incorporate future improvements in electronic technology.

I believe that the *Practical EHR* approach can help fulfill the promise of EHRs to provide effective technology that assists physicians in providing the best possible care to patients in a safe and cost-effective medical environment. In so doing, we not only move toward effectively closing the electronic chasm, but also make a significant contribution to closing the quality chasm as well.

References

1. Cox W, Love J. *The Best Investment a Nation Ever Made*. Washington DC. The American Highway Users Alliance; 1998.

2. Committee on Quality of Health Care in America, Institute of Medicine. *Crossing the Quality Chasm: A New Health System for the 21st Century*. Washington, DC: National Academies Press; 2001.

3. Kohn LT, Corrigan JM, Donaldson MS, eds; Committee on Quality Health Care in America, Institute of Medicine. *To Err Is Human: Building a Safer Health System*. Washington, DC: National Academies Press; 2000.

4. Kelly W. "Pogo Earth Day Poster 1970." http://www.pogo-fan-club.org/images/enemy%20low%20dens.JPG. Accessed March 20, 2007.

5. Brailer D. Framework for strategic action. Presented at What is the National Health Information Network (NHIN)? July 2004; http://world.std.com/, goldberg/hhsnhinfaq.pdf. Accessed March 20, 2007.

6. Dewey J. *On Experience, Nature and Freedom. Representative Selection.* Indianapolis, IN: Bobbs-Merrill; 1960.

Surveying Physicians' H&P: Challenges, Tools, and Standards

This section considers the paramount importance of the history and physical examination (H&P) component of electronic health records (EHRs) and the relationships among different levels of intellectual information stored and used in EHR systems. It explores the extraordinary potential for EHRs to promote the diagnostic medical process, the potential barriers blocking the path to fulfilling this potential, and an overview of goals for H&P record design enhancements that can eliminate these barriers and maximize benefits for physicians, patients, and the health care system as a whole.

chapter 1

What Physicians Want: The EHR at the Point of Care

In their presentations on system-wide adoption of electronic health records (EHRs), national health policy leaders focus on improving quality of care, increasing patient safety, and preventing medical errors. They also stress the cost savings that could result because access to patients' complete medical records should eliminate the ordering of "unnecessary tests, unnecessary X-rays, unnecessary doctor visits, and unnecessary hospitalizations."[1]

On the other hand, when physicians are asked to explain why they are considering EHRs for their own practices, they rarely raise these same issues. Most physicians believe that they are practicing high-quality care that protects patient safety, and that the tests, visits, and hospitalizations they personally order are medically (and/or medicolegally) indicated. At the same time, physicians and practice administrators are sensitive to external pressures from political leaders, medical societies, the Centers for Medicare & Medicaid Services (CMS), and/or private insurers for the adoption of EHRs. Although physicians acknowledge the increased convenience of having electronic access to outside medical information (eg, laboratory reports, radiologic studies, and records from hospitals and other physicians), this benefit alone usually does not provide sufficient motivation to justify the effort and cost to their practices. Nevertheless, in further discourse, most physicians who are currently investigating EHRs will raise significant issues that they believe are pertinent to improving the efficiency, quality, and compliance of their own medical practices. However, their reasons for considering purchase of an EHR system are distinct from the goals driving our current national agenda promoting adoption of EHRs.

FIVE MEDICAL PRACTICE PRIORITIES

"What do you want an electronic record to do for your practice that is better than your current system?" is a question that helps initiate discussions about the EHR decision process. This question commonly leads to a fairly extensive discussion, with physicians and administrators generally focusing on five major benefits they want for their practices from an EHR.

Access to Medical Records

For most physicians, the most attractive feature of EHRs is that they offer immediate access to all patient records at all times. Administrators recognize the amount of time and effort their staffs invest in keeping track of (and, all too often, in trying to track down) patients' paper charts. Similarly, physicians acknowledge that caring for a patient without having the medical chart available is a burden and a challenge for themselves and patients alike. Physicians cannot remember the details of every patient visit, and the medical record is critical for awareness of not only test data, but also of each physician's diagnostic thought process, which provides a roadmap for ongoing patient care. The appeal of this capability for real-time access is compounded for physicians whose group works in more than one office setting and for practices in which multiple physicians see the same patient during different visits (a common occurrence in current obstetric practice). In such situations, transporting or transmitting critical information stored in paper charts from one office to another creates an extra burden and increases the risk of misplacing charts among multiple settings.

Another advantage of EHR access occurs after hours, when a physician receives a call from or about a patient. Electronic access to the patient's record helps the physician recall the patient's medical issues and, thereby, provide the most appropriate analysis and response. Similar quality-of-care benefits occur when an on-call physician needs to address concerns from a patient he or she has never seen before.

Lower Cost Than A Paper System

Interestingly, most physicians and office managers have become aware that managing a paper-based medical record system requires a significant and ongoing investment. Yet, when asked for an estimate of the actual cost (eg, "How much does it cost, per physician per month, to run your paper record system?"), few practices have the answer. The breakdown on such costs includes the following:

- Chart materials, such as folders and labels
- Space occupied by actual charts
- Capacity for long-term storage of charts (practices are required to maintain their records for at least 7 years)
- Shredding costs for old charts (a cost that has increased significantly owing to Health Information Portability and Accountability Act requirements)
- Personnel costs

The most significant expense is personnel cost. Although it may initially seem that charts are primarily located, pulled, and returned to the files in association with patient visits to the office, in reality, these efforts in association with patient visits account for fewer than half the number of times that staff actually goes through this cycle. Charts are also pulled for filing laboratory test and X-ray reports, answering patient phone calls, responding to inquiries about specific patients from other sources (eg, other physicians, attorneys, and staff handling workers' compensation claims), and performing in-office tests and services by nonphysician staff (eg, X-rays, electrocardiograms, and stress tests).

Appendix A provides two worksheets for calculating an office's costs of operating its paper storage system. The first worksheet allows staff to track the amount of time spent pulling and refiling charts. The second worksheet combines all the costs and allows the staff to calculate the approximate cost per physician per month.

Costs of a Paper System

Several years ago, the front office staff in one practice tracked the amount of time spent retrieving and refiling charts during a 2-week period and found that this "routine" task required between 10 and 12 staff hours per physician per week. With the costs for materials and office space added in, the total was approximately $1,200 per physician per month in expenses.

However, a group of administrators in a similar specialty thought this estimate was too low. Estimates from administrators range from $1500 to $2500 per physician per month. It is important to note that costs for medical transcription are not included in estimates of costs for storing medical records in paper charts.

Solving the Evaluation/Management Compliance Challenge

Most physicians tend to view Evaluation and Management (E/M) compliance as independent of and disconnected from the patient care process. They therefore approach documentation and coding as an administrative step that is added on after providing patient care. In the current environment, in which E/M compliance is tied to reimbursement and the possible adverse consequences of external audits (by the CMS and private insurers), physicians seek and require a solution for E/M compliance.

An EHR system that can provide an effective and compliant E/M documentation and coding system will offer significant benefits for medical practices. Conversely, systems that fail to meet this requirement, thereby exposing practices to potential financial peril from E/M audits, present a powerful disincentive to their purchase and adoption.

Improved Documentation Efficiency and Enhanced Quality of the History and Physical

Although most physicians do not directly verbalize a concern about the quality of their existing medical record systems, the desire for increasing documentation efficiency and improving the quality and content of the history and physical examination (H&P) process and report reverberates through their questions and concerns about EHRs. For physicians, this means that an effective H&P report design has to guide physicians through the process of obtaining and documenting a high-quality, diagnostic H&P at the point of care. Furthermore, in this regard, some clinicians have specifically voiced concern about automated H&P data entry shortcuts in certain EHRs, which have the potential to compromise the quality of the H&P

Physician Assessment of the Importance of the Electronic H&P Report

Joseph Heyman, MD aptly summarized physicians' priorities for electronic records during his April 2006 presentation at the "Connecting Communities Learning Forum" in Washington, DC. Reflecting on earlier discussions of the value of EHRs for interconnectivity, interoperability, and health information exchange, Heyman emphasized, "the EHR first has to work as a medical record."

---

report by creating documentation that is nonindividualized, or "cloned." Many physicians also legitimately indicate that it is unacceptable if documenting the H&P in an electronic record requires more time than entering similar information into their accustomed paper records.

Improved Practice Productivity

Physicians are extremely concerned about short-term costs, long-term costs, and the potential return on investment for purchase or lease of EHR systems. In the current economic health care environment, which is commonly viewed by medical practices as being severely constricted, most practices are unable to justify significant economic purchases unless such purchases can promise a positive return on the investment.

IMPORTANCE OF ADDITIONAL EHR FEATURES

In addition to their primary requirements for EHRs, it is important to appreciate how physician practices assess the commonly highlighted beneficial features of EHRs, which also, coincidentally, form the centerpiece of interest for the Institute of Medicine book, *Crossing the Quality Chasm*.[2] These benefits include the following:

1. Health information exchange (HIE) between each physician's office and external medical facilities, including interconnectivity and interoperability with clinical laboratories, radiology offices, and pharmacies
2. Regional health information organizations and community health information organizations, providing HIE among multiple physicians' offices, hospitals, nursing homes, hospices, and/or patients' personal health records (as well as interconnectivity with laboratories, radiology offices, and pharmacies)
3. Clinical decision support software, including the following:
   a) Preventive care guidelines with automated recall functionality
   b) Disease management guidelines for common medical conditions
   c) Real-time connectivity to reference sources
4. Data mining capabilities
   a) Identifying patients with specific diagnoses
   b) Identifying patients taking specific medications
   c) Research protocol capabilities, including outcomes and risk management
   d) Functionality to facilitate "pay-for-performance" reporting
5. Communication with practice management software (or integrated systems)

Once these EHR capabilities are pointed out to physicians and practice managers, nearly all agree that they are valuable features that they would want in any EHR system they purchase for their practices. However, most also indicate that these features, however desirable, are not by themselves sufficient to justify the purchase of an EHR system. They are merely the *icing on the cake*. A medical practice investing in a *cake* wants the *icing* with it, but the EHR system must first satisfy all five priority requirements.

A Note on Document Management Systems

Document management systems are computer-based programs that store electronic images of paper and paper-like documents and audio files of dictation in labeled "folders" of each patient's documents. These systems provide immediate access to the images of paper charts, and they eliminate some of the costs of managing a paper-based medical record storage system. However, without enhanced design of paper forms, they fail to address physician needs for compliance, quality charts, and productivity. In addition, these systems could involve significant personnel time and cost for document scanning. Examples of functions of document management systems are the following:

- Scans handwritten paper documents, and saves dictated audio files into labeled patient folders

- Preloads an image of the physician's existing paper record onto the screen of a tablet PC. The physician handwrites notes directly on the screen, and the software saves an image of the handwritten form into labeled patient folders

Both of these designs are intermediate approaches, not true EHRs. By failing to provide for entry of digital information, they lack the potential for HIE, data mining and data management capabilities, and integrated clinical decision support. Because they do not provide the tools needed for crossing the quality chasm, they are not addressed further in this book.

ANALYSIS OF THE FIVE PRACTICE PRIORITIES

The ability to identify the major concerns of medical practices with regard to EHRs is an important first step in understanding a practical approach to the transition from paper records to an EHR system. It is equally important to analyze how the intrinsic characteristics of the electronic format and the designs currently used to accommodate those characteristics affect the ability of EHRs to meet physicians' needs. How EHRs function in real time for practicing physicians can be effectively explored by considering their data storage and retrieval characteristics separately from their data entry characteristics. Excellence in data storage and retrieval is an intrinsic feature of computer systems, whereby all data previously entered or programmed into the software can be accessed, organized, and retrieved, quickly and reliably. It is largely this capability that has aroused much of the enthusiasm by health policy analysts and strategists for EHR systems. Nevertheless, it is the data entry characteristics and requirements of software systems that are creating increased challenges for usability by physicians; for physicians' ability to record compliant, high-quality clinical documentation; and for facilitation of optimal patient care.

Priorities Related to Data Storage and Retrieval Characteristics

The first two listed medical practice priorities (immediate access to records at all times and reducing the cost of accessing records) relate to the proven data storage and retrieval capabilities of EHRs. Consequently, all well-designed EHR systems should fulfill both of these requirements. By transmitting information electronically, rather than by paper documents, EHRs provide immediate availability to patients' records at any office location through access to a computer terminal. With Internet access and secure connections, physicians can also retrieve patients' records from their homes, hospitals, and distant locations, such as at medical conferences.

Priorities Related to Data Entry Characteristics

The remaining three physician practice priorities (E/M compliance, improved quality of the H&P design, and improved practice productivity), which depend predominantly on the data-entry features of electronic records, have presented the most significant challenges to medical practices during their transition to EHR systems. Incorporating design and functionality features capable of overcoming these challenges will be a principal focus of *Practical EHR*.

Medical Practice Priorities and National Health Policy Priorities

Our health care and political leaders must recognize the importance of satisfying all five of the critical medical practice requirements for EHR design, and they should make a concerted effort to ensure that meeting these requirements becomes part of the national health information agenda. The design of EHRs must successfully address physician concerns if a rapid and successful adoption of EHR software throughout the health care system, as currently advocated, is to be achieved. Failure to meet the medical practice needs offers physicians valid reasons to resist adoption of EHRs.

THE HEALTH INFORMATION TECHNOLOGY LEXICON

One of the first challenges physicians encounter in considering EHR systems is understanding the extensive and overlapping terminology applied to various aspects of these systems and the interactions among them. This challenge is compounded by the fact that various authoritative sources commonly apply different definitions to the same terms. Furthermore, as the electronic environment evolves, new terminology is frequently introduced and older terms acquire different shades of meaning. This section does not purport to provide definitive explanations or a comprehensive collection of the current health information technology vocabulary. Rather, it provides an overview of a number of currently used terms so that readers will know how they are used throughout the book. This section also provides additional creative vocabulary that is needed to describe concepts presented in *Practical EHR* that are not included in common EHR descriptions.

General Electronic Record Descriptions

Electronic Medical Record (EMR) and Electronic Health Record (EHR)
EMR and EHR are two terms that are used interchangeably by different members of the medical and information technology communities to describe an electronic version of a physician's typical paper chart. Although there are no universally accepted definitions, it is generally acknowledged that electronic record systems employ digital entry, storage, and retrieval of information to create an electronic version of the physicians' medical record. This includes the clinical history and physical, laboratory reports, X-ray reports, copies of outside medical records, practice-patient correspondence, etc. These systems are searchable and often include ancillary programs for appointment scheduling, clinical decision support, data mining, and/or practice management functions. Nevertheless, some members of the information technology community have advocated

differentiating these two terms. They prefer to use *EMR* to describe fully functional systems whose information remains local, within the medical practice.

Using this classification, EHR is generally applied to systems that have additional features to permit interconnectivity and interoperability with programs and networks outside of a medical practice, such as clinical laboratories, hospitals, radiology offices, and nursing homes. The National Institutes of Health's report on EHRs also cites a definition from the Health Information Management Systems Society (HIMSS) that distinguishes EHR by its capability to "[support] other care-related activities directly or indirectly via interface—including evidence-based decision support, quality management, and outcomes reporting."* Because most electronic records currently available do include these advanced capabilities, *EHR* will be used throughout the book to describe systems that have all or most of these capabilities.

EHR Transformation

Transformation in the EHR context is the process of a medical practice transitioning from an existing paper-based medical record system to an EHR.

EHR Components

Electronic health records can be divided into a variety of components that interact to provide the various operating capabilities of each system. Their prevalence may vary among different systems, but most EHR systems include the majority of these components. Figure 1 illustrates a schematic of the internal and external relationships among various components of EHRs.

FIGURE 1.1

Relationships among the various components of electronic health records and external software systems.

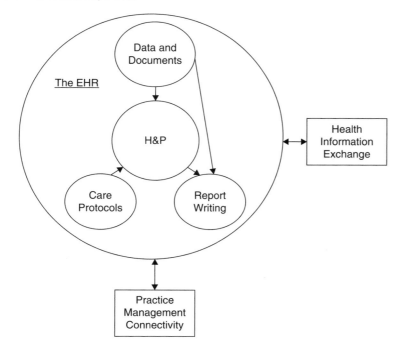

---

*National Institutes of Health National Center for Research Resources. Electronic Health Records Overview. Bethesda, MD: National Institutes of Health National Center for Research Resources; April 2006:5.

H&P Component

The H&P component comprises the longitudinal record of each patient's encounters with the physician. It is the documentation of the care provided, which is the basis of the physician's diagnostic process, and it includes the physician's evaluation of the probable causes of symptoms, the indicated diagnostic tests and treatments, and the ongoing assessment of the course of an illness and its response to therapy. As noted earlier in this chapter, this component is one of the major EHR requirements for physicians. As the foundation of the quality care process, a highly effective and easily used electronic H&P record should be the central feature of all EHRs in the marketplace. However, the inability of this feature to meet physicians' needs seems to be the most common source of failed transformation efforts and the central cause of the "Electronic Chasm," which will be discussed in coming chapters.

The Medical Diagnostic Process

This concept embodies the long-established approach taught to physicians as the ideal method for evaluating patients' problems and developing a valid differential diagnosis. Briefly, it emphasizes the importance of beginning an assessment by obtaining a thorough medical history. While obtaining historical information, the physician begins the process of figuring out a differential diagnosis and also develops an assessment of the severity and urgency of the medical condition. This step is followed by an appropriately thorough physical examination designed primarily to confirm or rule out probable diagnoses; the examination may also detect additional and/or unsuspected abnormalities. Next, the physician weighs the results of any available diagnostic studies against all possible diagnoses. Finally, the physician details his or her thought processes in the documentation of a differential diagnosis, further diagnostic tests, and management options for the patient.

However, it is the EHR components unrelated to the H&P component such as storage and retrieval features, interoperability, and clinical decision support that have drawn the most fanfare and the greatest attention to improving design and functionality. Thus, principal themes of *Practical EHR* include directing the attention of software designers and national policy leaders toward physicians' primary concerns for the medical record, identifying the current problems surrounding the H&P component, and offering realistic solutions.

Data and Documents Component

Just as with conventional paper charts, EHRs must be able to store and retrieve a variety of medical data and documents, including all correspondence related to each patient. How will these materials be entered and stored electronically? Although *scanning* with storage of visual images is an appropriate option for retaining correspondence and other printed documents, advocates for patient safety and cost-effectiveness promote *digital entry* and storage for laboratory diagnostic reports, including clinical laboratory results, radiology reports and images, and physiologic test results (eg, EKGs, stress tests, etc.). Ideally, laboratory data should enter into the appropriate section of each patient's medical record directly from the clinical laboratory facility through the HIE module. Once recorded, not only can the data be visualized by the clinician, but they can also be manipulated, graphed, tabulated, and searched. X-ray reports and images should also be loaded through the HIE module when possible, but these will be stored as digitized images.

Protocol Component

The protocol component of EHRs houses interactive programs that assist physicians with patient management. Typical programs include guidelines for preventive care and disease management. These guidelines are designed to help ensure that patients receive appropriate diagnostic and/or therapeutic interventions in accord with accepted standards of care. Other available protocol software relates to pharmaceutical management, providing the ability to cross-check prescriptions ordered against the stored lists of a patient's current medications and medication allergies to alert the physician of duplication, medication cross-reactivity, and/or potential allergic responses to a prescription.

Reports Component

The report-generating features of the software provide medical practices with the ability to mine digital data and create reports that assist in patient care, practice assessment, support of pay-for-performance protocols, and research projects. Ideally, an EHR system should arrive with preloaded functionality that can search clinical and financial records to compile a variety of standard practice information reports. These reports might, for example, enable a practice to identify lists of patients by specific diagnoses, treatments, medications, age, dates of appointments, laboratory values, and other variables. The EHR software should also provide the practice with the ability to create its own custom reports quickly and easily.

Internal Connectivity to the Practice Management System

Some EHR systems include integrated practice management components, whereas others may require an interface to an independent system. The primary benefit of this connectivity is to reduce or, preferably, eliminate requirements for duplicate entry of patient-related information into multiple software systems. Various analysts have placed different levels of the significance of fully integrated systems. However, only a relatively limited amount of information is shared between EHRs and practice management systems, such as patient demographics, referring physician lists, Current Procedural Terminology (CPT) and International Classification of Diseases, Ninth Revision (ICD-9-CM) codes, and patient scheduling.

Some EHR systems provide this connectivity by attempting to have physicians perform the "charge entry" function electronically, at the point of care, which involves identifying procedure codes and diagnostic codes on one of the EHR screens and then transmitting these data to the practice management system, where it can be used for billing purposes. Although assigning the physician to perform electronic charge entry is an attempt at saving time for the administrative staff, it may increase the physician's time. In addition, it is likely to create a significant compliance problem for these records, as discussed in Chapter 4.

External Interconnectivity and Interoperability (HIE) Component

Electronic heath record systems should have the ability to facilitate interconnectivity and interoperability with external electronic systems, including those of other medical offices, clinical laboratories, radiology facilities, pharmacies, third-party payers, and community and regional health information organizations. The information shared may include data, protocols (outcomes), and documents (eg, the H&P record).

EHR System Connectivity Details

Connecting to Clinical Laboratories

Sharing information between a physician's office and a clinical laboratory must be completed through a secure and standardized interface. There are two primary goals for such communications. (1) *Interconnectivity* allows the medical office to send requests for tests, potentially including diagnostic and/or clinical information. It also allows the laboratory to upload test results directly into the patient-specific sections of the EHR. (2) *Interoperability* adds another level of sophistication to this process by providing feedback between the two systems. It allows the laboratory computer to advise the physician's office if a patient did not have scheduled tests. Similarly, the EHR has the ability to automatically advise the laboratory's computer that the physician received and reviewed the results it had transmitted to the patient's chart in the physician's EHR.

Connecting to Radiology Centers

Just as with laboratory communications, this functionality promotes interconnectivity and interoperability between the physician's office and a radiology facility through a secure and standardized interface. It allows direct transmission of the physician's test orders and clinical patient information to the radiology facility, and it transmits radiology reports and images to the physician's office. Interoperability again allows interactive communication between the requesting physician's office and the radiology office. It provides feedback to the EHR, noting whether a patient arrives for a scheduled test, and feedback to the radiology computer that the physician received and reviewed the results.

Connecting to Pharmacies

Interconnectivity allows transmission of prescription orders from the EHR directly to the patient's pharmacy. Electronic communication eliminates potential problems caused by illegible handwriting, which may cause the dispensing of incorrect medications or instructing patients with incorrect dosages and frequencies. The interoperability feature allows the pharmacy's computer to advise the EHR that the patient has filled or renewed the prescription. It also provides the ability for the pharmacy's computer to notify the physician if a patient does not pick up his or her prescription.

Connecting to Communities

This feature enables interconnectivity among physicians and medical facilities within a geographic region, making it possible for them to electronically share clinical information and medical data. The benefits envisioned for these regional health information networks include providing knowledge of patients' medical conditions, diagnostic studies, and patient care data to other physicians and to public health agencies and medical researchers. This sharing of information also promises to reduce medical costs by decreasing or, ideally, eliminating duplication of services, procedures, radiology studies, and laboratory tests.

National Health Information Network

The goal of a national health information network is to provide connectivity among regional networks. By establishing secure and standardized interface connections among different regions, a national network would permit collection and analysis of data from all areas of the country. In addition, on a practical level, it promises to provide medical facilities with access to a patient's medical information when he or she is traveling.

SUMMARY

Medical practices' priorities when considering the acquisition of an EHR system focus on issues related to the needs of medical practitioners and practices, rather than on global concerns for reduced medical errors, increased patient safety, and decreasing overall medical care expenditures through efficiencies such as reduction or elimination of duplicate services.

Physicians generally agree on the benefits EHRs provide for improved access to their clinical records, which is an intrinsic element of the data storage and retrieval features of EHR software. However, physicians believe that such systems must also promote compliance and should optimize the quality of their H&P documentation. These needs relate to the data entry component of EHRs, which has created significant challenges for physicians, coders, and software designers. We can summarize this concept for physicians as a primary requirement that *EHR systems must be operable and interoperable.* Finally, medical practices look for EHR systems to provide a financial benefit, based on cost savings and a measurable return on investment, rather than an added economic burden. In other words, EHR systems must provide value to a practice, as well as clinical capability.

References

1. Remarks by Tommy Thompson, Secretary of the Department of Health and Human Services, The Willard Hotel, Washington DC; May 6, 2004. www.hhs.gov/news/speech/2004/040506.html. Accessed April 10, 2007.

2. Institute of Medicine (Committee on Quality of Health Care in America), "Crossing the Quality Chasm: A New Health System for the 21st Century." Washington DC: National Academy Press; March 2001.

chapter 2

Surveying the Electronic Chasm, Its Depth, and Its Causes

The extent to which available electronic health record (EHR) systems fail to meet the needs and expectations of physicians and medical practices defines the magnitude of the electronic chasm and our imperative to cross it. Reports in the information technology literature, observations by recognized national authorities, recognized limitations of software systems, and consistent insights from medical practices combine to create a three-dimensional picture of the ongoing challenges that accompany the adoption and use of EHRs. The following four steps are needed to address these concerns: (a) identify the major issues; (b) assess their impact on physicians, patients, and the provision of medical care; (c) evaluate the severity of each problem; and (d) consider a variety of acceptable solutions that can match the needs of different medical practices. Categorizing the challenges to the adoption of EHRs should lead to establishing a set of criteria that these systems must meet to fulfill physicians' accepted medical care standards and, thereby, eliminate the electronic chasm.

CHALLENGE 1: UNRELIABLE IMPLEMENTATION RESULTS

Observation: "Forty percent of all electronic record implementations fail."[1]

At the Second Health Information Technology Summit in 2005, Mark McClellan, MD, then the medical director of the Centers for Medicare & Medicaid Services, expressed concern and dissatisfaction with the fact that a large percentage of EHR system contracts result in failed implementation. That is, following purchase, training, and efforts to use the EHR system in their medical practice, physicians find that the systems are unsatisfactory and cease to use them.

Multiple sources have cited similar failure rates, and many publications and meetings state even higher rates. In April 2006, *CIO Magazine* reported, "The HHS [Health and Human Services] department itself has acknowledged that the failure rate for EHR system implementation is 30 percent to 50 percent. Some health-care network providers claim it is as high as 70 percent."[2] The significance of this problem has also been recognized by David Brailer, MD, PhD, the first National Coordinator for Health Information Technology. In July 2004, he released *The Decade of Health Information Technology: Delivering Consumer-Centric and Information-rich Health Care,*[3] his strategic framework report describing a 10-year national initiative to develop EHR systems and advance the adoption of health information technology (HIT). One of the stated strategies in Brailer's report to increase EHR use in clinical practice calls for using "support systems that reduce risk, failure, and partial use of EHRs."[3]

For *Practical EHR* standards, a failure rate of 40% or greater is unacceptable. Medical practices must invest significant time, expense, and disruption of normal processes when introducing an EHR system. To ask physicians to make this effort while facing a high probability of failure is unreasonable. This risk is compounded by the fact that neither vendors nor policy makers provide medical practices with a warning of the risks or with a guarantee or refund policy that will void a contract and return all invested funds if a system fails implementation owing to design problems, inability to meet physicians' medical requirements, and/or inability to meet reasonable benchmarks agreed on before purchase.

An overview of the failure rate of electronic implementation does not, however, tell the entire story. There is another smaller group of physicians who continue to use their EHRs, despite a low level of satisfaction with their features and their usability. When asked about their level of satisfaction, they unhesitatingly say "I hate my EHR." Further questioning consistently reveals that these physicians have no problems with the data storage features of their systems; instead, their dissatisfaction arises from data entry difficulties related to the features and functionality of the electronic history and physical examination (H&P) component. However, despite this dissatisfaction, many continue to use their systems because they appreciate the immediate access to their records and they are unwilling to throw away the significant financial investment they have made. Reports of such significant dissatisfaction are rare or nonexistent at HIT meetings and in the information technology literature. Yet when the topic is brought up with experts in an unrecorded conversation, none of the participants dispute that dissatisfaction with the H&P component is a significant problem.

EHR Implementation and Marriage

The implementation of EHR systems in the United States has a track record like marriage: it has about a 50% failure rate, but that does not mean that all of the other 50% are happy.

To reduce physician-software incompatibilities, it will be important to include a more constructive "courtship" phase, with physicians and coders defining their EHR design requirements; an "engagement" period, in which physicians conduct actual patient care trials to determine whether software systems meet their established benchmarks; and a possible "prenuptial agreement" to protect medical practice assets in the event of a failed "relationship."

In categorizing physicians who have implemented one of the current EHR systems, there seem to be three types of users, including those who:

- Discarded the system because of failed implementation
- Continued to use a system although it failed to meet many of the physician's important requirements
- Continued to use a system with which they are pleased

Physicians in the third category are critically important because some of them may act as endorsers for their software vendors. Medical practice groups investigating a particular software system should not only speak with these physicians about their EHR experiences, but also should ask to review charts the satisfied physicians created by using their EHR system. Ideally, the medical group should ask the physician to send a series of charts for patients with similar diagnoses, including records of several visits for the same patient. These records should, of course, be de-identified, and they should include a report of the evaluation and management (E/M) code submitted for each visit. This opportunity allows the group's coders (or a coding consultant) and physicians to review these charts. The coders should evaluate the documentation for E/M compliance, code levels compatible with medical necessity, and the possibility that "cloned" documentation fails to record individualized patient findings. The group's physicians should review the charts to determine if they provide meaningful individualized records that clearly define each patient's particular medical history, examination findings, clinical impressions, and management options.

It is important to find the reasons for failed implementations and physicians' reports of dissatisfaction. Physicians who have experienced these problems generally focus their concerns and their criticisms on the challenges they encounter when using the electronic H&P component to assist with patient care and to document patient encounters. Despite the fact that there are multiple EHR products on the market, from the physicians' perspective, most of these systems seem to generate similar obstacles. Identifying the underlying causes for these issues, which will be the focus of Part 2 of this book, should allow the formulation of effective strategies for avoiding them in the future and correcting those problems that already exist.

CHALLENGE 2: REDUCED EFFICIENCY OF ENTRY OF INDIVIDUALIZED NARRATIVE DATA

Observation: "Computer systems cost time on the front end. . . . They only save time on the back end."

The preceding quote, from a software systems analyst, describes one of the challenges of EHR utilization: data entry (the front end) can take additional time, while time savings are realized primarily when the data storage and retrieval components (the back end) are used. When physicians are responsible for entering all clinical information directly into the electronic H&P record, the time physicians spend on the front end (data entry) is increased in exchange for saving staff time on the back end (data storage and retrieval). This result directly contradicts the preference of medical practices to optimize the use of physicians' time for essential clinical tasks and to minimize their clerical responsibilities. Resolving this challenge, by introducing data entry options for EHRs that overcome this barrier and facilitate rapid entry of individualized clinical information, is a central focus of Part 3.

CHALLENGE 3: REDUCED PRODUCTIVITY FOLLOWING IMPLEMENTATION OF AN EHR SYSTEM

Observation: "Physicians implementing an EHR can anticipate a 20% to 30% decrease in productivity for the first 6 to 12 months."[4]

This observation was reported at the First Health Information Technology Summit, in 2004. The data were attributed to a report from the Institute of Medicine in 1997, *The Computer-Based Patient Record: An Essential*

Technology for Health Care,[4] which reported that there are "potential losses of productivity during transition to the system,"[4(p145)] and that, "one cost analysis of the implementation and operation of an automated ambulatory care medical record system found that the cost per patient encounter of a computer-based system was 26 percent greater than the direct costs associated with operation of a manual system."[4(p145)] Although this is an old assessment, published and anecdotal reports from current practices advise that this situation remains largely unchanged. A 2007 article in *Medical Economics* shared feedback on this topic from a small medical practice 3 months after implementation of an EHR system: "it still took Bedi an average of 30 minutes to see a patient, instead of the customary 10 to 15 minutes. As a result, he and Desai together were seeing only a few more patients than the 25 a day Bedi used to see by himself."[5]

In the current financially constricted economic environment, physicians and medical practices cannot afford months of reduced productivity. The questions that must be raised are the following: (1) What are the causes of the reduced productivity associated with EHR implementation? (2) What are the mechanisms that eventually permit a return to normal productivity (if that occurs)? (3) Are these techniques that eventually result in increased efficiency also compatible with physicians' quality and compliance standards? (4) How can we apply these mechanisms from the outset to eliminate the reduction in productivity? These questions are discussed in detail in Chapter 10, along with potential solutions.

Observation: "For outpatient practices . . . approximately 90% of the financial benefit accrues to payers and purchasers, though physicians must make the investment"[6]

This conclusion appears in the excellent 2005 article by Ash and Bates,[6] who reported their analysis of the financial impact of EHRs on physician practices and on our health system. While physicians and administrators commonly expect that improved access to data and increased interconnectivity may translate to an increase in income to cover the cost of their investment, the reality is that most of the anticipated savings from EHR adoptions seem to benefit everyone but the medical practices. It also underscores the fact that lack of a reasonable return on investment for medical practices is often cited as a significant barrier to their adoption of EHRs.

CHALLENGE 4: NONCOMPLIANT E/M DOCUMENTATION AND CODING

Observation: In 2006, the Medicare carrier for Connecticut warned physicians that "EMR software . . . may lead them to 'over document' and consequently 'select and bill for higher-level E/M codes than medically reasonable and necessary.' "[7]

One of the identified priorities of medical practices seeking an EHR system is a solution to E/M documentation and coding challenges. However, as illustrated by the quoted Medicare carrier, the Office of Inspector General, and multiple coding experts, the review of medical charts generated by EHRs demonstrates a significant frequency of noncompliant coding.

Several documentation and coding issues are at the root of this problem. Foremost among these issues is that most of the existing systems provide no assessment or guidance concerning medical necessity, despite the fact that the CMS emphasizes, "Medical necessity of a service is the overarching criterion for payment in addition to the individual requirements of a CPT code."[8] In addition, many of these software systems incorporate design and functionality features that are intrinsically noncompliant, such as the following:

■ Automated entry of clinical information

● Software that automatically inserts pre-composed generic "macros" or copies and pastes identical documentation from previous visits related to the medical history, examination, and/or medical decision making. Although this preloaded information may invite the physician to perform a small amount of modification, eg, typing a few additional words or filling in several blanks from a drop down "pick list," the software automatically pre-enters the majority of information. This functionality eliminates the requirement for physicians to obtain and/or document original information related to the present visit. It documents the software's ability to print the same information in case after case rather than documenting the patient's actual status at the time of the visit. All such preloaded information fails to meet compliance requirements for performing and documenting the patient's status on the date of the visit. It also permits and promotes "problem-focused" care, while using previously recorded information to justify submitting claims for "detailed" or "comprehensive" care, even when these higher levels of care may not have been performed and/or may not be medically necessary.

● Documentation by exception. This type of entry automatically pre-enters (or enters by a single mouse click) default documentation (ie, "negative" answers to a long list of medical history questions or "normal" responses for examination findings). It provides an inaccurate or false record because it indicates that the physician has actually asked the default questions or performed the listed examination elements, when that is not necessarily the case. This type of record lacks *individual* documentation by the physician that he or she actually provided this care. Commonly, such records present uniformly normal medical history responses and negative examination findings in case after case, for every patient and every visit. The only original information usually relates solely to the chief complaint; therefore, compliance review reveals that the care is problem-focused. In addition, this approach generates *comprehensive* levels of history and examination, based primarily on the automatic negative and normal entries. The submission of high E/M code levels occurs even in cases in which such extensive evaluation would not be medically necessary and/or may not actually have been performed. Under either circumstance, documentation by exception commonly leads to submission of inappropriately high-level E/M codes and, therefore, significant issues with compliance.

- Lack of capability for physicians to document all the elements of medical decision making. The *CPT®* manual describes three elements with a total of nine subcomponents of medical decision making. Current electronic H&P software components commonly fail to provide physicians with the ability to document four of these subcomponents (complexity of data, risk of presenting problems, risk of diagnostic procedures, and risk of management options). They also generally fail to help physicians separately document management options recommended and data ordered.
- Software that includes noncompliant coding methods
- Lack of documentation of nature of the presenting problem (the E/M system's measure of medical necessity)

Lack of E/M Compliance Is Not Unique to EHRs

The E/M compliance issue starts with the fact that a high percentage of physicians do not apply compliant documentation and coding principles to their paper records. In fact, audits of paper charts by the Office of the Inspector General during the last 10 years consistently show an error rate of approximately 80% in documentation, coding, and lack of consideration of medical necessity. When working with services that have five possible levels of care, a 20% success rate for coding is no better than random chance.

Therefore, in the past, software developers may not have had a reasonable paper-record model for E/M compliance. They also may not have created designs with the assistance of compliance experts or understood the relationship between compliance and the quality care process that physicians are taught to apply in the medical H&P.

As a result, current practice transformation efforts generally consist of providing physicians who are not E/M compliant with EHR software that contains noncompliant data entry features and/or noncompliant coding calculators. Under these circumstances, it is not surprising that the Connecticut Medicare carrier identified overdocumentation and submission of claims for higher levels of service than are medically necessary.

It is, therefore, critical for medical practices to understand that they cannot rely on EHR systems to "magically" resolve the E/M compliance challenge. Instead, they must address both parts of the issue: (1) training for physicians in using an effective and reliable E/M method and (2) evaluation of potential EHR systems before implementation (preferably, before purchase) to guarantee that they promote and ensure E/M compliance. When medical practices uniformly require E/M compliance as a condition for EHR purchase, vendors will assuredly respond with H&P component designs and data entry functionalities that meet this goal.

CHALLENGE 5: CHARTS WITH RESTRICTED DOCUMENTATION FEATURES CAN COMPROMISE QUALITY OF CARE

"The best HIT system in the world can't be effective without good content"[9]

In her keynote address at the Second Health Information Technology Summit, Carolyn Clancy, MD, director of the Agency for Healthcare Research and Quality, issued the preceding extremely important caution, which highlights the importance of the *data entry* aspects of EHRs. It reminds physicians, consultants, administrators, coders, and vendors of the potential pitfall inherent in all software systems: "garbage in = garbage out."

Leap of Insight

Clancy's concise analysis stands out as being nearly unique. It is one of the only statements that recognizes the pivotal importance of the *data entry* features of EHRs.

In general, HIT conferences and articles spotlight the benefits of EHRs in enabling the immediate availability of medical records, thereby fulfilling one of physicians' primary goals in adopting EHRs. However, it is important to understand that this *data retrieval* characteristic is not the result of sophisticated programming. Rather, this ability is an intrinsic benefit of software programs; they allow users to easily access and retrieve the information that has been entered into them.

In contrast, the creative and distinguishing features of each EHR need to include the ability to organize and mine these data and the ability not only to permit, but also to facilitate the entry of meaningful, individualized, descriptive patient information into the software, ie, high-quality medical H&P documentation.

Clancy's insight is one that all medical practices must put at the top of their EHR necessity list: The data entry features *must* help physicians efficiently provide and document a high-quality (and compliant) H&P. This capability is necessary to fulfill the "operability" requirement summarized in Chapter 1: "the EHR first has to work as a medical record."

All physicians appreciate the value of having optimal *data storage and retrieval* features for their medical records because all have experienced the discomfort of having to care for an established patient when his or her old record is not available, whether the record is "missing" in the office, the patient is being seen in an emergency department setting, or the physician is answering an urgent phone call after hours. Working in the intellectual vacuum of not having patients' medical records available not only deprives physicians of the knowledge of previous *data,* more important, it deprives them of the documentation of previous diagnostic impressions and the thought processes that led to those clinical judgments. Physicians accustomed to using a well-documented chart are also deprived of the recorded treatment blueprint, which lists not only their recommended primary treatments, but also contingency plans if the treatments do not yield optimal outcomes.

Observation: Charts that do not permit or require entry of individualized (ie, narrative) data give the impression of being cloned.

Comments from three physicians, in unrelated practices and using three different EHR systems, summarize the clinical impact of suboptimal data entry features for physicians seeking to provide high-quality care:

- From a physician in a large group practice: "When I review the charts in our EHR, they are all *vanilla.*"
- From a physician in the military health system: "When I read my records [on the EHR], I can't get the *flavor* of the patient."

■ From a physician in an academic center whose department is next in line to convert to the EHR: "When I look at the charts from the department that just converted to our new EHR, I can't tell anything about the medical condition of the patients."

The medical record should be the physicians' most powerful diagnostic tool. Obtaining and documenting the individual course of each patient's illness, the unique examination findings, and the medical decision-making process leading to diagnostic impressions and therapeutic options are the foundation of quality patient care. Software designs that impede an optimal data entry process restrict documentation of medical options and encourage a shortcut approach to clinical care that promotes similar diagnoses and similar care for all patients with similar symptoms. Limiting the extent of data entry by including pre-entered text, limited-vocabulary pick lists, and/or copy and paste functions handicaps physicians' ability to document and, similarly, their ability to perform in-depth inquiries into the individual features of each patients' illnesses. Yet, it is often attention to such details that distinguishes the medical excellence we are striving to achieve from "average" or even sub-optimal care. In other words, data entry shortcuts discourage physicians from providing detailed evaluations and individualized medical care.

Practical EHR underscores an essential data entry prerequisite for any EHR system to be considered operable and capable of promoting high-quality care: the design and function of the H&P component must help physicians obtain and document the essential elements of the H&P in a manner that enables them to carry out the "medical diagnostic process" individualized for each patient and each visit.

CHALLENGE 6: EXCESSIVE TRAINING TIME FOR THE ELECTRONIC H&P COMPONENT

Observation: Physicians and EHR companies commonly report that at least 3 months, and up to 6 months, are needed for physicians to learn to effectively use the H&P component of an EHR.

Physicians and coders experience ongoing difficulty with data entry designs that promote the use of preloaded generic documentation, copy and paste functions, and/or pick lists for the H&P component. Coders recognize that these designs create cloned documents, which fail to meet compliance requirements for individualized documentation specific to each visit. Physicians struggle to fulfill a requirement of creating a standard macro that can fit all patients with each common presenting complaint. Most (fortunately) find this process to be alien to their training, realizing that every patient has unique features and that it is only through obtaining and documenting the unique medical history and detailed examination findings for every visit that they can increase the probability of identifying correct diagnoses and selecting optimal management for each patient.

Physicians are comfortable with the medical diagnostic process they learn early in medical school for performing and documenting a high-quality H&P. Even though the time constraints of the current economic environment have compelled compromises in how most residents and practicing physicians currently document their paper-based medical charts, they all recall the method of performing and documenting a comprehensive H&P.

When provided with tools that permit effective and efficient documentation of the H&P, physicians are able to incorporate such an approach into their patient care with only a brief learning curve.

How Quickly Do Physicians Learn to Use a System Compatible With Their Medical Training?

Experience with the medical records constructed on a foundation of E/M compliance (labeled "intelligent medical records"[10]) in written format (with or without dictation) has consistently demonstrated a brief learning curve for physicians. When record interfaces are designed on the principles of the comprehensive H&P taught in medical school, learning to use them can be analogous to riding a bicycle for the first time in 20 years. Generally, physicians can expect to be using these structured forms comfortably within 1 to 2 hours, with the added benefits of working quickly and having complete E/M compliance.

UNDERLYING CAUSES OF THE ELECTRONIC CHASM

Given the momentum of the movement toward EHRs, plus the reliability and effectiveness of computers for storing and retrieving information in general, we can assume that if current EHR designs were also capable of meeting physicians' requirements for an effective electronic H&P record, these systems would already have been widely and successfully adopted by medical practices. The fact that this has not occurred is evidence that most existing software designs do not adequately meet these needs.

Multiple overlapping factors seem to contribute to the differences between physicians' H&P requirements and the design features of currently available software systems. One of the greatest challenges, experienced by physicians and software designers, is the difficulty reconciling the desire for increased efficiency (ie, speed) of data entry with the requirements to ensure compliance and promote quality care. For physicians, this challenge has its origins during medical school and residency training. Although most medical students are taught how to perform and thoroughly document a high-quality, comprehensive H&P, medical school generally fails to provide tools that enable E/M compliance or *efficient* documentation. As a result, graduating students and residents lack the means to use their H&P skills optimally, under the time constraints of current medical practice environment. "Not only have medical schools failed to incorporate the skills of E/M documentation and coding into their curricula, they have also generally not equipped their students with anything more sophisticated than a pen and a blank sheet of paper as their sole means of collecting and documenting patients' healthcare information. The medical student can obtain and document the comprehensive H&P he or she was taught with this primitive technology, but it requires an inordinate amount of time (as much as 60 minutes per patient)."[10(p19)]

However, as all medical practitioners unfortunately realize, time demands and the economic constraints created by existing reimbursement policies necessitate that physicians perform and document patient care in a maximum of 10 to 20 minutes per encounter. As a result of not being provided with effective and compliant medical record tools during their training, most physicians have unfortunately reacted by deleting significant portions of the comprehensive H&P from their care and/or documentation. This omission can lead to more problem-focused care, even for patients with complex illnesses, and can result in less effective diagnosis, suboptimal treatment, and increased costs, all of which are symptoms of what the Institute of Medicine identifies as the "quality chasm."[11]

Medical Necessity and Compliance

The disconnect between the levels of care documented and the relative severity of patient illness has been fostered by the traditional approach of teaching E/M coding and documentation to practicing physicians that largely fails to take into account the critical element of medical necessity. As a result, the approach has been unsuccessful in providing physicians with a reliable method for achieving compliance. Consequently, most physicians "remain uncomfortable with their coding and documentation skills."[10(pxvi)] Formal E/M audits of their paper records reveal a high percentage of *problem-focused* documentation, even for patients who have high-severity illness that warrants *comprehensive* care.

As a result of their enforced migration away from a high-quality, compliant medical record that is matched to the severity of patient illness, most physicians find themselves unable to define the precise features that should be mandatory in the H&P component of EHRs. They remain unhappy with EHR design features that restrict their ability to document a thorough and individualized H&P, even though they may not recognize that these limitations are a consequence of inadequate functionalities and/or design elements.

Software Design Emphasis

The attention to long-range EHR benefits generated by *Crossing the Quality Chasm*[11] has inspired a *top-down* approach to EHR priorities, putting the spotlight on what happens to data once entered rather than on how the record itself impacts care and the caliber of the clinical information documented. Owing to this widespread attention to EHR's "data out" features, plus the relative lack of demand from medical practices for quality standards for the "data in" features, it is likely that software designers have been unable to appreciate the importance of incorporating E/M compliance and medical necessity parameters into the foundation of the electronic H&P component. As a result, the pressures for increased documentation speed have not been counterbalanced and controlled by standards for compliance and the requirement for individualized documentation for each patient and each visit. Just as current software systems have made significant strides toward improving interconnectivity and interoperability, they must also act on physicians' requirements for a solid foundation design that meets criteria for compliance, usability, promotion of quality care, and data integrity.

PRACTICAL EHR GOALS, REQUIREMENTS, AND STANDARDS FOR SUCCESS

The primary cause of the *electronic chasm* can be localized to the design and functionality of the H&P component of EHRs. Imperfections in this central feature of EHRs can negatively affect the quality of health care that physicians provide and the integrity of the clinical data they are able to record. Our mission is to set goals for eliminating the causes of this chasm and to establish protocols for effective design and successful implementation of the H&P component. The goals to achieve this mission include the following:

1. Implementation success: 100% of EHR implementations should be successful. Ensuring such results requires a shared responsibility and a cooperative effort among physicians, coders, and vendors for design compliance, planning, and physician training.

2. Efficiency success: Design and functionality of EHR systems must facilitate completion of the care and of compliant documentation for a medically indicated *comprehensive* new patient visit (ie, CPT code 99204 or 99205) in *not more than 15 minutes of a physician's time.*

    ■   The 15-minute time factor results from calculating the amount of time being reimbursed for comprehensive E/M care when comparing current Medicare payment for practice expenses with physicians' current true practice costs.

3. Productivity success: There should be no decrease in practice productivity on implementation of an effective EHR system. Ensuring seamless EHR implementation without loss of time or productivity requires not only software that proves to be usable and efficient, but also appropriate planning and training of physicians and administrative staff.

4. E/M compliance success: Electronic health records must incorporate compliance-based design and functionality, thereby guiding physicians to provide and document an appropriate level of care during every medical encounter, based on consideration of medical necessity.

    ■   The design of EHR systems must also eliminate all features that intrinsically allow and/or promote noncompliant documentation.

5. Quality care success: Electronic health records must provide for documentation of free-text narrative descriptions in all sections of the H&P component that require input of *individualized* patient clinical information.

    ■   The design of EHR systems must also eliminate all features that provide preloaded clinical narratives with generic clinical descriptions.

    ■   The record of each medical visit should be patient-specific, visit-specific, coherent, and cohesive. On review of the record, another physician (or an attorney) should easily be able to understand the patient's medical condition, the physician's diagnostic process, and the planned course for subsequent evaluation and treatment, including the ability to identify and characterize the unique symptoms and findings that distinguish each patient from the norm because these may affect treatment choices and/or modify outcomes.

6. Training success and efficiency: For physicians who are well-trained in using an effective paper record, training for use of the basic clinical information input features of a well-designed EHR should require no more than 8 hours of a physician's time for software customization and learning.

> **Reasonable Expectations**
>
> All of these listed requirements and standards for data input features of EHRs (ie, implementation success, efficiency, sustained productivity, E/M compliance, quality care, and rapid training) have been achieved with high-quality paper systems, based on data input by writing, with or without added dictation. Physicians have a right to expect the EHR to be at least as successful. In addition, EHR developers should be able to build on this successful foundation and match or exceed the achievements of paper records.

SUMMARY

The current electronic chasm results from two sources. One obstacle to successful transformation to EHR systems is physicians' general lack of success in meeting compliance principles in their existing paper records. This is combined with a failure of medical software designers to create H&P data entry designs built on principles of compliance, medical necessity, and documentation of *individualized* clinical care.

Implementation of an EHR should meet all of the optimal standards that physicians should apply to introduction of any medical record technology, regardless of its format. These standards include usability, efficiency, E/M compliance, promotion of individualized quality care, and data integrity. In addition, physicians need to be ensured of implementation success and that they will be able to maintain or increase productivity (for physicians who do not currently overcode) without interruption after their practices implement an EHR.

Fulfilling these goals will require a combination of physician training for use of compliant records plus modifications to the design and functionality of the existing electronic H&P record. Software systems must facilitate efficient documentation, while also ensuring E/M compliance, consideration of medical necessity, and promotion of individualized clinical documentation. A cooperative effort among physicians, coders, administrators, and EHR developers is needed to help medical practices achieve a seamless and successful transformation to EHRs.

References

1.   McClellan M. CMS Quality, Efficiency and Value-Based Purchasing Policies: The Role of Health Information Technology Summit. Presented at: the Second Health Information Technology Summit; September 9, 2005; Washington DC.

2.   Charette R. What happened to do no harm? *CIO Magazine.* April 1, 2006. www.cio.com/archive/040106/keynote.html?page=1. Accessed April 23, 2007.

3.   eHealth Initiative Policy Landscape Archives. www.ehealthinitiative.org/initiatives/policy/archives.mspx. Accessed April 23, 2007.

4.   Dick RS, Steen EB, Detmer DE, eds; Committee on Improving the Patient Record, Institute of Medicine. *The Computer-Based Patient Record: An Essential Technology for Health Care, Revised Edition.* Washington, DC: National Academies Press; 1997.

5.   Terry K. Implementing an EHR: Going live is no snap. *Med Economics (online).* July 6, 2007. Available at: www.memag.com/memag/article/articleDetail.jsp?id=438100&sk=&date=&%0A%09%09%09&pageID=2. Accessed July 10, 2007.

6.   Ash J, Bates D. Factors and forces affecting EHR system adoption: report of a 2004 ACMI discussion. *J Am Med Inform Assoc.* 2005;12:8-12.

7. Vogenitz W. EMR and E/M: beware of software's potential to upcode. *Part B News.* May 1, 2006. www.eclinicalworks.com/2006-05-01-pr2.php. Accessed May 15, 2007.

8. Centers for Medicare & Medicaid Services. Selection of level of evaluation and management service. *Medicare Claims Processing Manual.* Chapter 12:section 30.6.1. www.cms.hhs.gov/manuals/downloads/clm104c12.pdf. Accessed April 23, 2007.

9. Clancy C. Keynote address. Presented at: the Second Health Information Technology Summit; September 9, 2005; Washington, DC.

10. Levinson SR. *Practical E/M: Documentation and Coding Solutions for Quality Patient Care.* Chicago, IL: AMA Press; 2005.

11. Committee on Quality of Health Care in America, Institute of Medicine. *Crossing the Quality Chasm: A New Health System for the 21st Century.* Washington, DC: National Academies Press; 2001.

chapter 3

Quality Care, the Medical Diagnostic Process, the Physicians' Medical Record, and E/M Compliance

Providing patients with high-quality care must be the highest priority for all physicians. Achieving this objective requires a combination of superb training, dedication, insight, curiosity, and sophisticated tools to assist and guide physicians through the complex thought processes of clinical diagnosis and optimal treatment. To establish acceptable standards of effectiveness for electronic health records (EHRs), a reasonable description of "quality care" should first be developed. This insight will help define the structural and operational features that EHRs must provide during the patient evaluation process to help physicians consistently achieve the quality care goal.

QUALITY CARE

Since the Institute of Medicine's publication of *To Err Is Human*[1] and *Crossing the Quality Chasm*,[2] numerous national organizations have attempted to define *objective* criteria for measuring the predominantly *subjective* topic of quality care. There are two measures currently being applied in "pay-for-performance" programs that provide financial incentives for practicing in a prescribed manner:

1. Following established guidelines for preventive care services, such as obtaining diagnostic mammograms and colonoscopy after defined ages

2. Following established guidelines for management of previously diagnosed chronic illnesses, such as congestive heart failure, diabetes, and asthma

Although the ability to follow established guidelines *under appropriate circumstances* certainly meets a standard of care, it is not, by itself, sufficient to be considered providing "quality medical care." Simply following guidelines in case after case can often be more an administrative task than a medical one. For example, nonphysician clinical staff (facilitated by an EHR when available) should be able to monitor a practice's diabetic patients to ensure they adhere to guidelines for obtaining appropriate blood tests every 3 months. The staff should also review the laboratory results to monitor patients' health status, bringing patients with suboptimal status to the attention of physicians.

The *quality* part of medical care is far more sophisticated and more difficult to measure, which is likely why we have no universally accepted measures for it. For purposes of this book, the concept of medical quality starts with the physician making the correct diagnosis. Certainly no physician or patient would categorize care as quality if a physician were to perfectly apply the guidelines for asthma treatment to a patient whose true diagnosis was later found to be lung cancer or chronic obstructive pulmonary disease.

Similarly, to promote true quality, physicians must not treat such codified guidelines as a restrictive box, but rather as a base platform on which to build their recommendations for care. In other words, after making an accurate diagnosis for a particular patient but before initiating a treatment protocol, a physician should also consider whether care under a particular guideline might be inappropriate for the particular patient owing to comorbidities, genetic problems, medication side effects, drug incompatibilities, and/or any of a myriad of contributing factors that might alter or modify the indicated treatments and anticipated benefits. True quality also calls for physicians to promptly determine which patients are not having an optimal response to a "standard" protocol and then analyze whether a different evaluation or treatment approach might be warranted that might prove more efficacious for the individual circumstances. In other words, such medical guidelines should *facilitate* physicians' medical evaluation and clinical judgment, not replace it. Physicians' abilities to make these medical determinations in a consistent and reliable manner are the cumulative result of years of ongoing training and experiential learning. All physicians should strive to apply this "medical diagnostic process" throughout every patient encounter. It includes not only determining the cause of each patient's complaints, but also assessing his or her response to treatments and taking into account what more could be done to promote optimal health, all while appreciating the whole spectrum of each patient's medical and biopsychosocial circumstances.

Although a major part of the *science* of medicine involves identifying the general disease category (ie, diagnosis) appropriate for each patient, a significant part of the *art* (and quality) of practicing medicine involves applying this diagnostic process, which helps to identify the distinctive aspects of each patient's medical issues and to determine when a patient's care warrants additional or atypical evaluation and/or management.

A Philosophical Question

Imagine the response of the great diagnostician, Sir William Osler (the first professor of Internal Medicine at Johns Hopkins Hospital), if a student had asked the philosophical question: "Which is the most important element of medicine, science or art?" Undoubtedly, the esteemed professor would have uttered the one word answer: "Both."

By their nature, software programs enable systematic approaches and, thereby, facilitate the scientific component of the medical profession. Designers need to exercise caution that EHRs facilitate, rather than eliminate, individualized diagnosis and treatment that impart the artful component of health care.

During their first 2 years of medical education, students focus on the science of medicine, concentrating on how to place each patient's illness into an appropriate diagnostic category. Although physicians must diligently nurture and update their scientific knowledge and thought processes throughout the remainder of their careers, the didactic teachings and ongoing educational efforts that follow these first 2 years also incorporate the *art* of identifying the features that *individualize* each patient's clinical concerns and make them special. It is this aspect of medical care that helps physicians discover when a patient's condition calls for an insightful, nonstandard diagnosis and/or treatment. Many physicians recall from their student years the admonishment of several of the best clinical professors that patients are the best teachers. Mentors use this statement to underscore the importance of listening carefully to each patient to detect any subtle or distinguishing features of the illness that make his or her own symptoms and/or findings atypical. These additional insights allow physicians to make correct diagnoses more frequently and to individualize each patient's care. They also expand physicians' knowledge of diseases and their ability to provide better care to future patients.

The introduction to *Practical E/M* observes[3(pxv)]:

"As clinicians, *quality of care* is our central theme. It is the reason we chose medicine as a career, and it should be a driving principle for the way we practice and for our growth as physicians. It would be possible to write a book far larger than this one with the sole purpose of attempting to define all the parameters of 'quality of care.' In the interest of brevity, let's simply accept a basic assumption that the provision of quality care calls for physicians to (1) make the optimal effort to determine correct diagnoses, (2) in the most timely manner possible, and (3) institute the optimal therapies to address patient problems, with (4) a minimum number of complications. Quality care also involves identifying patients' risk factors, providing preventative counseling and interventions, and maintaining a good physician-patient relationship. Finally, consideration of cost-effectiveness has become an additional and important component of quality care in today's environment."

Three more elements might be added to this summary description of quality care: (1) selection of only tests that are appropriate to confirm or deny the probable diagnoses derived from a high-quality history and physical examination (H&P), (2) prompt recognition of circumstances calling for medical consultation, with timely referral to a physician who has the appropriate training and expertise for the individual patient's medical concerns, and (3) the ability to use guidelines appropriately and to go beyond automated responses to patient symptoms and diagnoses, incorporating into each individual patient's care the consideration of cultural differences and personal preferences in order to determine the program of care that is in the best interest of each patient (ie, the care that is "best" for a particular person is not always what is generally considered the "best" treatment for all patients who have the same illness).

THE MEDICAL DIAGNOSTIC PROCESS AND QUALITY CARE

The medical diagnostic process, which has been taught to medical students in fundamentally the same way for at least 50 years (probably far longer), is the cornerstone method that physicians apply in pursuit of quality care. In the first step of this approach, physicians gather all of the relevant clinical (H&P), laboratory, and diagnostic test information. They then correlate, analyze, and compare this information with their understanding of the natural course of various diseases to derive appropriate diagnoses and treatment options. Of course, as physicians increase their experience and skills, the elements of obtaining high-quality information and deriving accurate diagnostic impressions become interwoven. This maturation of diagnostic thinking with increasing expertise is well described in the widely used reference for performing the clinical H&P, the *Bates' Guide to Physical Examination and History Taking*, which advises physicians "as you gain experience, your thinking [of clinical reasoning and decision making] will begin at the outset of the patient encounter, not at the end."[4]

The common protocol for this process begins with obtaining (and documenting) an in-depth medical history at the beginning of a patient visit. The history-taking concludes when the physician decides that he or she has sufficient information about the patient's background and the course of the patient's illness to be secure in the probable accuracy of a preliminary differential diagnosis, which includes a preliminary appraisal of the severity of the patient's condition. Next, the physician performs a physical examination, the primary purpose of which is to confirm, disprove, and/or expand on the physician's history-based clinical impressions. The examination also provides the opportunity for the physician to find additional or unsuspected abnormalities that may be contributing to the patient's current problems or that may be unrelated. Next, the physician reviews any available laboratory data or related records. At this point, the physician prioritizes the differential diagnoses in order of probability and/or severity. Next, he or she determines whether any diagnostic studies are warranted for further verification of these clinical impressions, selects appropriately indicated treatments and/or consultation requests, and counsels the patient about all of this information. In addition, during and/or immediately after a patient visit, the physician must document this entire diagnostic process in the patient's medical record to facilitate effective care for the patient in the future.

The Pivotal Role of the Medical History in the Diagnostic Process

The medical history consists of information related to past medical history (PMH), social history (SH), family history (FH), review of systems (ROS), chief compliant (CC) and history of the present illness (HPI). The PMH, FH, and SH are often abbreviated collectively as the PFSH.

From the outset of their clinical training, physicians are taught that a comprehensive and effective medical history is the most reliable diagnostic tool in their armamentarium and a key factor in a successful patient encounter. In fact most physicians are told in medical school that obtaining a good medical history from the patient will most often lead them to determine the correct diagnosis most of the time, before they even examine their patients.

Setting Our "Quality" Goal for Medical History

I was a second-year medical student, sitting with my classmates in a course called "Introduction to Clinical Medicine." I had not yet even taken a medical history or examined a patient. Yet I vividly recall the highly respected internist and diagnostician who, when explaining the importance of obtaining a thorough medical history, set forth the standard of using the medical history to correctly diagnose the cause of medical problems "95% of the time."

Although reaching this level of diagnostic skill seemed a goal beyond human possibility at that stage of my career, our training is designed to lead all of us to a high degree of success in deriving reasonable and accurate medical diagnoses at the conclusion of our encounters with patients.

In compliance terms, a *comprehensive* medical history includes a *complete* PMH, SH, FM, and ROS, as well as an extended HPI. However, in clinical terms, this is just a starting point for obtaining a thorough medical history, which calls for more extensive exploration of the PFSH than the minimal number of questions needed to satisfy compliance requirements. The process of obtaining a medical history can be greatly facilitated, and made far more efficient, by designing medical record forms (or electronic screens) preloaded with baseline medical history inquiries. Without the physician present, well-designed forms give patients the ability to document preliminary positive and negative responses related to all elements of the medical history other than the HPI.

STRUCTURED MEDICAL RECORDS AND THE PROMOTION OF QUALITY PATIENT CARE

Although most physicians understand that the documentation in the medical record should be a reflection of the quality of care they provide, few appreciate the complementary insight that the depth and extent of the care they provide is very much influenced by the quality of the medical record they are using. Just as the medical diagnostic process provides physicians with the cornerstone for providing quality care, the design of the medical record must provide physicians with the stable structure needed to support that cornerstone.

The Comprehensive Care H&P

Medical students are taught how to perform the medical diagnostic process by being provided with the structure of a *comprehensive* H&P. Students learn this process and incorporate it as an integral element of their care by accurately documenting this entire process in the form of a *structured* medical record:

- Complete medical history, including
  - Thorough HPI, including CC
  - PMH
  - SH
  - FH
  - Complete ROS
- Comprehensive physical examination (or level of examination appropriate for the severity of illness)
- Review of all relevant medical data
- Differential diagnosis
- Diagnostic studies to be obtained
- Primary and secondary treatment options
- Subsequent care plans

Designs for the H&P record that include all of these elements allow and encourage physicians to carry out and document the diagnostic process. Designs that partially eliminate or substitute preloaded data for original documentation may compromise the diagnostic process and the integrity of the information recorded in the clinical record.

Addressing the Need for Higher Efficiency

The current time-limitations in both medical training and medical practice require physicians to need and seek more effectively designed electronic medical record tools than the traditional tools. Adding structured documentation to the electronic medical record serves two purposes. First, it helps physicians follow the diagnostic process and complete all the appropriate components of the H&P. Second, intelligently designed medical record templates can decrease the time required for documenting a comprehensive care record while maintaining the integrity and usefulness of the clinical information.

Practical EHR defines documentation efficiency as increasing speed of documentation without loss of quality care, be E/M compliant, and preserve data integrity. Physicians must exercise caution in evaluating these medical record tools to ensure that they do not introduce any associated loss or distortion of portions of the H&P structure. Improper changes to records may impair the diagnostic process and negatively affect the quality of care.

Medical Record Structure and the Comprehensive Medical History

Eliciting and recording a PFSH and ROS can be time consuming. Nonetheless, almost all physicians already employ a standardized list of questions in compiling an inventory of the patient's past experience with illnesses and symptoms. Incorporating these questions into the structure of the medical record in accordance with compliance guidelines, ensures that a complete PFSH and ROS is obtained for every initial visit and significantly increasing the efficiency of the entire PFSH and ROS process. With an optimal design, physicians can have all the preliminary information of a complete PFSH and ROS obtained and documented with minimal investment of their time.

Modifying the Order of Obtaining Components of the Medical History

Traditional training for obtaining the medical history instructs medical students to begin a patient encounter by asking about the CC and the HPI. Only after completing this task does the physician inquire about the PFSH and ROS. However, following this traditional sequence may, under the time stress of current practice economics, create an inclination for physicians to obtain an abbreviated PFSH and/or ROS or none at all. This tendency is further exacerbated by the fact that most physicians, on completing the HPI, have already formed a working differential diagnosis, and they are eager to move forward with the physical examination to confirm their impressions.

One of the many benefits of integrating evaluation and management (E/M) compliance guidelines into the structure of the EHR has been the introduction of structured medical history questionnaires. This tool encourages physicians to modify the order for obtaining the medical history, while also removing the incentives for haste. During initial visits, before seeing the physician, patients complete survey forms that document their PFSH and

ROS and indicate their reason for the visit (ie, the CC). As a result, physicians have a thorough picture of these history elements *before* obtaining the HPI. This change in the traditional order of obtaining the medical history not only allows physicians to move forward with their care at the conclusion of the HPI, it also adds a subtle but significant change in how patient's problems are analyzed. The effect of this reordering is that physicians can implement a more holistic approach because they have a mental impression of the patient's overall health care picture as the context, *before* beginning an investigation of the current problems.

Puzzling

When confronted with 500 scattered pieces of a jigsaw puzzle, what is the first thing we do? We look at the picture of the completed puzzle on the front of the box. By doing so, we can accomplish our task much more effectively and efficiently, because we have an understanding of the whole image before we attempt to put the fragmented pieces back together.

Similarly, understanding a patient's overall health picture before analyzing the individual parts leads to far more effective care than attempting to figure out what is wrong before understanding the patient's health context. For purposes of the scientific analysis of a medical problem, individualization of care, and effective communication with patients, approaching an encounter from this holistic perspective is extremely beneficial.

For example, while obtaining the HPI of a person with a recent onset of respiratory symptoms, understanding that the patient has a family history of asthma; has excessive dust in the house related to recent remodeling; just traveled to an exotic Asian location; has a long history of throat clearing, postnasal drip, and heartburn; and/or has an unexplained 20-pound weight loss provides a far more valuable starting point for the HPI than knowing only the CC of "3 weeks of cough."

Medical Record Structure and the Physical Examination

Most experienced physicians can perform a comprehensive examination that is appropriate for their own specialty in a remarkably efficient manner. However, without a structured medical record, it can actually require significantly greater amounts of time to document all aspects of this examination, particularly all the normal findings, than it takes to perform it. Additionally, it is unreasonable to require physicians to memorize all the E/M guidelines that provide the medically indicated extent of examination associated with each level of care. In nonstructured records, this combination of barriers commonly leads either to documentation that is less extensive than the care performed (recording only the abnormal findings and bypassing the relevant normal findings), or in care and documentation that are both less extensive than medically warranted by the severity of a patient's illness.

Incorporating a structured physical examination design can address both these issues, facilitating rapid documentation of normal findings and providing guidance to ensure that appropriate levels of exam are performed and recorded.

Medical Record Structure and Medical Decision Making (MDM)

Even though physicians apply sophisticated reasoning to develop a differential diagnosis and weigh a broad spectrum of treatment options, it is common for physicians who use an unstructured record to document only one, most likely diagnosis and the final treatment option. In addition to potentially failing to fulfill compliance criteria, this simple documentation also fails to record the physician's thought process in evaluating the patient's pathology. This can result in a relatively problem-focused and linear approach to patient care, which can also impair the quality of patient care over time.

Incorporating an effectively structured MDM design not only facilitates documentation that meets the challenging compliance aspect of this component of care, it also promotes documentation of a more extensive differential diagnosis and of a variety of treatment options. This additional information facilitates ongoing care by clarifying the thought processes underlying the physician's diagnostic and therapeutic decisions.

Katrina's Health Impact

"Katrina's Lingering Medical Nightmare," a September 2005 article posted on Time Magazine's web site, has surveyed some of the serious medical damage inflicted by Katrina's destruction of existing paper medical records. It reports, " 'Not having a portable medical record has been a massive challenge,' says Mark Clanton, a deputy director of the National Cancer Institute, of the tens of thousands of patients dispersed around the country and needing access to doctors and drugs. . . .[T]here is no doubt that many cancer patients displaced by Katrina—the region has 7,600 participants in experimental trials, with many thousands more receiving conventional care—have had delays or disruptions to treatment, in some cases with devastating consequences." In assessing the challenges and compromises resulting from the efforts to care for patients in the absence of their medical documents, the article concludes "[the] lesson learned is the need for a national database of electronic medical records. "We're all aware of the issues of protection of privacy, and that's an absolute requirement," says John Gallin, director of the National Institutes of Health Clinical Center. "But I consider this one of the top priorities for the health care delivery system in this country."[17]

The Role of the Medical Record in Ensuring Data Integrity

To assist physicians in providing quality care, the data entry features of the record must facilitate clinical documentation in a manner that allows any physician to understand the purpose and details of that care when they review the record. The H&P record should include the particular details of each patient encounter. It must not produce records that are *generic*, with entry of similar or repetitive documentation for visit after visit and patient after patient.

The Importance of *Meaningful* Clinical Documentation

During compliance reviews of a series of visits by diabetic patients, I encountered clinical records that listed only a series of laboratory results followed by modification of the insulin dosages. They provided no documentation of medical history or physical examination. Not only did these charts fail compliance criteria, they also failed to provide meaningful clinical documentation. It was not possible to judge how well or how sick each patient was feeling.

The same frustration can occur when either a physician or an auditor reviews a "cloned" electronic (or transcription) record that is compiled by entering preloaded generic information related to history, examination, and/or medical decision making or by repeated copying and pasting of near-identical information from one visit to the next.

Meeting the implementation goals for EHR systems requires more than just the availability of clinical documentation; it requires the documentation of *meaningful* information, individualized to each patient and each visit and reflective of the physician's diagnostic process during each encounter. A well-designed clinical record must support and record the physician's thought process, not supplant it.

E/M COMPLIANCE, THE MEDICAL RECORD, AND THE DIAGNOSTIC PROCESS

In October 1991, the American Medical Association (AMA) and the Health Care Financing Administration (HCFA, the precursor to today's Centers for Medicare & Medicaid Services, or CMS) trained a selected group of physicians and auditors to educate physicians in the use of the soon-to-be introduced E/M documentation and coding system. The instructors presented E/M as a new system that was replacing the existing time-based coding system for cognitive care. (Under the previous system, physicians coded a 5-minute established patient visit as level 1, a 10-minute visit as level 2, a 15-minute visit as level 3, and so forth.) Most or all who attended these sessions probably interpreted the E/M system as an administrative invention, developed for reimbursement purposes, which has become a prevailing belief among physicians. Nevertheless, the E/M system is beyond administrative invention because there are similarities between the CPT E/M codes and the *Bates' Guide to Physician Examination and History Taking*. This is neither unexpected nor unwarranted because the *Bates' Guide* has been a primary reference in medical schools for many years and has contributed to the clinical diagnostic techniques of many practicing physicians. As such, the E/M codes should reflect clinical practice to appropriately capture physician work and efforts in patient care.

Careful research demonstrates that the E/M codes are codification of the standard diagnostic process taught to physicians during their training. The descriptions in the *CPT* manual mirror the H&P methods and the diagnostic principles taught in the *Bates' Guide*. Table 3.1 shows the similarity between the *Bates' Guide* and the three E/M "key components" (history, physical examination, and medical decision making) and the E/M emphasis on medical necessity. The *Bates' Guide* describes the "nature of the patient's problem," which is the equivalent of the *CPT* manual's "nature of the presenting problem(s)' that represents medical necessity and that can be recommended as a "mandatory fourth factor" in documentation and coding.[5]

TABLE 3.1

Comparison of *Bates' Guide* and *CPT* E/M Terminology and Principles

Section of Medical Record	*Bates' Guide* Description[4]	*CPT* Description[a]
History of present illness (HPI)	"A complete, clear, and chronologic account of the problems prompting the patient to seek care." Includes seven features: location, quality, quantity or severity, timing including duration, setting [ie, context], aggravating and relieving factors, associated manifestations	"A chronological description of the development of the patient's present illness from the first sign and/or symptoms (ie, duration) to the present. This includes a description of location, quality, severity, timing, context, modifying factors, and associated signs and symptoms."
Past medical history	Medical illnesses, surgical procedures, obstetric/gynecologic, and psychiatric conditions; and immunizations (allergies and medications included in HPI)	Prior illnesses and injuries, surgical procedures, hospitalizations, medications, allergies, immunizations, and dietary status
Social history	Occupation, last year of schooling, home situation, significant others, stress, life experiences, leisure activities, religious affiliation, activities of daily living, exercise, diet, and alternative health care practices (use of tobacco, alcohol, and drugs <u>included</u> in HPI)	Employment, occupational history, marital status or living arrangements, use of drugs, alcohol and tobacco, level of education, sexual history, and other relevant social factors
Family history	Age and cause of death of each immediate relative; record of hereditary conditions in the family	Health status or cause of death of parents, siblings, and children; specific diseases related to problems in the HPI or ROS; diseases of family members that may be hereditary
Review of systems (ROS)	Questions about symptoms in 16 body systems	Questions about signs and symptoms in 14 body systems (the same systems as in the *Bates' Guide*, but with skin and breast combined into one system and cardiovascular and peripheral vascular combined into one system)
Medical decision making	Data reviewed, impressions, treatments, and data requested	Data reviewed, impressions, treatment options, data requested, and complexity of data and three levels of risk
Medical necessity	Considered the "nature of the patient's problems"	Considered the "nature of the presenting problems"

[a] American Medical Association. *Current Procedural Terminology* (*CPT*)® 2007. Chicago, IL: American Medical Association; 2006.

Using Compliance as the Building Block for an Effective Electronic H&P

For physicians, learning that the E/M coding system is actually a *codification* of the method they were taught in medical school as the basis for quality patient care shatters the perception that the E/M system is nothing more than an administrative burden. It allows physicians to replace this negative interpretation with a constructive approach, transforming the compliance guidelines into sophisticated medical record tools capable of integrating documentation and coding principles into the quality care process. This insight not only justifies and reinforces the rationale for building medical record design and functionality on the foundation of E/M guidelines, it also explains why using records designed in this manner facilitates the diagnostic process and optimal patient care.[6]

This chapter has portrayed a medical care paradigm that establishes quality care as the paramount goal for success, the traditional medical diagnostic process as the cornerstone for attaining that goal, and an effective medical H&P as the mortar stabilizing that cornerstone. The final element required for success is a solid foundation on which to build this effective H&P. Although it comes as a surprise to most physicians, this solid foundation is built by using the guidelines of CPT's E/M codes as the basis for the design and the functionality of an effective electronic H&P component.

Traditionally, E/M coding has been presented to (and interpreted by) physicians as if it were an unrelated administrative chore, added to a medical visit after providing patient care and then documenting that care. When approached in this manner, the E/M "rules" have proven complex and impractical for physicians to memorize or apply. The result has been consistently poor compliance, demonstrated repeatedly since the introduction of E/M coding in 1992, as poor results for compliance audits (approximately 80% rate of incorrect coding, documentation, and/or compatibility with medical necessity[7]).

It therefore makes sense to reengineer the approach to E/M and the clinical record. Instead of asking physicians to memorize the considerable collection of E/M rules and guidelines and apply them at the conclusion of a patient encounter, the *Practical EHR* approach incorporates the rules into design components of the clinical H&P record. It thereby allows physicians to integrate documentation and coding into the patient care process, mobilizing E/M compliance principles to actually support and guide quality care.

The Logic of Building the Medical Record for Compliance

In 2002, Edward Miller, MD, dean and chief executive officer of the Johns Hopkins Hospital, Baltimore, MD, in an editorial in the *Hopkins Medical News* entitled "Compliance and Creativity" described the benefits for compliance *and* quality care when his institution had to respond to a complication that occurred during a research protocol. He acclaimed the value of building medical and scientific protocols on compliance principles and the ensuing benefits for improving and enhancing the institution's research programs. His summary of the hospital's experience was that "the solution to the 'problem' of compliance is to see compliance as a solution."[8]

It first became possible to build a medical record using E/M compliance principles in 1995, when the AMA and HCFA developed and published the first set of "Documentation Guidelines." These guidelines added *quantitative* values to the *qualitative* E/M descriptors for the medical history published in the *CPT* manual. The extended documentation guidelines, published in 1997, added quantitative values for CPT's physical examination descriptors. Using these history and examination guidelines, plus proposed quantitative guidelines for medical decision making, has made it possible to successfully design compliant paper medical records.[9] Using clinical records designed this way helps physicians efficiently perform (and document) medically appropriate levels of care while also using the medical diagnostic process. Applying a similar approach to the design for an effective H&P component in EHRs promises to fulfill physicians' requirements for high-quality clinical records that facilitate effective care while ensuring compliant documentation.[10]

OBSTACLES TO OVERCOME

When considering optimal design and functionality for the electronic H&P, physicians and software developers should benefit from realizing how and why most physicians abbreviate the comprehensive H&P process they learned in medical school.

Time

All medical schools seem to train students to perform a comprehensive H&P and to follow the medical diagnostic process. Unfortunately, however, little if any attention is given to E/M compliance, and the only medical record tools generally provided to medical students for documentation are a pen and a blank sheet of paper. When using such primitive technology, almost regardless of the skill and efficiency a physician may have in *providing* comprehensive care, the documentation process is so prolonged that the completion of each patient encounter commonly requires an hour or more, most of which is consumed recording all the documentation free hand.

This time frame for patient care is, of course, incompatible with the volume of patient responsibilities physicians experience during their residency and under the economic requirements of medical practice. This conflict between the goal of appropriately comprehensive care and the demand for speed sets the stage for physicians to seek a faster mechanism for evaluating patients and documenting care. Because most physicians, during their training, have not been exposed to compliant medical record tools that can facilitate performing and documenting a *comprehensive* H&P in a highly efficient time frame, they are generally forced to use more *problem-focused* documentation.

Although this approach saves time initially, physicians may not be consciously aware that deleting portions of the H&P can influence them to constrict or eliminate portions of the care they provide, thereby compromising the diagnostic and treatment processes. The mandate for *Practical EHR* is to eliminate the need for such a choice, by creating electronic H&P components capable of combining efficient documentation with appropriately comprehensive care and compliant documentation.

How Physicians Can Detour Off the Road to Comprehensive Care

I recently presented these practical EHR concepts as part of a physician users' group meeting sponsored by an EHR company. The discussion highlighted EHR software design approaches capable of providing efficiency and comprehensive care. One physician who approached me after the discussion was shaking his head in amazement at this new perspective. He had not considered the powerful influence of medical record design on his own approach to patient

continued

care, and he was surprised that he could not remember at what point he had lost his comprehensive care record and adopted less effective shortcuts.

I reassured him that my own personal experience had been similar. I know exactly when I had stopped using a comprehensive H&P; it was after completing my residency training and when starting private practice. I used the comprehensive care and documentation format throughout medical school and residency training, eventually refining my efficiency so that I could accomplish this task in about 45 minutes. However, when I entered private practice, my associates handed me blank 5 × 7 inch index cards and told me to use these for documentation, while seeing five or six patients per hour. So, I started using these small forms and defaulted to problem-focused care (an HPI, a brief PMH and SH, an effective examination of the head and neck, and impressions and treatment recommendations confined to the patient's presenting problem), without even a consideration of what I was losing.

It was 19 years later, shortly after introducing compliant E/M documentation forms into my practice, when the metaphorical light bulb went on in my consciousness. With new, sophisticated paper template forms built on E/M compliance, my return to practicing comprehensive care happened automatically, as easily as if I had gotten on a bicycle after not riding for 19 years. These forms provided two sides of documentation on 8 × 11-inch paper for established patients and four sides for new patients. And I continued to care for five to six patients per hour, comfortably. It was only after I discovered a design that added efficiency to the type of medical record I had used during my student and residency years that I became aware of what I had lost.

Reimbursement

Under the current reimbursement model, physicians have far less time available for individual patient care than is called for by our own guidelines for "typical" time spent in providing care, particularly for patients with high-severity illness (Table 3.2).

TABLE 3.2

Time Designated as "Typical" by CPT Descriptors for Higher Levels of E/M Service

Type of Service	Level of E/M Care	"Typical" Visit Time,* min
New	99202	20
patient, office or other	99203	30
outpatient visit	99204	45
	99205	60
Established	99212	10
patient, office or other	99213	15
outpatient visit	99214	25
	99215	40
Outpatient consultation,	99242	30
new or established patient	99243	40
	99244	60
	99245	80
Initial hospital care	99221	30
	99222	50
	99223	70

continued

TABLE 3.2

Time Designated as "Typical" by CPT Descriptors for Higher Levels of E/M Service, cont'd.

Type of Service	Level of E/M Care	"Typical" Visit Time,* min
Subsequent hospital care	99231	15
	99232	25
	99233	35
Inpatient consultation	99252	40
new or established patient	99253	55
	99254	80
	99255	110

* CPT provides different descriptions for the "time" guidelines for different types of services. "Intraservice times are defined as **face-to-face** time for office and other outpatient visits and as **unit/floor** time for hospital and other inpatient visits."[16] CPT's E/M section provides a detailed explanation of this distinction.

The severely restricted payments from Medicare, Medicaid, and managed care programs provide insufficient reimbursement to cover medical practice costs associated with the time designated for these levels of care, particularly for physicians using conventional medical record tools.

The Reimbursement Dilemma

The current payment level for the practice expense and liability insurance for code 99205 is approximately $72 under the CMS conversion factor.[11] Because most physicians' actual overhead expenses range between $200 and $300 per hour, this level of payment covers only about 15 minutes of care for these seriously ill patients.

Unfortunately, a threefold or fourfold increase in the Medicare conversion factor is highly unlikely at present. The challenge, therefore, is to create designs that enable comprehensive care to be performed and documented (compliantly) in approximately 15-20 minutes.

Problem-Focused Approaches

It is worthwhile to examine some of the less-than-comprehensive (and also noncompliant) approaches that physicians encounter during their training and experience, including the following:

■ Instructions for their medical licensing examination
■ SOAP (subjective information, objective information, assessment, plan) notes
■ Dictated H&P report

The Medical Licensing Examination and Problem-Focused Care

It appears that the imperative to truncate care and documentation occurs even during medical school. In fact, this pruning of the diagnostic process to problem-focused care has become a requirement for junior and senior medical students to successfully complete the "clinical skills" component of their national medical licensing examination. During this section of the examination, students encounter a series of trained actors, each portraying a patient with a single medical abnormality. The directions for the examination provide a total of merely 25 minutes to complete and document a medical history, physical examination, and extensive differential diagnosis and evaluation plan for each patient. For medical record tools, the students are "provided a clipboard, blank paper for taking notes, and a pen."[12] Despite the fact that performing and documenting comprehensive care with these limited tools requires about 60 minutes, the examination permits no use of time-saving structured documents. Instead, to complete the care within the allotted time frame, the students are instructed to perform their evaluation "by asking this patient *relevant* questions and performing a *focused* physical examination."[12]

The instructions for the licensing examination also limit the extent of medical history elicited, by instructing "the elements of medical history you need to obtain in each case will be determined by the nature of the patient's problems."[12] This approach contradicts physicians' training in the diagnostic process, which builds on the premise that obtaining a comprehensive medical history is necessary for physicians to understand the full scope of a patient's illness and, thereby, to determine the nature of the patient's problems.

The Medical Licensing Examination Message and the Standard of Care

The US Medical Licensing Examination reinforces the time dilemma by prohibiting the use of sophisticated and compliant documentation forms. Under this limitation, it must choose between speed and appropriate levels of care, and it chooses speed as the means for students to pass the examination. The message of the licensing examination to medical students is that problem-focused history and problem-focused examination are appropriate care, even for patients with high-severity illness (eg, carcinoma).

However, this message contradicts the standard of care established by physicians and their specialty societies in the E/M section and clinical examples section of the *CPT* manual. These criteria specifically indicate that patients whose nature of presenting problem(s) are moderate to high or high warrant a *comprehensive* medical history and a *comprehensive* physical examination (in addition to moderate or high-complexity medical decision making) to meet the standard of care.

SOAP Notes and Problem-Focused Care

As residents and medical students seek to reduce the time they spend performing and documenting an H&P, many discover and adopt the truncated H&P structure of a SOAP note, or its equivalent. In this protocol, a physician summarizes a patient's subjective information (ie, medical history), objective information (ie, physical examination), assessment (ie, clinical impressions), and plan (ie, diagnostic testing ordered and/or treatments instituted).

A Brief History of SOAP

Lawrence Weed, MD, introduced the problem-oriented medical record (POMR) in 1968.[13]

The following year, he introduced the SOAP note concept as a means of organizing the chart for progress notes (SOAP was not offered as a structure for an initial patient encounter).[13] Review of his writing indicates that Weed's purpose for this approach was not to diminish the importance of documenting a high-level H&P.[14] Rather, it was to add a structured problem list and action plan into the documentation of every medical record.[15]

Some medical schools now teach students to use the SOAP framework for initial patient encounters. However, the professors teach that "subjective" includes the PMH, SH, FH, and ROS, in addition to the HPI, and "objective" still requires performing and documenting a comprehensive physical examination. In other words, this teaching approach superimposes the shorthand of a SOAP framework onto a comprehensive H&P.

Even though the SOAP note concept could theoretically include the elements of a comprehensive H&P, as commonly used today it encourages and guides physicians to perform and document problem-focused care. For example, an HPI alone is sufficient to satisfy the SOAP note's requirement for obtaining and documenting subjective information. Consequently, the medical histories found in most medical records structured in this manner contain nothing more than an HPI (or even just a CC). Similarly, in practice, physicians most often document a problem-focused examination to satisfy the requirement for objective information, a single diagnosis to satisfy their documentation of an assessment, and one management option to indicate their plan. The SOAP method, as commonly used, therefore, has the potential to erode the comprehensive care that forms the support structure for the medical diagnostic process.

Despite Weed's original description of the SOAP approach, the current reality is that when physicians use this architecture for their H&P, it guides them to provide problem-focused care. Its use also fails to incorporate documentation of numerous elements of the H&P required for E/M compliance (including complexity of data ordered and reviewed; level of risk of presenting problems; level of risk of diagnostic procedures recommended; level of risk of management options recommended; and the nature of the presenting problem(s)), which appeared 23 years after SOAP was introduced. Therefore, use of the SOAP note as the model for an H&P commonly results in noncompliant levels of care and documentation.

Dictation

When they enter practice, many physicians elect to reduce the time of documentation by using dictation, which is generally faster than writing for several sections of the H&P. However, dictation has a number of drawbacks. In addition to the considerable extra cost to pay for transcription, the time requirements still remain too great for physicians to complete comprehensive care and documentation in the amount of time available. As a result, the H&P report is often abbreviated, with audits commonly identifying documentation of less extensive levels of care than warranted by the severity of patient illness.

There are additional practical issues that may occur when physicians use dictation as the only format for H&P documentation. Owing to time constraints, many physicians delay some or all of their dictations until the end of the day, when not only must they invest personal time to complete their work, but they also are likely to have forgotten significant portions of encounters completed hours before. In addition, they lack the additional time to review each transcribed H&P report to ensure accuracy of the transcription, even though they are required to sign the documents to meet compliance and medicolegal requirements. This can also increase potential quality concerns.

Eliminating Detours to Problem-Focused Care at Their Origin

To Err Is Human[1] and *Crossing the Quality Chasm*[2] have heightened everyone's awareness of the importance of medical records in promoting high-quality care and patient safety. This spotlight creates our opportunity and focuses on our responsibility to design EHRs in a manner that reinforces and promotes the comprehensive care all physicians are trained to perform. We hope that this renewed focus will also lead to introducing such tools (in paper and/or electronic format) into medical education curricula. While medical schools effectively train medical students to provide appropriate levels of comprehensive care using the medical diagnostic process, they also need to give them a set of tools that provides them with the ability to apply these principles under the demands of medical practice. It will be far easier to give students the tools that will keep them on the "right" road than it will be to try to rescue (and reeducate) them after they have detoured off of it.

SUMMARY

Quality care continues to be the top priority for physicians. It also occupies the center of attention for policy makers, whose goals include reducing medical errors and increasing patient safety, and for payers, who advocate that quality care is the most cost-effective care. From their initial medical school course for the introduction to clinical medicine, physicians learn and understand that their medical record documentation should be an accurate reflection of the patient care they have provided. Understanding the truth of the complementary concept, that the depth and extent of patient care provided is a reflection of the medical record tools used, provides powerful insight into the critical importance of effective design of the electronic H&P.

There is a strong interrelationship among E/M compliance, the comprehensive H&P, the medical diagnostic process, and facilitating quality care. Understanding that the CPT's E/M system is a codification of the comprehensive H&P and of the diagnostic process (as described in the standard reference text, *Bates' Guide to Physical Examination and History Taking*[4]) provides EHR designers with a solid foundation on which to construct effective H&P component design and functionality. While solving the problem of compliance, this approach helps and guides physicians to implement the medical diagnostic process, which in turn promotes quality care.

Einstein and E/M Compliance

One of Albert Einstein's insights about the atomic bomb was his observation, "The release of atomic energy has not created a new problem. It has merely made more urgent the necessity of solving an existing one."[15] This same logic can be applied to the impact of EHR systems on the urgency of solving the problem of creating an H&P component that provides documentation efficiency while also facilitating comprehensive care and E/M compliance.

Fortunately, integrating E/M compliance principles into medical records stored on paper has provided such a solution. The task now is to duplicate this success with the design features of medical records stored electronically.

References

1. Kohn LT, Corrigan JM, Donaldson MS, eds; Committee on Quality Health Care in America, Institute of Medicine. *To Err Is Human: Building a Safer Health System.* Washington, DC: National Academies Press; 2000.

2. Committee on Quality of Health Care in America, Institute of Medicine. *Crossing the Quality Chasm: A New Health System for the 21st Century.* Washington, DC: National Academies Press; 2001.

3. Levinson SR. Introduction. In: *Practical E/M: Documentation and Coding Solutions for Quality Patient Care.* Chicago, IL: AMA Press; 2005:xv.

4. Bickley LS, Szilagyi PG. *Bates' Guide to Physical Examination and History Taking.* 8th ed. Philadelphia, PA: Lippincott Williams & Wilkins; 2003.

5. Levinson SR. Features of the E/M coding system and the *Documentation Guidelines.* In: *Practical E/M: Documentation and Coding Solutions for Quality Patient Care.* Chicago, IL: AMA Press; 2005:35-48.

6. Levinson SR. The practical E/M experience for physicians at the point of care. In: *Practical E/M: Documentation and Coding Solutions for Quality Patient Care.* Chicago, IL: AMA Press; 2005:57-62.

7. Office of the Inspector General, Bureau of Internal Audit. Office of the Inspector General Compliance Audit of 1997***

8. Miller ED. Compliance and creativity. *Hopkins Medical News.* Winter 2002. www.hopkinsmedicine.org/hmn/W02/postop.html. Accessed June 17, 2005.

9. Levinson SR. Intelligent medical record format option 1: written (paper) and transcription. In: *Practical E/M: Documentation and Coding Solutions for Quality Patient Care.* Chicago, IL: AMA Press; 2005:171-178.

10. Levinson SR. Intelligent medical record format option 2: electronic health records. In: *Practical E/M: Documentation and Coding Solutions for Quality Patient Care.* Chicago, IL: AMA Press; 2005:179-200.

11. American Medical Association. Medicare RBRVS: The Physician's Guide. Chicago, IL: AMA Press; 2004:440.

12. United States Medical Licensing Examination Web site. www.usmle.org/step2/Step2CS/Step2CS2007GI/description.asp. Accessed March 25, 2007.

13. NHS Information Authority. Briefing paper: problem oriented medical record (POMR) and SOAP. CEN WGII, Prague, October 7, 1999. www.prorec.it/documenti/EPR_EHR/NHS-Update-POMR-SOAP.doc [p 1]. Accessed March 25, 2007.

14. Weed LL. *Medical Records, Medical Education, and Patient Care.* Cleveland, OH: Case Western Reserve University Press; 1969:14.

15. Einstein A. Empyrean Web site. www.empyrean.ca/words/quotes/einstein.html. Accessed March, 25 2007.

16. American Medical Association, *Current Procedural Terminology* (*CPT®*) 2007, Professional Edition. Chicago, IL: AMA *Press*; 2006: 5.

17. Bower, A. "Katrina's Lingering Medical Nightmare." September 22, 2005. Available at: www.time.com/time/nation/article/0,8599,1107826,00.html. Accessed June 30, 2006.

chapter 4

Information Integration:
Data, Protocols, and Process

Analyses of future health system benefits deriving from electronic health records (EHRs) focus primarily on the accessibility of *data*. Specifically, data stored electronically should be readily available, not only to the patient's physician, but also to other physicians, pharmacies, laboratories, radiology facilities, insurers, and even organizations that want to use this information to extract statistics for evidence-based medicine studies and the development of best practice protocols. The elements that health policy experts most often designate in the category of *patient data* are, however, largely confined to a collection of *objective* patient-specific information, including demographic information, dates of visits, procedure codes, diagnosis codes, medications, laboratory and X-ray results, and vital signs.

Another touted benefit of EHRs is the ability to provide clinical decision support for physicians at the point of care. This support results from adding programs with recognized protocols for care into EHR software. These protocols help physicians promote quality care by providing preventive care guidelines and disease management guidelines, both of which also fall into the category of objective information, for patients whose diagnoses have already been established.

The third category of information integrated into EHRs is the medical diagnostic process. Unlike data and protocols, the diagnostic process requires a more complex *subjective* approach, because evaluating and managing the care of patients requires a flexible and individualized response to each patient and each medical issue, rather than a preset or automatic algorithm for care. This aspect of care, along with the ability to document its details and nuances, is of paramount importance to physicians providing quality care. The ability to facilitate the diagnostic process and document it effectively should be two of physicians' primary criteria for successful EHR design and functionality. However, reviews of current literature and presentations on EHR benefits by policy leaders and software developers present few, if any, claims for EHRs being able to facilitate the diagnostic process. Therefore, it is important to highlight the need for software vendors to develop designs that assist physicians in obtaining a meaningful history and physical examination (H&P) and in deriving accurate diagnoses in order for EHRs to achieve true success as valuable assets for helping physicians to help patients at the point of care.

Achieving these goals calls for EHRs to offer all three classes of information to physicians: *data*, *protocols*, and *process*. Each of these categories contributes a distinct and constructive type of knowledge to the provision of patient care. Although their benefits and use partially overlap, they also form a sophisticated information hierarchy for helping physicians provide optimal quality care.

- **Data**: The evaluation of data helps physicians make correct diagnoses and monitor their patients' responses to treatments.

- **Protocols**: The application of protocols may contribute to preventive care, to evaluation for selected diagnoses, and/or to implementation of guidelines for treatment and ongoing care, particularly related to chronic conditions.

- **Process**: The diagnostic process is the essential element of care that includes finding and synthesizing clinical information from a patient's H&P, data, and protocols. It is the critical method physicians apply for identifying correct diagnoses and treatments, monitoring patients' responses to therapy, and providing ongoing care. It is important to note that the diagnostic process is also the approach that physicians use to combine the science and the art of medical care.

Because access to data and the application of protocols rely on the inherently effective *storage and retrieval* features of EHRs, many current systems have successfully incorporated these features into their software. On the other hand, integration of the diagnostic medical process depends on the *clinical data entry* capabilities of EHRs. However, because data entry capabilities remain problematic, integrating this highest level of medical record information remains a challenge in most EHR systems.

DATA

Current literature and promotional materials concerning EHRs reveal an overwhelming focus on data, which is the most straightforward level of information recorded in medical records. A partial list of the types of information categorized as data includes patient demographic information, laboratory results, radiology reports and images, reports and images of the results of diagnostic physiologic tests (eg, electrocardiogram and pulmonary function tests), lists of medications, lists of allergies, and lists of *International Classification of Diseases, Ninth Revision, Clinical Modification* diagnostic codes. EHRs offer recognized advantages for storing, retrieving, mining, measuring, correlating, sending, and sharing these types of information.

Data Input

Physicians order diagnostic studies, such as laboratory and radiology tests, as one component of performing the H&P. However, entering the results of these studies and most other types of the aforementioned data into an EHR generally should not require additional time on the physicians' part. The office's administrative staff should enter patient demographic information, a step that could be further streamlined by online registration for patients who are able. For maximum efficiency, system designs should allow nursing staff or patients to document lists of their allergies and medications, which can be entered in the software directly or indirectly. The ideal method for entry of reports and images from clinical laboratories, radiology offices, and physiologic studies is direct electronic uploading into the appropriate sections of the EHR. This feature requires interconnectivity between a physician's office and each type of diagnostic facility, so that orders to obtain studies can be transmitted from the office to the facilities and complete results of the studies can be transmitted from the facility directly back to each EHR.

Using Data

Physicians utilize use most electronically recorded data to assist with evaluation and management (E/M) related to patient encounters. The data can contribute to confirming probable diagnoses and selecting the management options for individual patients. At the onset of the investigation of a new problem, physicians ideally obtain directed laboratory and radiologic tests to confirm or refute their initial clinical impressions. Later in the course of an illness, these tests are commonly used to help monitor a patient's progress and provide early detection of further problems.

Most of the data entered into clinical records are objective. To some, it might seem as if the results of clinical tests could simply be taken at face value and applied by nonphysicians or even by computers to make clinical diagnoses or medical management decisions based on statistical probabilities alone. However, such an approach would reflect only the science of medicine, not the art, which requires interpretation of these data by physicians. Because each patient's medical profile introduces multiple variables, physicians' assessment of clinical test results may appropriately vary for different patients or in different circumstances. Combining the science and art of medicine is needed to provide the individualized care that patients require and that our health system seeks as a basis for quality care.

Are *Data* the Paramount Feature of Medical Care?

During a discussion about the challenges that EHR designs can create for physicians in performing and documenting compliant E/M services, one executive of a medical software company commented that "physicians just have to get the H&P out of the way as quickly as possible—they get their answers from the data."

His understanding of health care was clearly that diagnosis and treatment are all science and no art. However, the paradigm for quality care is that the effective H&P provides physicians with a differential diagnosis, with a high probability of accuracy. In most cases, the added diagnostic tests fill the role of confirming and providing greater detail of the physicians' impressions or, occasionally, disproving them. This method is the medical diagnostic process, which allows physicians to characterize not only the type of illness a patient has, but also to identify the features that distinguish his or her problems. These individual characteristics may, in turn, call for different evaluation and/or treatment from that of other patients with a similar diagnosis.

In other words, data should supplement physicians' clinical impressions, not supplant them. Data are important building blocks of excellent care, but they are not the total structure. Data must be combined with recognized management standards and, most important, with a physician's experience and judgment to achieve personalized care based on clinical expertise rather than automated generic care based solely on laboratory test results.

The role of EHRs should be to help physicians implement the medical diagnostic process and enhance it with available data and protocols, not to replace physician expertise with automated responses based solely on laboratory findings and statistically based protocols.

Data Evolution

Many of the sophisticated tools physicians rely on today for confirming diagnoses and monitoring care did not exist 25 years, 10 years, or even 5 years ago. Furthermore, how and when we use these tests, and sometimes even how we interpret their results, undergoes continual reevaluation and change. For example, the laboratory values considered "normal" for cholesterol and low- and high-density lipoprotein levels have changed dramatically during the last 20 years, and they promise to keep evolving as we increase our understanding of the relationship between blood levels of these substances and vascular occlusion, cellular health, and side effects of medications.

Because most data enter EHRs as information sent from outside sources, the EHR's ability to accept and report data is a passive recording function. Therefore, although data may evolve over time, any changes to the type of data or to ranges for normal values will be made by the reporting facilities and included in their reports. Such changes should not require significant modifications of the EHR software.

PROTOCOLS

The ability to provide clinical decision support is one of the highly praised benefits that EHRs can provide to the practice of medicine. This feature involves incorporating software programs that present recognized guidelines to assist physicians in patient management. The guidelines should be built on currently accepted standards of care, particularly standards that are evidence-based. Such protocols can be used to identify patients with indications for specific tests or treatments, based on appropriate timing and/or clinical indications. This valuable input may occur not only at the point of care, but also in response to predetermined schedules or medical circumstances. Presently, there are two types of protocols being advocated and implemented: preventive care guidelines and disease management guidelines.

Preventive Care Guidelines

Preventive measures improve patient health by providing reminders of when particular patients should be scheduled for diagnostic tests. These guidelines are in accord with evidence demonstrating that obtaining such studies assists with early diagnosis or prevention of serious illnesses. Examples of such regularly scheduled tests with proven health care benefits include mammography, electrocardiograms, and colonoscopy. Software usually provides multiple ways of alerting practices to remind patients when the time is appropriate for them to undergo these studies. The common modalities include pop-up reminders that appear when the physician views a patient's chart (eg, during a visit or a phone call with the patient or with entry of laboratory data) and providing monthly printouts of patients who should be contacted and advised that the appropriate time has arrived to obtain these studies. Because the results of studies obtained in this manner are entered in these patients' medical records, EHRs should also have the capability to identify patients who were advised of the need for a study but did not obtain it. The software can then print a list of the patients so that the practice may recontact them and remind them to obtain the indicated care or find out why they did not obtain it.

Disease Management Guidelines

Disease management measures help physicians implement guidelines for diagnostic testing and for the management of acute and chronic illnesses. These protocols assist with scheduling patient visits at appropriate intervals and scheduling tests in a timely manner. They may even suggest management strategies based on clinical findings or test results indicating that a patient might benefit from further intervention. Current measures of this type being implemented in electronic environments include management of cardiovascular conditions (such as hypertension, coronary disease, and congestive heart failure), diabetes, and asthma.

Protocol Input

Physicians must select the protocols they want loaded into their software and integrated into the disease management approach. They should consider protocols that are relevant to their own specialty and then evaluate which, if any, of the accepted guidelines reflect their own criteria for providing optimal care. Most of the currently recognized protocols apply to primary care specialties, such as family practice and internal medicine. However, most specialty societies are working diligently to develop measures appropriate to the specialty.

Using Protocols

Protocols can ensure that patients with particular diagnoses receive appropriate testing and follow-up care in a timely manner. Disease management guidelines can also facilitate increased use of clinical extenders (eg, nurse practitioners, physician assistants, nurses, and/or medical technicians) to assist in monitoring of patients with chronic conditions.

These significant benefits of using protocols should, however, be accompanied by comparable precautions. Applying a protocol for what later proves to be the wrong condition can delay accurate diagnosis and effective medical management. The foundation for quality care remains the identification of correct diagnoses in a timely manner, a goal that requires physicians to use the more sophisticated level of medical reasoning embodied in the diagnostic process.

In addition, physicians should understand that every patient is unique and more than a statistic. Therefore, before implementing a generally accepted protocol for a specific patient, the physician must analyze whether it is appropriate for the patient's individual circumstances or if the patient's associated conditions or personal needs might call for protocol modification or even rejection. One of the challenges EHRs must overcome is how to facilitate input and subsequent storage of this unique medical information in a manner that accurately reflects the physician's analysis of patient factors that influenced selection and implementation or modification of protocols.

Finally, regardless of whether it is a physician or an extender who is monitoring patients with a protocol, it is critically important that the patients be reassessed at each visit to ensure that they are responding optimally to the management guidelines. This reassessment helps physicians identify patients who should undergo modification of their existing regimen and/or have further evaluation to seek additional or alternative factors affecting their medical status.

As the use of guidelines to provide clinical decision support expands, it is important that physicians and policy makers view protocols as a platform, or starting point, for care, rather than as a confining box that limits the application of individualized care, insight, and creativity. Although guidelines, including evidence-based guidelines, broadly outline a current standard of care, physicians must recognize that *standard* care is the first tier of excellence rather than the final one. Physicians should treat guidelines as a starting point for care, not as a final or automatic management plan. Furthermore, such standards are not written in stone. Some clinical conditions create exceptions to the use of a given protocol. Furthermore, protocols are continually changing on the basis of new observations and new studies. Therefore, they must be continually reassessed and updated.

The Role of Clinical Judgment in Going Beyond a Protocol

Before the introduction of childhood vaccination for *Haemophilus influenzae*, acute epiglottitis was an infrequent but life-endangering airway disease in young children. In children who contracted this infection, severe throat pain developed, along with associated rapid swelling of the soft tissues of the epiglottis, which could obstruct the passage of air through the vocal cords and cause death. Patients commonly arrived at the emergency department in airway distress, with difficulty breathing and significant stridor. The standard protocol in the early 1970s for dealing with this situation was an emergency call to the ear, nose, and throat specialist, who would always take the patient immediately to the operating room, secure the airway with an endotracheal tube, and perform a tracheostomy. This procedure ensured safe breathing through the tracheotomy, which was removed after the patient's condition responded to antibiotics. In the late 1970s, this protocol evolved to include the alternative of avoiding tracheostomy by leaving the endotracheal tube in place for 3 days.

Given the severity and risk of the infection, this protocol for childhood epiglottitis remains highly appropriate. Yet, on two occasions, I was able to diagnose children with this infection before it had compromised their airways. Under this circumstance, it was reasonable to bypass the normal treatment protocol. Instead, it was safe and appropriate to avoid implementing the "standard" trip to the operating room with surgery (or prolonged intubation) by using appropriate antibiotics and personally monitoring the children (with emergency equipment at hand) for 3 or 4 hours, until their fever and pain had completely resolved.

The extreme to which the potential utilization and value of protocols could potentially be overstated can be seen in Mark D. Smith's (MD, MBA) summation of his interview of Clayton M. Christensen, Harvard Business School professor, in the California HealthCare Foundation's March 2007 issue of *Health Affairs*. According to Smith, Christensen proposes that "in the same way Intel turned the art of computer design into a 'rules-based activity,' we are now turning the diagnoses of increasing numbers of diseases, possibly even cancer, into rules-based activities. This shift would allow for lower-cost nurses and medical assistants to take over the treatment of these diseases from higher-cost physicians."[1] Although what Christensen really said was that ". . . what Intel did, as it integrated forward, was that it commoditized computer design, and it made the design of a computer *almost* [emphasis added] a rules-based activity,"[1(pw293)] it still demonstrates the potential hazards (vs pitfalls) of shifting away from a critically important human interaction between physician and patient by delegating excessive and unchecked responsibility to protocols. In the interview, Christensen also advocated a possible commoditization of physicians and investing "more in diagnostics so that you actually don't need expensive physicians and you don't need expensive hospitals to provide the 85–90 percent of health care events that arise in the lives of typical people."[1(pw293)] The critical flaw in this perspective is that we require a physician's knowledge and experience to know for certain which individual is having a relatively insignificant headache and which individual is in the 15% of patients who require immediate sophisticated intervention. Those 15% of patients with critical disease, who could be permanently harmed by protocols designed for the other 85% of patients, will not be comforted by the knowledge that physicians have been commoditized. Protocols must be positioned to assist physicians, not replace them. Similarly we must order our priorities to understand that while cost-saving is an important goal, it must not be attained at the cost of sacrificing appropriate and quality care to each and every patient.

The reality of cost-effective medicine aside, the importance of quality health care and the care of a patient can never be equated to designing computers. To identify the circumstances under which a given protocol should be implemented, modified, or avoided and to accommodate each patient's unique characteristics, medical protocols require the supervision of trained physicians to identify and address the differences among patients as well as their similarities. Unlike computers, a patient's H&P changes over time, and it is precisely this organic and living history that has to be taken into consideration each time a patient is seen and evaluated, ultimately affecting the diagnosis at each visit. Although science predominates in technology and medicine, it is the coupling of science with the art of medicine that allows physicians to identify and prioritize individual differences in order to customize E/M care appropriately for each patient.

A reasonable paradigm for optimal use of protocols begins with making correct diagnoses, which may be challenging because of complex or atypical symptoms, examination findings, and/or laboratory results. Next, a physician must select a potentially appropriate treatment protocol and assess whether the individual patient is a good candidate for this protocol or has contraindications. Finally, as treatment progresses, quality care requires that a physician continually reevaluate this initial decision during follow-up visits, modifying treatments and even diagnoses in accordance with the patient's responses. This continual reassessment distinguishes quality medical care from routine treatments that would be dictated purely by laboratory data and systematic application of protocols.

Although protocols offer great advantages by standardizing proven approaches to a variety of medical problems, their maximal value occurs when they are used to support and supplement good clinical judgment, not to replace it. Protocols are limited by an intrinsic one-dimensional design approach—they generally consider the evaluation and management of only one medical issue because of the nature of the studies they are based on. Because of this limitation, they are inadequate for incorporating a second dimension of multiple coexisting and interacting medical problems or a third dimension of a patient's psychological, environmental, and/or social milieu. It remains each physician's responsibility to identify the circumstances that warrant modification or replacement of a given protocol to facilitate quality care and maximize patient safety and favorable outcomes.

Protocol Evolution

Protocols progressively evolve, and they generally do so at a relatively rapid pace. Changes in guidelines and standards of care are based on external influences, such as new technology and physicians' discovery of improved approaches. For example, the guidelines for frequency of mammograms after age 50 years have been modified on the basis of improved statistical information and with improved detection equipment. Protocols may also evolve as a result of modifications to data standards, through the introduction of new studies (eg, the use of hemoglobin A_{1C} to assist in diagnosis and monitoring of diabetes) or by changes in interpretation of existing studies (eg, the ongoing evolution of standards for the normal level of serum cholesterol and its subcomponents).

Protocols and Optimal Care

In 2005, the *New York Times* published an entertaining and insightful op-ed article written by Abigail Zuger, MD, entitled "When Is a Doctor Too Old? Or Too Young?[2] that considers the relationships among physicians' ages, the type of medical records they use, and the quality of their documentation. One of her observations was that older physicians, owing to their experience, appreciated that "after witnessing enough changing fashions in medical care, a doctor generally learns that most 'best practices' are evanescent."[2]

We therefore need to practice continual reassessment of our existing protocols, so that they can evolve or be replaced as we test them against new knowledge and new experiences.

The ongoing reevaluation and improvement of protocols provide a positive contribution to medical quality. Physicians expect and seek for standards of care to evolve as knowledge, experience, and technology all improve. Although EHRs offer the opportunity of integrating new and modified protocols into each physician's medical practice, it remains the responsibility of physicians to search for ways to improve on existing protocols. It should also be the duty of software providers to be certain that all protocols integrated into their software are updated in a timely manner and without undue cost to physicians as these changes occur.

PROCESS

The medical diagnostic process is represented in the E/M codes physicians use when providing patient care. As noted throughout the book, this process should be the central element of every patient visit. It involves actively obtaining a patient's medical history and performing an appropriate physical examination. It also includes the medical decision making component, which integrates the results of the H&P, consideration of the severity of the patient's medical status (ie, nature of the presenting problems), counseling, and coordination of ongoing care. This process also specifically integrates the other categories of information in the medical record, including analysis of patients' existing diagnostic data and determination of need for additional testing. It also includes assessment of the appropriateness of protocols and ongoing analysis of their success in fulfilling a patient's medical requirements. Because the diagnostic process integrates clinical data and medical protocols into patient care, it is the most complex level of information addressed in EHRs.

As described in Chapter 3, the Current Procedural Terminology (CPT®) E/M codes and guidelines accurately capture the way medical schools teach the diagnostic process to physicians. Therefore, incorporating compliant E/M design and functionality into medical records in general, and into the electronic H&P component in particular, should not only help physicians document accurately, it should also provide a road map for following the diagnostic process and increase the efficiency and effectiveness of patient care.

However, to date, the concept of incorporating E/M compliance principles, including consideration of medical necessity, into H&P component design has drawn insufficient attention from software developers, presenters at national health information technology (HIT) meetings, and authors of HIT publications. Yet, in all likelihood, the ability to integrate compliance and the diagnostic process into the electronic H&P component will have a significant impact on the clinical effectiveness of EHRs and on physicians' adoption rates.

Diagnostic Process Input

Taking a medical history, performing a physical examination, and documenting the medical diagnostic process appropriately occupy most of physicians' time and effort during every patient encounter. Effective provision and documentation of this care benefits from medical record designs capable of meeting multiple important criteria, including the following:

1. **Promotion of quality care:** the ability to guide and promote the diagnostic process and facilitate accurate documentation of this care; the paramount criterion for any medical record

2. **Usability:** to provide a medical record structure compatible with the principles of care and documentation taught to physicians so that they can use it intuitively while caring for their patients

3. **E/M compliance:** capable of meeting current standards of care and documentation established by medical societies, as published in the *CPT* manual and Documentation Guidelines

4. **Efficiency:** allowing provision and documentation of appropriate levels of care within the restrictive time frames currently available, without loss of quality or compliance

5. **Integrity of clinical information:** facilitating entry of visit-specific information that reliably records all significant patient history, exam findings, and decision making in a manner easily interpreted during subsequent encounters, reliable for medical studies, and effective for liability protection

6. **Promotion of appropriate productivity:** based on providing, documenting, and coding levels of care warranted by the severity of patient illness at the time of each visit

In reviewing the relationships among these six criteria, it is noteworthy that medical records with design and functionality that incorporate E/M coding compliance, efficiency, and usability should significantly promote quality care, information integrity, and appropriate levels of practice productivity.

Despite the acknowledged importance of creating compliant medical records, evidence demonstrates that, to date, a significant number of EHR systems have fallen short of meeting standards for compliance and for promoting the diagnostic process:

1. In May 2006, the publication *Part B News* cited internal documents at the Office of the Inspector General that called for a "fraud alert" regarding *noncompliance* of E/M documentation and coding produced by using EHRs.[3]

2. In May 2007, the Foundation of Research and Education of the American Health Information Management Association issued a call for public comment on proposals it sent to the Certification Commission for Healthcare Information Technology (CCHIT) to enhance and expand fraud management through software in EHRs. Among the concerns stated in this report are the existence of several data entry designs intended to increase speed of entering clinical information that, when used as instructed, are susceptible to creating generic and noncompliant documents. As examples of this problem, the report voices concern that "the use of defaults, templates, copying and other tools . . . *could be subject to fraud or abuse* [emphasis added]."[4] It also identifies fraud issues related to E/M coding software in current systems.

3. During consultations across the country, physicians and clinical staff have repeatedly reported problems with EHR *usability*. Many administrators report that one of their greatest frustrations in implementing EHRs is that implementation often requires many months for physicians to adjust their care to the data entry characteristics of the EHR.

4. Many physicians and staff also report problems with lack of documentation *efficiency* for the H&P, reporting it takes considerably longer for them to enter patient-specific clinical details directly into software than it would to write or dictate the same information. On the other hand, many design efforts to increase the speed of documentation have also sacrificed the ability for physicians to enter descriptions that are specific to each patient and each visit. These documentation shortcuts may endanger not only compliance, as noted earlier, but also the quality of the physician's diagnostic process and the integrity of the clinical information recorded.

5. *Quality* problems may arise from these same design problems, such as software that reproduces identical clinical information from previous visits and/or creates documentation by uploading macros with preentered generic clinical information instead of visit-specific descriptions. Documentation created in this manner lacks individualized descriptive information, making it more challenging to appreciate the true course of each patient's illness.

Using the Diagnostic Process

Although the use of information related to data and protocols is based on the reliable data storage and retrieval capabilities of EHRs, physicians' ability to use the diagnostic process and record their findings and interpretations depends on the design and functionality features of the electronic H&P component. It is, however, these design features that have created significant challenges for physicians. The critical issue for software design arises from the difficulty of facilitating physicians' provision and documentation of comprehensive care in a relatively compressed amount of time. Even though medical software will accurately store and retrieve the clinical information the physician enters, a problem arises if the software fails to facilitate the documentation of high-quality, encounter-specific clinical information, which can lead to the recognized potential pitfall of all software systems: "garbage in, garbage out."

During the question period following her keynote address at a 2006 national conference on health information exchange, Carolyn Clancy, MD, director of the Agency for Healthcare Research and Quality, was asked her opinion regarding the need for a national standard for EHR designs that will promote efficient input of quality clinical information. Clancy observed "I do think there is some groundbreaking work needed at the fundamental level for clinical information, including work that needs to be done to make this [ie, input of medical history and physical information] easy and useful."[5]

Standards for Recording Clinical Data

Clancy's recommendations for improved clinical content can be implemented by requiring software companies to apply a standard for effective design of the clinical record. Fortunately, the CPT E/M system provides the recognized standard for documenting the H&P. Because this system is a codification of how physicians are trained to carry out the diagnostic process and to record their care, the next logical step is to establish E/M compliance as a standard, or prerequisite, for the design features of the electronic H&P component.

The groundwork for meeting this requirement is, in fact, already in place. The CCHIT's Final Ambulatory Functionality Criteria for 2007 require that "the system shall provide the ability to select an appropriate Evaluation and Management code based on data found in the clinical encounter."[6] Recognizing the need to include "appropriate" E/M functionality is a valuable first step. However, this general statement should be expanded and enforced. This calls for specifying designs that meet all parameters of E/M documentation compliance, including consideration and documentation of medical necessity and elimination of potentially noncompliant design features, that CCHIT has already identified[5] and that will be analyzed in greater detail in Part 2 of this book.

The medical diagnostic process described in the *Bates' Guide to Physical Examination and History Taking*[7] is is appropriately similar to related portions of the *CPT* manual: the E/M chapter at the beginning of the book and the "Clinical Examples" section in Appendix C. In practical terms, this process begins with the physician obtaining a thorough medical history, which leads to the development of an initial differential diagnosis and a preliminary assessment of the severity of the patient's medical problems. The physician next performs a physical examination to the extent warranted by the severity of illness. After this, he or she reviews available data (eg, previous records, laboratory results, and X-ray results), finalizes a differential diagnosis, considers management options for the illness, and orders any indicated additional tests or procedures needed to confirm or rule out the possible diagnoses.

Finally, the physician should accurately and thoroughly record all these findings, impressions, diagnostic possibilities, and management plans in the medical record. This documentation is of critical importance for each patient's future care, whether by the same physician or by others.

"Why" as Well as "What"

Lawrence Weed, MD, is a noted authority on medical records. In the 1960s, he introduced the problem-oriented medical record concept and the SOAP (subjective information, objective information, assessment, plan) note for subsequent care visits. He also wisely observed, "It's not sufficient just to know what was done. It's a very incomplete record if we don't know why it was done."[8]

Weed's insight underscores the importance of reporting not only the findings and plans, but also the highlights of the physician's thought process and reasoning, which are shown by listing other potential diagnoses and alternative treatments. This documentation, which parallels E/M guidelines, provides the physician (and other future caregivers) with a full perspective of the basis for clinical decisions and recommendations. It facilitates ongoing management, as well as reassessment when indicated. In addition, this insight may provide a physician with support during claims review, audits, and even in the event of medical liability actions.

Evolution of the Diagnostic Process

During the last 40 years, physicians have experienced an ever-increasing pace of breakthroughs in medical science: newly discovered diagnoses, new tests, new treatments, new procedures, new protocols, and even a multitude of new medical specialties. Yet the critical principles that guide and inspire physicians remain constant: dedication to patient care and caring, commitment to excellence, allegiance to medical ethics, and the medical diagnostic process. The structure and method taught now for performing and documenting a thorough and effective H&P continues to follow the same principles of the medical diagnostic process taught during the 1960s and 1970s.

A physician examining a medical record from the era of Sir William Osler would expect to see documentation of the patient's medical history, the physical examination, one or more diagnostic impressions, and plans for care. Over time, refinements have divided the medical history into six elements[9]:

- Chief complaint: concise statement, in the patient's words, of reason for the patient's visit
- Past medical history: medical illnesses with which the patient has been previously diagnosed
- Social history: environmental factors potentially affecting the patient's health and well-being
- Family history: hereditary factors potentially affecting the patient's health and well-being
- Review of systems: survey of possible signs and symptoms that may provide insight into the patient's presenting problems and reveal possible additional or impending medical issues
- History of present illness: chronological description of the course of the problem(s) concerning the patient on the date of the medical encounter

Also during the last 40 years, there have been two noteworthy refinements to the structure of the medical record and the diagnostic medical process. In the late 1960s, Weed's *Problem Oriented Medical Record (POMR)*[10] provided an increased focus on the impressions section and stressed the importance of a comprehensive listing of all of the patient's medical and medically related problems, with appropriately documented plans for each problem. This record structure guides the physician to incorporate a comprehensive vision of each patient's health status. Weed continued his focus on the impressions and plans sections during subsequent care with the introduction of the SOAP note structure for documentation of follow-up visits.

The next noteworthy medical record change arrived in 1992, with the American Medical Association's introduction of the E/M system for documentation and coding of medical records.[9] This approach does not alter most of our long-established medical record architecture, but rather codifies and quantifies the standard H&P design and the diagnostic medical process. It includes the same medical history (with chief complaint, past medical history, social history, family history, review of systems, and history of present illness), physical examination, and medical decision making (data reviewed, clinical impressions, management plans, and data ordered). The E/M system introduces two material innovations to the H&P. First, it relates the extent of cognitive care to CPT codes and, thereby, to levels of reimbursement. Second, to help categorize the complexity of medical care, it calls for formal consideration (and documentation) of several elements of the diagnostic process that had not previously been documented in medical records. These elements include the following:

- Complexity of data requested and/or reviewed
- Risk of the presenting problem(s)
- Risk of diagnostic tests
- Risk of management options
- Nature of the presenting problems, a measure of medical necessity

Unfortunately, medical student education and most formal E/M training programs do not identify the importance of actually *documenting* these five elements. Yet, by incorporating these elements into the structure of effectively designed records, adding such documentation requires little time and effort on the part of the physician, and it is one of the keys to making E/M compliance an integral and user-friendly component of patient care.[11,12]

Since its introduction, applying E/M principles while caring for patients has, unfortunately, presented significant challenges for physicians. The combination of factors responsible for this difficulty includes the following: (1) the lack effective tools that would allow physicians to incorporate E/M principles into the care processes, (2) absence of E/M training in medical schools and residency programs, (3) noncompliant E/M auditing approaches, and (4) punitive rather than educational audits by Medicare and insurers.

Early in medical school training, nearly all physicians are taught and closely supervised for performing and documenting *comprehensive* H&Ps. Since 1974, for many students this training has commonly been based on the principles in the *Bates' Guide,*[7] which parallels E/M coding and documentation. Despite their training, most physicians leave residency and enter practice routinely performing and documenting *problem-focused* or *expanded problem-focused* levels of care during the majority of patient visits. This approach often is used even for patients whose severity of illness warrants significantly higher levels of care, as indicated by specialty societies in Appendix C of the CPT manual.[9] Medical school graduates commonly enter the "real world" with insufficient training in CPT coding principles, little familiarity with CPT's documentation requirements, and a lack of awareness of the E/M Documentation Guidelines. In most cases, they have not received the methodology, tools, and/or experience to have the ability to provide compliant and comprehensive care in the limited time that most have available for each patient visit.

Medical Schools and E/M

It is worthwhile to briefly explore what happens to physicians as they progress from initial clinical experiences in the first or second year of medical school through the culmination of medical school and then into their residency years.

In the course on the "introduction to clinical medicine," students learn and practice the comprehensive H&P, which is the embodiment of the diagnostic medical process. During this time, instructors carefully scrutinize care and documentation by students to ensure that they master these core elements of quality medical care. However, as tools to document their care, instructors provide and permit students to use nothing more sophisticated than a pen and a blank sheet of paper. With such rudimentary tools, as most physicians accurately recall, the time necessary for performing and writing down the care involved in an initial encounter requires approximately 60 minutes.

Although there is significant value in learning comprehensive care from the ground up, including gathering information and building patient relationships, this is a time frame that does not realistically prepare students to practice quality medicine under real-world circumstances, in which reimbursement supports only 5 to 15 minutes of care. At a reasonable point during training, instructors should be able to introduce structured forms that speed the documentation effort without disrupting effective performance of a comprehensive H&P. (Such forms should provide a framework of commonly asked questions and examination components while requiring students to enter all findings and encouraging them to expand on these basic elements.) This type of transition would allow students to obtain the same quality (and quantity) of information in a shorter time.

Following this introductory course, supervision and scrutiny of medical record documentation generally diminishes. Once formal clinical responsibilities begin, with the increasing pressures of greater patient responsibilities and overwhelming amounts of information to learn, students find they no longer have an hour to devote to each patient encounter. Under such duress, because they have not been trained using efficient and compliant documentation tools, they gradually trim their comprehensive H&P, learning and introducing shortcuts to care and documentation. This trimming process continues throughout the residency years, as time constraints increase, emphasis on the importance of comprehensive documentation diminishes, and staff assessment of the quality of the resident's medical record fades.

E/M COMPLIANCE, THE DIAGNOSTIC PROCESS, AND MEDICAL RECORD SOLUTIONS

Since 1995, The *Practical E/M* approach[13] (published by the AMA Press in late 2005) has provided effective tools and a functional method to facilitate the diagnostic process for practicing physicians who use conventional medical records. The solutions of *Practical E/M* for achieving an effective medical record in the E/M era include the following: (1) formally including nature of the presenting problem as an integral component of the medical diagnostic process, (2) incorporating documentation of ancillary medical decision-making elements (data complexity and the three levels of risk) and the nature of the presenting problems into the H&P, (3) integrating E/M principles into the customary medical diagnostic process so that documentation and coding become an intrinsic component of patient care, and (4) designing a structured medical record framework ("Intelligent Medical Record") that functions intuitively for physicians while ensuring compliance and maximizing efficiency.

There are two additional goals for successfully incorporating effective E/M concepts into patient care. The first is that these principles should be introduced during the earliest stages of clinical education and maintained during residency training so that they become integrated into physicians' usual practice patterns as part of the medical diagnostic process that they complement. The second is the substance of this book, which is to incorporate all of the elements of this practical solution into the H&P design of electronic records. When medical practices make it a priority to seek out and purchase EHR software systems that incorporate these principles, they will be using designs that help them bridge the electronic chasm and achieve a smooth and seamless transition into the new world of EHRs.

SUMMARY

With improvements in science and technology, medicine is experiencing a rapid evolution in the means of diagnosing illness and providing treatment. As a part of this evolution, EHRs can facilitate these advances by supporting effective use of three classes of information: data, protocols, and the diagnostic process physicians use to evaluate patients.

Examples of *data* include clinical laboratory reports, radiology reports and studies, and physiologic test reports and studies. Care *protocols* may include clinical decision support tools, such as preventive care schedules and disease management guidelines, as well as patient education sheets. The significant advantages of EHRs in improving use of these two types of information during patient care have justifiably drawn the spotlight from advocates of EHRs. These two information categories provide *objective* patient information, which is often entered from sources extrinsic to the physician's interaction with patients and then applied to patient care. Their use, therefore, relies on the data storage and retrieval functionality of EHR software. Because this type of functionality is readily programmed in electronic systems, using EHRs to enhance care with improved use of data and protocols is commonly described at HIT conferences as "picking the low-hanging fruit."

However, effective use of improved access to data and protocols for clinical decision support must build on a solid foundation of established medical principles. This foundation for providing high-quality care is the medical diagnostic process. It is the method by which physicians integrate clinical history, physical examination, data, and protocols to accurately determine severity of illness, derive correct diagnoses, and implement optimal treatment options. The fundamental principles of this diagnostic process, which have been taught relatively unchanged to medical students for many decades, provide the consistent intellectual basis for supporting and properly using rapid improvements in health care. This process is the core concept physicians rely on for promoting quality care.

Unlike test results and protocol information, which rely solely on objective information, the diagnostic process uses objective patient findings and subjective interpretations of information elicited during interaction with patients at the point of care. Successful integration of the medical diagnostic process into EHR design demands an appreciation of these complex information elements and necessitates data entry software that can accommodate these requirements. These demands require software designers to move into the more challenging realm of "high-hanging fruit." Facilitating the development of designs that successfully incorporate all the elements of the diagnostic process into the electronic H&P component in a compliant format is the purpose of Part 2 and Part 3 of this book.

The Role of the Diagnostic Process in Achieving Quality Goals

Although a variety of organizations and stakeholders have offered their impressions of what constitutes "quality health care," we have no universally accepted definition of this concept. In *Crossing the Quality Chasm*,[14] however, the Institute of Medicine directly relates enhancing quality of care to creating designs that facilitate the processes physicians rely on, stating:

> "Substantial improvements in quality are most likely to be obtained when providers are highly motivated and rewarded for carefully designing and fine-tuning care processes to achieve increasingly higher levels of safety, effectiveness, patient-centeredness, timeliness, efficiency, and equity."

It is therefore essential that EHR designs for the electronic H&P must also be capable of supporting this finely tuned care process.

References

1. Smith MD. Disruptive innovation: Can health care learn from other industries? A conversation with Clayton M. Christensen. *Health Aff.* 2007;26:w288-w295. doi: 10.1377/hlthaff.26.3.w288. *California Health Care Foundation*, March 13, 2007.

2. Zuger A. When Is A Physician Too Old? Or Too Young? *New York Times.* February 8, 2005.

3. Vogenitz W. EMR and E/M: Beware of software's potential to upcode. *Part B News.* May 1, 2006. www.eclinicalworks.com/2006-05-01-pr2.php. Accessed December 15, 2006.

4. Office of the National Coordinator for Health Information Technology, US Department of Health and Human Services. In: Recommended Requirements for Enhancing Data Quality in Electronic Health Record Systems: Final Report. June 2007: 46. Available at: www.rti.org/pubs/enhancing_data_quality_in_ehrs.pdf. Accessed December 14, 2007.

5. Clancy C. Presentation at national conference on Health Information Exchange; April 11, 2006; Washington, DC.

6. CCHIT Ambulatory Functionality 2007 Final Criteria. March 16, 2007:41. www.cchit.org/files/Ambulatory_Domain/CCHIT_Ambulatory_FUNCTIONALITY_Criteria_2007–Final–16Mar07.pdf. Accessed June 7, 2007.

7. Bickley LS, Szilagyi Peter G. *Bates' Guide to Physical Examination and History Taking.* 8th ed. Philadelphia, PA: Lippincott Williams & Wilkins; 2004.

8. Versel N. Dr. Weed's software cure. www.bio-itworld.com/hitw/emag/070104/289. html?terms=Dr.+Weed%e2%80%99s+software+cure. Accessed June 7, 2007.

9. American Medical Association. *Current Procedural Terminology (CPT®).* Chicago, IL: American Medical Association; 2007.

10. Weed LL. *Medical Records, Medical Education, and Patient Care.* Cleveland, OH: Case Western Reserve University Press; 1969.

11. Levinson SR. Documenting the nature of presenting problem. In: *Practical E/M: Documentation and Coding Solutions for Quality Patient Care.* Chicago, IL: AMA Press; 2005:119-126.

12. Levinson SR. Documenting medical decision making. In: *Practical E/M: Documentation and Coding Solutions for Quality Patient Care.* Chicago, IL: AMA Press; 2005:137-158.

13. Levinson SR. Intelligent medical record format option 1: written (paper) and transcription. In: *Practical E/M: Documentation and Coding Solutions for Quality Patient Care.* Chicago, IL: AMA Press; 2005:171-178.

14. Committee on Quality of Health Care in America, Institute of Medicine. Executive summary. In: *Crossing the Quality Chasm: A New Health System for the 21st Century.* Washington, DC: National Academies Press; 2001:1-22.

Analyzing Prevalent Electronic H&P Design Characteristics

Having narrowed our focus to exploring the critical role of the electronic history and physical examination (H&P) in meeting the goals of physicians and medical practices, this section explores the breadth and depth of issues that can create barriers to success. Identifying these issues will provide a starting point for establishing the fundamental principles of electronic health record design and functionality required to meet physicians' needs for the H&P component of EHRs.

NOTE: Following completion of Part 1, readers are offered two options for choosing the next section of the book to read.

- If you wish to follow the step-by-step examination of usable, complaint, and effective H&P designs, read the analyses in Parts 2 and 3 before concluding with Part 4's investigation of an approach to successful practice transformation.

- If you wish to focus first on effective medical practice strategies for evaluating, preparing for, and verifying EHR systems prior to implementation (or effectively addressing problems with an existing system) you may prefer to skip directly to Part 4's discussion of Practice Transformation and Health Information Transformation, before returning to explore the critical design and functionality features presented in Parts 2 and 3.

chapter 5

Assessing Potential Barriers
to Success With Electronic H&P

Medical practices encounter a series of challenges in their efforts to eval-uate and implement electronic health records (EHRs). As an initial step, the physicians and administrative staff must select a knowledgeable and appropriate evaluation committee, which proceeds through stages that should include the following:

- Identifying current medical record issues they want and need to address
- Determining if an electronic system will address these issues
- Anticipating new issues that an electronic system may introduce and existing issues it may affect or exacerbate
- Planning a strategy to avoid or limit such complications
- Weighing costs and benefits, both economic and noneconomic
- Evaluating software packages, selecting a vendor, and negotiating a contract
- Preparing the practice for EHRs
- Implementing the EHR system
- Establishing protocols for ongoing monitoring and improvement

Although these issues affect all aspects of a medical practice, *Practical EHR* focuses specifically on refining and optimizing the history and physical examination (H&P) component of EHRs, particularly its impact on how physicians practice and on their provision of patient care. A physician's first mandate is to perform the medically indicated level of individualized care during each patient encounter. A second mandate is that the information the physician enters into the record must be a true reflection of the care pro-vided. Therefore, a prerequisite for any medical organization investigating the purchase of an EHR system should be to verify that the systems it con-siders must have the ability to provide its physicians with functionality that complements the diagnostic process plus an effective format for efficiently documenting a comprehensive H&P.

Organizing EHR Priorities

A large hospital in the Southwest had just begun the second year of a 5-year project for implementing an EHR system. The phases for introducing each element of the inpatient EHR system assigned the physicians'

continued

clinical notes as the final element to be integrated—at the end of the project—because *how* the clinical notes would be integrated had not yet been determined.

Current software designs have generally failed to provide an optimal solution for the H&P component. However, because this component is an indispensable feature of an EHR, a medical organization should verify that the vendor's H&P design will meet the physicians' criteria for quality, usability, and compliance before accepting a particular system and its introduction into patient care.

Medical organizations, physicians, administrators, information management specialists, and professional coders offer few if any concerns related to the data storage and retrieval functions of EHRs. Their most significant difficulties and/or frustrations with EHRs relate to the electronic H&P component. The issues range from a variety of efficiency and data entry challenges that arise while physicians are caring for patients to concerns by physicians, coders, and compliance specialists about records that guide physicians to create nonspecific generic documentation and/or fail to meet compliance criteria.

When significant problems are identified, the first step in addressing them is to ask "why," and then to analyze the factors creating the problems so that they can be successfully addressed and eliminated. This second section of *Practical EHR*, therefore, examines the current state of issues surrounding the electronic H&P component. The current chapter begins examining these challenges and their overall impact on physicians and their potential for success with EHRs. The following four chapters peel back these issues, layer by layer, to reveal the obstacles that software designers must overcome to create systems that meet physicians' needs during the patient care process. Identifying the source and the scope of these issues should lay the foundation for proposing and then implementing solutions that can rectify them.

SURVEYING THE CURRENT ELECTRONIC H&P LANDSCAPE

The five features of EHRs identified as "physicians' requirements" for success all involve the H&P component of medical software programs. The first two priorities—immediate access to medical records and reducing costs compared with using a paper system—relate to the *data storage and retrieval* features of EHRs. Many well-designed electronic systems successfully fulfill these two requirements.

The remaining three priorities—evaluation and management (E/M) compliance and related quality of care, quality and efficiency of documentation, and optimal productivity—all depend on the design and functionality features of the electronic H&P and physicians' ability to document meaningful clinical information in this portion of the EHR.

The goal in this section of the book is to identify existing electronic H&P features whose structure and/or function are inadequate to meet these last three requirements or have the potential to interfere with accomplishing them. These consequences may result from problems intrinsic to the design or from designs that fail to protect against physicians using the software incorrectly, intentionally or unintentionally. The mission is to ensure that the next generation of EHRs acknowledges each of the problematic features and corrects or eliminates them, thereby supporting the final three medical practice priorities.

Problematic Electronic H&P Designs

There is evidence that significant problems exist with the conventional design of electronic H&P and its data entry functionality. First, authoritative sources cite a 33% to 50% failure rate for electronic record adoption.[1,2] In addition, a variety of sources have reported that physicians should anticipate a decrease in productivity during the first 6 to 12 months of EHR implementation.[3,4] Finally, as noted in Chapter 4, Clancy recommended additional effort to facilitate the ease of entering clinical information and to ensure that this information is clinically useful.[5]

Despite these compelling observations, I have found no published reports or presentations that identify these as the causes for implementation failures or reductions in productivity. However, physicians and administrators who have experienced these problems indicate that they frequently result from challenges physicians experience in using the electronic H&P. Their focus is on efficiency issues and/or difficulties creating individualized descriptions and compliant documentation.

The concerns with documentation are reinforced by the fact that in the last several years, multiple authoritative sources have identified significant compliance problems following reviews and audits of physicians' documentation in electronic H&P records.[6-9] A review of some of their conclusions not only underscores the gravity of this issue, but it also focuses attention on some of the major compliance and quality-care problems that need to be addressed.

Articles by Gustin

In her series of articles in 2006 entitled "What You Don't Know About Electronic Health Record Clinical Progress Notes and Paper Templates Could Be Creating Compliance Risk," compliance expert Georgette Gustin noted that many EHRs have documentation features and coding software that promote "increased potential for upcoding."[6] She further quotes the Trailblazer Medicare carrier's "concern that the computerized programs may default to a more extensive history and physical examination than is medically necessary… [for] the patient's condition on the specific date of service."[10] These articles also introduce the critical issue of EHR "cloning," which is described in multiple publications and compliance reviews. Gustin describes *cloning* as "each entry in the medical record for a patient that is worded exactly like or similar to the previous entries. Generally, it is most often found in the form of pre-printed or template-type notes."[10] Cloned records can be found not only for multiple visits of the same patient, but also when notes for many different patients are nearly identical, varying by only two or three words or phrases. Many EHR software systems advocate (and some require) physicians to use "templates" or "macros" as the basis for their documentation of medical histories and/or physical examination findings. However, when these macros contain preentered clinical information, such as a generic medical history or normal examination findings, the documentation is cloned.

Gustin emphasizes that cloned documentation violates "one of the key fundamentals of documentation, coding, and billing [which] is that the clinical care be patient and date specific."[6] She further cites a Cigna Medicare carrier's conclusion that "Cloned documentation does not meet medical necessity requirements for coverage of services rendered due to the lack of specific, individual information. Further, cloning of documentation will be considered *misrepresentation* of the medical necessity requirement for coverage of services."[10]

Problems Created by Cloned Documentation

Certain elements of the medical H&P report require patient-specific and visit-specific *narrative* information to describe and distinguish the individual and unique features of a patient's medical circumstances. Cloned documentation substitutes preloaded information, which precludes the physician from obtaining or documenting a true narrative description for these critical sections of the record, which are integral to accurately performing the diagnostic process.

Physician Rhymes with Musician

Once while attending an annual jazz festival with close personal friends, one of them discovered a flyer for *Downbeat* magazine that highlighted an old quotation from the renowned jazz composer Charles Mingus:

"Once you achieve technical facility, you're either a musician or you're not. You're either a creative person or a stenographer."

This insight for musicianship parallels concerns we should have for electronic medical record designs that substitute standardized verbiage for the insights available to physicians who approach the history, examination, and clinical assessment individually for each patient. Cloned documentation tends to reinforce the "stenographer" approach to patient care. Although physicians' education begins with teaching the standard methodology of evaluation and care, it also stresses that this must be only a starting point, not a final destination. While a majority of patients will respond to a formulaic approach, a significant number will not. Physicians' training includes learning the art of identifying which patients and problems call for going beyond a standard approach and how to provide it. The electronic H&P design must facilitate this benefit, not obstruct it.

The sections of the medical H&P record for which preloaded macros are most commonly substituted for free-text narrative descriptions include the following:

1. History of present illness (HPI): The *Bates' Guide to Physical Examination and History Taking*[11] describes this component of the medical history as a "complete, clear, and chronological account of the problems prompting the patient to seek care. The narrative should include the onset of the problem, the setting in which it has developed, its manifestations, and any treatments."[11(p4)] Cloned documentation fails to fulfill this requirement because it is clearly not possible to preprogram the timeline of the course of each patient's specific illness.

2. Addressing patients' positive responses to questions in the review of systems (ROS): Each positive clinical symptom or sign for the ROS indicates the existence of potentially significant illness. The physician

must evaluate each of these positive responses to determine if it is a contributing factor to the presenting problems or an additional potential medical problem. This effort requires the same type of medical history taking, narrative documentation, and diagnostic process as the HPI.

3. Abnormal findings of the physical examination: Detailed descriptions of the variations from normal are also patient specific and visit specific. Painting an accurate picture of the findings allows physicians to reliably follow the course of a patient's illness and response to therapy.

Cloned Documentation, Compliance, and Quality Care

When a coding auditor reviews 5 or 10 or 15 records generated by an EHR system and the charts all read identically except for a few words in each record, the auditor has no choice but to conclude that all of this documentation, except for the few differing words, was the product of a software system's capability to mass produce the same information over and over. In the face of such findings, an auditor is required to conclude that the only medical care supported by the documentation relates to the words that are different. As a result, this limited amount of individual documentation generally substantiates only problem-focused care during every patient encounter. An auditor would be compelled to reach the same conclusion if a physician documenting an H&P used a rubber stamp with a few blanks for individualization of information on a paper record.

Medical record tools that sacrifice individualization for speed can impede individualized care and documentation. Physicians cannot rely on automated documentation to convey an accurate picture of a patient's health or medical concerns. Another physician reading cloned medical records is forced to discredit all elements that read the same on every chart.

Cloning contradicts one of the basic tenets of quality health care that all physicians learn early in training: "no two patients are alike." Although there may be many similarities among patients with a given chief complaint, not all have the same diagnosis and not all should receive the same treatment. Identifying—and documenting—patients' individual differences allows determination of accurate diagnoses and optimal treatments.

A senior coder at an academic medical center described working with one physician to design H&P macros for more than 11 months, with continued dissatisfaction of the physician because the standardized forms were unable to accurately describe the individual features of each patient's illness. The software support team suggested making more and more macros, but this approach also was unsatisfactory. The physician and coders understood that, when used as intended, the use of macros failed to meet quality and compliance standards.

Publication by *Part B News*

The May 1, 2006 issue of *Part B News* headlined the compliance warning "EMR and E/M: Beware of Software's Potential to Upcode."[12] The newsletter staff obtained a draft of an internal document from the Office of the Inspector General, which they described as seeming to be a preliminary national Medicare fraud alert, warning government and law enforcement agencies about the "use of medical documentation software programs in a manner that results in the upcoding of Office Evaluation and Management Services."[12] This article voiced concern about EHR systems that use "copy and paste" functions as a documentation mechanism that can result in cloned records. This software capability allows a physician to duplicate information from a previous encounter and insert it into the documentation for the current encounter, although such identical documents cannot certify that the physician actually repeated the elements of history or examination. Copy and paste functions also fail to confirm that there was a medical indication on the date of the visit to perform the elements of the H&P that are copied and pasted. The article specifically discussed a document from a Medicare carrier that "warned providers in Connecticut that EMR software, by automatically filling in stored information from separate chart notes, may lead them to 'over document' and consequently 'select and bill for higher-level E/M codes than medically reasonable and necessary.'"[12] It is important to note that the article also stated that "providers can't hide behind ignorance."[12] Improper documentation and coding occurs when physicians use such software as it is designed to be used, not necessarily out of malice or fraudulent intent: "[providers] didn't know but should have known they were submitting false claims."[12]

Presentations by Rappaport

Bruce Rappoport, MD, is highly qualified, not only as a physician and a certified coder, but also as a compliance consultant and medical director (Broward Health, Fort Lauderdale, FL). In 2006 and 2007, he presented a program entitled "Electronic Medical Records—Friend or Foe"[7,8] at the annual conference of the American Academy of Professional Coders. Dr. Rappoport is a strong advocate for the health care benefits of EHRs, emphasizing the positive features of data access, clinical decision support, computerized physician order access, and interconnectivity. He is equally insightful about the importance of physicians identifying and addressing potential compliance, quality care, and data integrity problems in the design and functionality of the electronic H&P, including his observations that:

- EHR programs that rely solely on templates and do not allow for free text integration can give rise to pattern documentation. Pattern documentation often lacks individualized, patient-specific supporting information that supports medical necessity for services provided. Limitations on free text ability can lead to quality and compliance concerns.

- Documentation for each patient encounter that is worded exactly like or very similar to the previous entries is considered cloning. Medical necessity is not supported when documentation is not specific and individualized for each encounter.

- Coding based solely on bullet points without consideration of medical necessity is noncompliant. The *Medicare Claims Processing Manual* stresses that medical necessity is the overarching criterion for payment.[13] EHR programs that base their evaluation and management coding determinations solely on meeting documentation guidelines without integration of medical necessity should not be used.

- There is a significant concern over complacency by physicians when an EHR program can autopopulate medical information from prior visits that is not verified for accuracy and updated by the provider before the encounter is completed.

Recommendations in *Practical E/M*

Practical E/M: Documentation and Coding Solutions for Quality Patient Care[14] considers the same E/M compliance concerns and adds recommendations for promoting visit-specific information and achieving compliant EHR documentation. For all components of the H&P record that call for individualized narrative documentation, such as the HPI and abnormal findings of the physical examination, the software must permit physicians to enter free-text descriptions. In addition, these systems should assist physicians by replacing designs that have the potential for creating cloned or otherwise noncompliant records with designs that provide guidance for compliant care and documentation.

Analysis by Linker

At the Fourth Health Information Technology Summit in March 2007, Robin Linker, a certified professional coder, an experienced auditor, and a highly respected leader and educator in the health care industry, spoke on compliance issues physicians have experienced when using EHRs.[9] One of her copresenters, Michael Barr, MD, vice president, American College of Physicians, discussed physicians' concerns with patient care issues that can arise from the use of certain EHR software features.[9]

Linker presented the results of reviews of a number of physicians' charts created with EHR products, which she performed at the request of a state medical board. The board was responding to complaints from patients who noted that their clinical records differed significantly from the care they had received.[9] Her analysis of the EHRs revealed that the electronic software inserted "pre-canned [sic] EHR template language" into every chart. The cloned documentation made it "difficult to determine the actual services rendered, due to extensive duplication of the records."[9] As a result of these audits, the physicians were required to make refunds to payers of more than $100,000.

Linker's conclusions provide authoritative insight into the compliance and quality issues that can arise when EHR features fail to require and facilitate *individualized* documentation for every patient and every encounter:

■ The providers submitted high-level E/M codes (levels 4 and 5) for 98% of patient visits.

■ Audit results proved cloning (copying and pasting as well as canned macros) was used in documentation in a majority of records.

■ Although the charts presented comprehensive documentation in every case, there seemed to be no consideration of the NPP or determination of appropriateness of the submitted codes.

■ Medical necessity for performing the documented comprehensive H&P was nonexistent, and the level of care sometimes conflicted with the information in the HPI.

■ There were no differences in notes for the different patients other than in some portions of the HPI and parts of the plan and medical decision making.

■ The EHR analysis proved the existence and use of canned documentation.

> ### How Could These Medical Practices Not Have Noticed Such Overcoding?
>
> Two goals of physicians in purchasing EHR systems are to create compliant medical records and to increase productivity. Unfortunately, many physicians lack training in compliance and, in particular, have not been made aware of the overriding importance of medical necessity in determining appropriate levels of service. It must be assumed that the physicians and practice administrators noticed and were aware that they were submitting an increased frequency of high-level codes. Having said that, it is likely that they were relying on their EHR software systems to ensure compliance (even though the licenses for most systems include disclaimers regarding coding compliance).
>
> ### A Pivotal Role for Coders
>
> Physicians are ultimately responsible for their own documentation and coding, regardless of the method they use to record their care. However, based on the analyses showing that certain EHR software designs may not meet E/M care and documentation compliance requirements, medical practices cannot presume that software developers have incorporated fully compliant designs. Therefore, it would be wise for practices to include coding professionals as members of their EHR evaluation and implementation teams, which would allow them to identify and address noncompliant designs and help ensure that the physicians are able to use the system in a manner that fulfills compliance criteria.

Linker's cautions about potential design problems in the current generation of EHRs underscore the compliance risks created by cloned documentation and by the failure of these EHRs to require physicians to consider and document levels of medical necessity. Such systems also present the danger of providing physicians with a process that allows entry of clinical information that does not reflect a patient's true medical status, which may lead to noncompliant upcoding and "potentially falsifying the patient record without [physician] realization of participation or the consequences of false claims."[9] Linker stated that physicians should select the level of service based on medical necessity and that the care given must be justified in the documentation. She also stated that software systems "should remove all [potentially] fraudulent documentation features, ensuring that templates contain only structure but not substance (ie, preloaded clinical information)."[9] These statements reflect and underscore the compliance principles of *Practical EHR*.

CCHIT Identifies Noncompliant Data Entry Designs

In January 2007, the Certification Commission for Healthcare Information Technology (CCHIT) officially recognized the existence of significant problems with noncompliant techniques for documenting the H&P. At that time, it issued recommendations compiled by the research institute, RTI International, and requested public comment on those recommendations.* This

---

*This organization compiled its report under the sponsorship of the Office of the National Coordinator for Health Information Technology. It convened the Model Requirements Executive Team (MRET), a volunteer panel of experts including providers, payers, informatics experts, law enforcement professionals, and data quality professionals. Their charge was "to develop model requirements to prevent medical claims errors and detect potential health care fraud." http://ehrantifrauddev.rti.org/

report resulted from a study to determine the use of health information technology (HIT) in enhancing and expanding fraud management. To develop these proposals, "FORE [the Foundation of Research and Education of the American Health Information Management Association] convened a multi-stakeholder group of experts, the National Executive Committee (NEC), to identify the best opportunities to strengthen the fraud management capability of a nationwide interoperable HIT infrastructure."[15] By building on CCHIT's existing 261 functionality criteria for EHR certification, this project identified EHR design elements that, when used by physicians as intended, provide the opportunity for fraudulent documentation and coding. These issues were refined and finalized in the final report, issued in May 2007 by the Office of the National Coordinator for Health Information Technology. Among the six current CCHIT criteria that address the H&P component, the NEC identified the following EHR design and functionality elements that have the potential for creating fraudulent documentation (ie, intrinsic noncompliance):

- In the section that addresses "Documentation Process Issues," the final report cites the variety of data entry mechanisms available for documentation of the H&P, including discussion of problems that can arise from the use of "automated machine-entered default information; pre-created documentation via form or template; copy/import of an object including date/time user stamp of original author; and copy forward previous note contents. . . ."[16] The report concludes that these are "legitimate benefits of using an automated system and can be extremely helpful if used correctly; however, the tools can also open the electronic health record systems (EHR-S) up to fraud or abuse."[(p4-10)]

- The report's section on "Evaluation and Management (E&M) Coding" addresses the acceptable limitations of functionality related to E/M coding. First, it acknowledges, "It is appropriate for EHR-S to calculate an E&M from the encounter data that has been entered and to indicate the basis for that calculation."[(p4-11)] The report continues with a warning that "[i]t is not appropriate to suggest to the provider that certain additional data, if entered, would increase the level of the E&M code."[(p4-11)] However, following input during the comment period, the final RTI report appropriately modifies this conclusion by recognizing that the restriction on providing physicians with E/M documentation guidance "does not apply to prompts for additional documentation for E&M levels already achieved, *for medical necessity* [emphasis added] or for quality guidelines/clinical decision support."[(p4-11)]

- By identifying compliance problems and potential fraud issues that are intrinsic to some of the design features of currently available EHR systems, CCHIT's findings provide a critical first step toward acknowledging the need to correct these deficiencies. Unfortunately, rather than recommending that defective data-entry feature of EHRs be corrected, CCHIT recommends that EHRs incorporate additional features, which essentially act as an audit of a physician's encounter data "to indicate the basis for that calculation."[(p4-11)] To confuse the situation even more, MRET's rationale in the Final Report suggests that ". . . it is not appropriate to suggest to the provider that certain additional data, if entered, would increase the level of the E&M code. The wording of the current CCHIT requirement, although unintended, could be interpreted to suggest the latter."[(p4-11)] Ultimately, this still leaves practices open to uncertainties, possibilities of upcoding and audits—all of which would subject them to potentially severe financial penalties for using their EHRs as designed and intended by the developers.

An Alternative Action Plan to Address Noncompliant Documentation Shortcuts

It would have been more appropriate for the NEC to conclude that these documentation shortcuts are *inappropriate* design elements that may interfere with compliance and with what should be the primary role of EHRs, which is to help physicians provide individualized patient care and maximize quality and patient safety. Therefore, the report's proper conclusion should be that the inclusion of these inappropriate design features in an EHR would be cause for denial of certification by CCHIT.

OVERVIEW OF ELECTRONIC H&P CHALLENGES

Compliance and Quality Challenges

As discussed in Chapter 3, the correlation between the principles and language in the *Bates' Guide to Physical Examination and History Taking*[11] and the "E/M Services Guidelines" section of the *Current Procedural Terminology (CPT®)* manual[18] provides powerful evidence that following E/M compliance guidelines promotes quality medical care. Including the role of the clinical examples in Appendix C[18(pp423-454)] and the *CPT* manual's E/M descriptors[18(pp9-33)] reinforces this relationship, advising physicians to provide levels of care warranted by the severity of each patient's medical problems at the time of his or her visit.

However, as noted, some features of EHRs that are intended to promote more rapid entry of clinical information also have the potential to permit and even encourage noncompliant documentation. Such features may also negatively affect the quality of care a physician provides by limiting the ability to document patient-specific and visit-specific information.

From the Patient's Perspective

When patients see their physicians because of a medical problem, they want individualized evaluation and treatment that match their personal health and needs, not nonpersonalized "copy and paste" care based on preloaded clinical information and treatment plans.

No two patients are identical, and it is physicians' professional responsibility to identify the differences and similarities among patients. Software tools must facilitate this philosophy of care, not interfere with it.

Usability Challenges

Many medical practices experience prolonged time frames for physicians to create generic macros (which may promote noncompliant documentation) and learn to use them in documenting care. Because the established and proven model for performing a H&P requires care and documentation customized to each specific visit, adapting to software designs that use preset documents may create an uncomfortable choice for physicians—taking too much time to accurately document individualized care or using shortcuts for rapid documentation, which might compromise the rigorous diagnostic process. Overcoming this challenge calls for H&P designs that can replicate physicians' familiar diagnostic process and promote efficient documentation of individualized care. Such designs should shorten the EHR learning curve for physicians and significantly increase the rate of successful EHR adoption.

Efficiency Challenges

The quality and compliance challenges physicians face are exacerbated by the time limitations for care imposed by the economic constraints of our health care system. To increase efficiency, data entry systems (in any format—written, dictated, or electronic) must incorporate design tools that increase the speed of the documentation process. Moreover, electronic systems are able to introduce more powerful tools and more options for H&P documentation than structured paper charts or dictation templates. However, software designers must exercise great care in the structure and functionality of these H&P programs because they influence physicians' interactions with patients and documentation of the encounters. In all formats, physicians require that designs permitting speedy documentation must not compromise quality, compliance, or usability of their H&P process and record. Therefore, designers must ensure that tools that increase efficiency also facilitate the diagnostic process and maintain the ability of physicians to record detailed individualized descriptions that will provide a valid record of the patient's condition and care.

Of course, efficiency is not an element of compliance. In fact, an examination of the contributory factor *time* that CPT guidelines designate as "typical" indicates that providing complex levels of care is assumed to be a time-consuming (ie, "inefficient") process (see Table 3.2, Chapter 3). Similarly, asking patients about their goals for care reveals that they are seeking more time and attention from their physicians, not less, particularly when they are very ill. Efficiency enters the medical record equation primarily as a result of economic factors in our present health reimbursement system. Analysis of the relative value units for E/M services and current Medicare and insurer conversion factors reveals that current payment levels provide payment for only approximately 30% of the time allotted as typical for these services. In practical terms, "efficiency" is an *economic* requirement for success in using medical records, rather than a quality criterion. A major challenge for EHR designers is helping physicians achieve high levels of compliance and quality while providing increased levels of efficiency.

Productivity Challenges

As with the external pressures for efficiency, the call for optimal productivity is the result of economic constriction created by reimbursement rates far lower than would be provided under a realistic resource-based system. A caution, which applies to physicians, administrators, and software developers, is that *overcoding is not an acceptable remedy to underpayment by insurers.* These are individual issues that should be addressed independently of each other. Software that fosters overcoding, which generally occurs as a result of failing to address medical-necessity concerns and through the use of noncompliant designs, is not only noncompliant, but as noted in the reports by the Office of the Inspector General and CCHIT,[12,16] it can expose physicians using such practices to charges of fraud and subject them to severe financial penalties.

Practical EHR's goal for productivity is that EHR coding functionality should follow the compliance principle of helping physicians perform and document the level of care warranted by the NPP at the time of the visit. This approach promotes quality (by ensuring that patients are provided an appropriate extent of history, examination, and decision making) and compliance (by ensuring that codes are submitted at the appropriate level for the severity of illness and for the care provided). Productivity is maximized to the extent that guidance, based on E/M's NPP, ensures that physicians provide, document, and code for the level of care that is medically indicated for the severity of each patient's medical condition at the time of the visit.

The Goldilocks Rule

The conventional E/M approach emphasizes only the three "key components": the levels of history, examination, and medical decision making. This emphasis leaves physicians and auditors primarily comparing the level of code submitted with the level of documentation, without initial consideration of the risks of morbidity, mortality, and/or loss of function inherent in the patient's illness. For example, when a claim shows a level 3 code, but documentation supports only level 2, an auditor may conclude that either the chart has been overcoded or underdocumented. These interpretations are two sides of the same coin.

However, the *Practical E/M* method[19] recognizes the NPP as a "mandatory fourth factor." Coders using this approach first compare the code selected with the NPP to determine whether there has been overcoding (coding at a level higher than warranted by the NPP) or undercoding (coding at a level lower than warranted by the NPP). The conventional comparison of level of documentation with code selected becomes a second step, which determines whether there is underdocumentation (the three key components are insufficiently documented to support the submitted code) or adequate documentation for the selected code.

Physicians following this method are advised to employ the "Goldilocks Rule": when compared with the identified and documented level of NPP, the level of care selected (ie, E/M code) should be "not too high and not to low but just right." By using this approach, neither overcoding nor undercoding should occur.

Data Challenges

Medical records must record objective data, which is quantitative or rigidly defined, and subjective data, which is qualitative or descriptive. Objective data can more readily be searched and analyzed than subjective data, and policy makers who cite the benefit of using EHRs to promote health information exchange concentrate primarily on the value of sharing objective data. This type of medical information includes patient demographic information, laboratory and radiology test results, vital signs, patient allergies, patient medication lists, CPT codes (procedures billed), and ICD-9 CM (diagnoses submitted with claims).

Subjective information encompasses clinical details, such as the HPI, descriptions of abnormal examination findings, and detailed clinical impressions. Documenting the richness and variety of this category of information warrants and requires the use of narrative free-text. Owing to the greater ease of analyzing objectively entered data, some software designs have eliminated the use of free-text in some sections of the H&P by requiring physicians to compile clinical descriptions from multiple series of limited preselected vocabulary pick-lists, using a mouse to "point and click" to sequentially select words or phrases and create a pseudonarrative. This approach is arduous and extremely inefficient, and the resulting description lacks the breadth and depth of free-text—albeit it is easier to search the descriptive sections of such medical records, the descriptions are less satisfactory. Software designs should not compromise data integrity in an effort to improve search capabilities.

PLACING H&P DESIGN ISSUES ON THE EHR ENHANCEMENT AGENDA

The *Practical EHR* approach recognizes the importance of identifying non-compliant data entry designs, such as those recently reported by CCHIT.[16] It also advocates that all such faulty designs be eliminated from EHRs rather than simply monitoring their use, which is an approach that ultimately helps Medicare and insurers to extract financial retribution instead of correcting the flawed functions. Physicians must be able to rely on their medical records to facilitate quality patient care, without fear that using the software as instructed could result in compliance and fraud concerns. The RTI report's contention that these documentation shortcuts, which are designed essentially to increase speed of documentation, "are benefits of an automated system"[15] is not a valid reason for the continued inclusion of designs that permit noncompliant, imprecise, or fraudulent documentation. Physicians and information management professionals should require that software systems protect them from these electronic H&P problems through the use of designs that ensure compliance and quality, not interfere with it.

One of the cardinal rules of H&P design in EHRs must be that electronic systems cannot forgo quality care, compliance, and/or usability in an effort to increase speed.

SUMMARY

Current EHR designs successfully address medical practice goals related to data storage and retrieval. However, physicians, coding experts, the Office of the Inspector General, and the CCHIT have identified certain design features of electronic H&P components that may guide physicians to perform care and documentation that fail to satisfy E/M compliance standards. These features may also fail to meet physicians' desires to have EHRs that promote and reflect high-quality individualized clinical care. To address this concern, one of the cardinal rules of H&P component design in EHRs should be that electronic systems not compromise quality care, compliance, and/or usability in an effort to increase speed of care and/or documentation.

Instead, to fulfill physician requirements for the electronic H&P component, EHRs must incorporate designs that facilitate compliance and clinical effectiveness while also meeting the efficiency requirements of the current health care environment. Achieving this goal requires inclusion of tools and functionality that provides guidance on proper consideration of medical necessity, and it also mandates elimination of all design features that offer the potential for noncompliant or potentially fraudulent documentation.

References

1. McClellan M. CMS Quality, Efficiency and Value-Based Purchasing Policies: The Role of Health Information Technology. Presented at: the Second Health Information Technology Summit; September 9, 2005; Washington, DC.

2. Chin T. Avoiding EMR meltdown: how to get your money's worth. *AMA News.* December 11, 2006; 49(46): Business Section.

3. National City. Going paperless: do electronic health records hold value for your practice? 2007, www.carenetsystems.com/pdf/EHR%20White%20Paper.pdf. Accessed July 23, 2007.

4. National Quality Forum. CEO Survival Guide™ to Electronic Health Record Systems: Tools for Executives Q & A. 2005. www.nqfexecutiveinstitute.org/ executiveinstitute/ehrs_qanda.cfm. Accessed July 23, 2007.

5. Clancy C. Keynote address. Presented at the Third Annual Connecting Communities Learning Forum; May 11, 2006; Washington, DC.

6. Gustin G. What you don't know about electronic health record clinical progress notes and paper templates could be creating compliance risk, I: the compliance department needs to be involved in the selection and implementation process. *J Health Care Compliance.* January-February 2006:57-59.

7. Rappoport B. Electronic medical records: friend or foe. Presented at the Annual Conference of the American Academy of Professional Coders; April, 2006; St. Louis, MO.

8. Rappoport B. Electronic medical records: friend or foe. Presented at the Annual Conference of the American Academy of Professional Coders; April 18, 2007; Seattle, WA.

9. Linker R, Levinson S, Barr M. Meeting E/M Compliance & Quality Care Standards with the Next Generation of EHRs. Presented at the Fourth Health Information Technology Summit; March 30, 2007; Washington, DC.

10. Gustin G. What you don't know about electronic health record clinical progress notes and paper templates could be creating compliance risk, II: being proactive can help your organization identify coding and documentation concerns. *J Health Care Compliance.* March-April, 2006: 45-47. Available at: www.trailblazerhealth.com/pub/sentinel/2002/02-2.pdf. [1] Ibid, Part II, March–April, 2006, pp. 45–47, Cigna citation: www.cignamedicare.com/docs/Medicare_Bulletin/idaho.htm. Accessed July 23, 2007.

11. Bickley LS, Szilagyi PG. *Bates' Guide to Physical Examination and History Taking.* 8th ed. Philadelphia, PA: Lippincott Williams & Wilkins; 2004:4.

12. Vogenitz W. EMR and E/M: beware of software's potential to upcode. *Part B News,* May 1, 2006. www.eclinicalworks.com/2006-05-01-pr2.php. Accessed May 15, 2007.

13. Centers for Medicare & Medicaid Services. Selection of level of evaluation and management service. *Medicare Claims Processing Manual.* Chapter 12:section 30.6.1. www.cms.hhs.gov/manuals/downloads/clm104c12.pdf. Accessed May 15, 2007.

14.   Levinson SR. Intelligent medical record format option 2: electronic health records. In: *Practical E/M: Documentation and Coding Solutions for Quality Patient Care.* Chicago, IL: AMA Press; 2005:179-200.

15.   RTI International Anti-Fraud Model Requirements. http://ehrantifrauddev. rti.org/Home/tabid/36/Default.aspx. Accessed July 23, 2007.

16.   Office of the National Coordinator for Health Information Technology (ONC). Recommended Requirements for Enhancing Data Quality in Electronic Health Record Systems. www.rti.org/pubs/enhancing_data_ quality_in_ehrs.pdf. Published May 2007. Accessed July 23, 2007.

17.   Office of the National Coordinator for Health Information Technology, US Department of Health and Human Services. 4.2.5. Requirement 5: evaluation and management (E&M) coding. In: Recommended Requirements for Enhancing Data Quality in Electronic Health Record: Final Report. May 2007:47. www.rti.org/pubs/enhancing_data_quality_in_ehrs.pdf. Accessed July 23, 2007.

18.   American Medical Association. *Current Procedural Terminology.* Chicago, IL: American Medical Association; 2007.

19.   Levinson SR. Practical E/M methodology. In: *Practical E/M: Documentation and Coding Solutions for Quality Patient Care.* Chicago, IL: AMA Press; 2005:49-56.

chapter 6

Toolkit for Analyzing Electronic H&P Software

Whether medical records are stored in paper files or electronic records, physicians have long experienced challenges in meeting the health care system's standards for documentation and coding compliance. For electronic health records (EHRs) to successfully supplant paper medical charts, they must satisfy physicians' documentation requirements. To achieve this, it is mandatory that they meet standards for evaluation and management (E/M) compliance.

EVOLUTION OF THE CURRENT E/M COMPLIANCE PARADOX

Following the 1992 introduction of the E/M coding system and extensive training sessions conducted by instructors from the former Health Care Financing Administration, "friendly" audits (ie, without financial penalties) of physicians' paper records revealed a higher than acceptable rate of coding errors because of inadequate documentation and/or lack of medical necessity.

Similar findings have been reported by the Centers for Medicare & Medicaid Services (CMS) in a letter dated June 1, 2000, from Thomas Scully, CMS Administrator, which "notified Medicare physicians that CPT codes 99233 and 99214 for evaluation and management services had accounted for a significant portion of the FYs 1998 and 1999 coding errors."[1] These inaccuracies were documented and reported again in the OIG's analysis and review of Fiscal Year (FY) 2001 Medicare fee-for-service claims, as outlined in the February 15, 2002, memorandum and final report from Inspector General Janet Rehnquist to Thomas Scully, Administrator of CMS. Included in the report are tables that review audit results for fiscal years 1996 through 2001; these demonstrate error rates ranging between 31.3% and 56.6% for code 99214 and error rates from 30.8% to 54.6% for code 99233.[1*]

Regardless of the format used, medical records have continued to demonstrate E/M compliance problems. As a result, software developers have faced a dual challenge: lack of a reliably compliant medical record model among practicing physicians and low demand from most physicians for development of such a model. The low demand from physicians can be attributed to the fact

---

* Further, the description of the review of the documentation for these codes suggests the findings are based solely on the three key components (history, examination, and/or medical decision-making), without additional consideration of medical necessity.

that E/M compliance audits of small practices are rare. In contrast, large medical groups that have undergone compliance audits and university centers that have been the subject of Physicians at Teaching Hospitals (PATH audits)* are highly sensitive to requirements for E/M compliance and the need for an active compliance program in their organizations.

Given the economically dictated time constraints for patient care and the resultant medical record shortcuts used by many physicians as a result of those constraints, it is unfortunate that physicians in training and in practice have rarely been introduced to the alternative of using *compliance-based* H&P forms. These are structured records that are capable of facilitating comprehensive care in the same amount of time needed to perform and record problem-focused care when using a written or dictated note composed entirely of free-text. Although in the last several years many practices have incorporated forms to facilitate documentation of initial patient visits, scrutiny of these efforts generally exposes compliance deficiencies for one or more components of E/M care. Most frequently, the charts are missing required documentation related to medical decision making and medical necessity. They may also employ suboptimal designs for portions of the medical history and physical examination. These same deficiencies are common in EHR software presently in the marketplace.

Early EHR Designs and E/M Compliance

In early EHR systems, E/M coding was not addressed. The design features of these early EHR systems usually lacked sufficient E/M documentation elements to permit physicians to document a comprehensive history, a comprehensive examination, and/or complex medical decision making, all of which are required to document and code correctly. The software also failed to provide for evaluating and documenting medical necessity. In other words, even when used to their full capacity by physicians caring for patients with severe illness warranting level 4 or level 5 care, these early systems lacked the ability to guide and facilitate compliant levels of care and documentation. Regrettably, these problems persist in many current electronic H&P designs.

The E/M Compliance Paradox

The current perceptions of physicians and EHR vendors about E/M documentation and coding demonstrate that neither party has been willing or able to comfortably assume responsibility for E/M compliance. The EHR companies contend that physicians should be responsible for correct documentation and coding. They confirm this point of view by including instructions and license agreements advising physicians that they have the ultimate responsibility for coding correctly, even when their systems include

continued

---

* Many of these audits, which were conducted by the Office of the Inspector General (OIG), resulted in significant financial penalties for universities and/or their physicians. The first OIG audit of this type was at the University of Pennsylvania and concluded in 1995. In that review, an audit of 100 charts showed significant compliance issues (approximately half of which related to improper E/M code levels). Based on extrapolation of the findings, the physicians reached a settlement with the OIG for a penalty of $30 million.

a software "coding engine." Physicians, on the other hand, assume that their EHRs are providing all the necessary H&P components for compliant documentation and are able to guide them to code correctly.

The resolution to this conundrum requires a dual approach. First, physicians should insist on H&P designs that allow them to document all the components of E/M services (including medical necessity) and EHR programming and functionality that provide guidance for meeting the standards for compliant care, documentation, and coding. Second, physician preparation for using EHRs should include training in E/M compliance principles because the ultimate responsibility for compliance rests with physicians.

MEDICAL RECORD DESIGN ELEMENTS

The seven components of E/M coding[2] dictate five medical record sections that must be successfully addressed to create E/M compliant medical records:

- Medical history, consisting of subsections for chief complaint, past medical history, family history, social history, review of systems (ROS), and history of the present illness (HPI)
- Physical examination
- Medical decision making, including subsections for data reviewed, clinical impressions (ie, differential diagnoses), treatment options, data requested, complexity of data reviewed and/or requested, risk of presenting problems, risk of diagnostic tests, and risk of treatment options
- Nature of the presenting problem(s)
- A section that considers the combination of three contributory factors: counseling, coordination of care, and time

Practical E/M[3] introduced a set of tools for analyzing the general design and functionality of each subsection of the H&P report, which can be applied to gaining insights into electronic record design. These three analytical tools include (1) consideration of the different types of *interface* between the medical record and the person entering the data, (2) identification of the options for *data entry personnel,* and (3) the choice of *formats* available for entering and storing clinical information.

Interface

The term *interface* describes the design structure that an electronic H&P offers to physicians for documenting clinical information. Selecting an appropriate interface for each section of the record directly impacts physicians' efficiency for documenting clinical findings, the potential for data input by nonphysicians, and the ease with which physicians can access and use the information entered.

There are two distinct medical record interface categories, each with significantly different strengths and weaknesses.

- A *graphic user interface* provides the person entering information with a preprinted list of questions or descriptions from which to select appropriate responses (eg, a survey of possible medical illnesses in the past medical history section of the H&P screen or form). A second variation expands on this option by also allowing the entry of brief written responses to specific predetermined questions.

■   A *narrative* interface presents a blank section of the form that permits recording of detailed free-text information. This type of interface is most effective for portions of the medical visit that call for analog (expository) documentation (ie, an individualized history of the patient's present illness).

Optimal medical record design should present the type of interface that is best suited to the information-gathering requirements of each subsection of the H&P component. Each physician's H&P document can further be customized as appropriate for different specialties and individual physician preferences, provided that the fundamental compliance and quality care requirements are maintained.

Graphic User Interface

The graphic user interface allows efficient documentation of data that can be expressed in a concise, straightforward manner. It presents structured clinical elements that have been pre-entered into the H&P design. The person recording clinical information can enter information rapidly, by indicating whether each element is present or absent. There are several design options for graphic presentation, including:

1.   Check-boxes to record *yes* or *no* or *normal* or *abnormal* responses
2.   Blank lines for concise answers
3.   Selection lists for designating specific choices

A graphic user interface that combines check-boxes and blank lines is particularly useful for several sections of the history elements of medical records. The check-boxes provide an efficient tool for clinicians or patients to enter positive and negative responses rapidly in sections for the past medical history, family history, social history, and ROS. Check-boxes are similarly effective for efficiently documenting whether the physician's findings for each element of the physical examination are normal or abnormal. This type of interface, which is illustrated in Figure 6.1, ensures compliance with CPT® coding because it requires the person entering medical history information to review and actively document a *yes* or *no* response for each question.* In addition, the adjacent blank lines provide the ability to document further details when appropriate. This design can be applied to electronic screens and to paper documents, and this interface allows patients to complete their own documentation. Therefore, it must use straightforward language that permits patients to easily understand and reply to the individual questions. Chapter 12 explores the various data entry tools available to EHRs that allow patients to document the appropriate elements of their own medical history.

---

* As opposed to noncompliant graphic designs, such as 1) "default" documentation, which provides pre-entered negative or normal responses that the physician may (or may not) choose to modify to accurately reflect findings; and 2) graphic interfaces that suggest that the *lack of documentation* indicates a negative response (even though a nonresponse could equally indicate a question was not asked or a body area was not examined). An example of the second problematic design would be an interface that has only a single check-box next to each statement, where the box should be checked for a positive response, but otherwise left blank.

F IGURE 6.1

Past Medical History: Check-Boxes (Sample Design). Example of graphic user interface, combining check-boxes and short answers for documentation of past medical illnesses (diagnoses). The checked boxes and *italicized* response illustrate the appearance of a completed partial form.

Past Medical History			
Please check the "Yes" or "No" box to indicate if you have any of the following illnesses; for "Yes" answers, please explain.			
	Yes	No	
Diabetes	☐	☒	
High blood pressure	☐	☒	
Thyroid problems	☒	☐	*low thyroid diagnosed in 1999, treated with thyroid pills*
Heart disease/cholesterol problems	☐	☒	
Allergy problems/therapy	☐	☒	

By using a similarly designed interface for the physical examination component of the H&P, a physician documenting his or her findings can, by rapidly checking the appropriate box, indicate an impression of *normal* or *abnormal* for each body area examined. (Specific details of abnormal findings must be added in a narrative section.)

Software designers must respect two design principles to ensure compliance and the entry of quality information when incorporating the checkbox graphic interface. First, the preloaded template must contain structure but not substance. In other words, each check-box is programmed to appear blank; it is then individually completed as *positive* or *negative* (or *normal* or *abnormal*) during the visit. Any preloaded responses are considered noncompliant because they record information the software "memorized." A graphic interface that reports preloaded responses (ie, documentation by exception) has the potential to create documents that do not accurately reflect the patient's responses and/or examination findings.

The second quality and compliance factor that needs to be respected when using graphic interface designs is that physicians must investigate any positive responses in greater depth and document the details of that investigation. For example, when a patient reports a positive history of thyroid disease or a symptom of chest pain, effective care and compliance require the physician to elicit and record more detailed information. This additional information enables the physician to form an assessment regarding whether the patient's past illness or additional symptoms are clinically significant and, therefore, require further evaluation, regardless of whether they might be contributing to the patient's presenting complaint. Similarly, evaluating and documenting an abnormal finding during the physical examination calls for providing a more detailed description than a preliminary impression indicating, eg, "lung sounds, abnormal." The additional narrative documentation of this abnormal examination finding should create a verbal picture (or, in this example, an auditory description) that is precise enough for another physician to readily interpret what is wrong with the patient (eg, "diffuse moist inspiratory rales throughout the right lower lung field; remaining areas clear to auscultation"). In addition, the extent of this description should be sufficient to allow a physician who is reexamining the patient in the future to knowledgeably compare the findings on the two separate dates and determine whether the abnormality is stable, improving, or becoming worse.

A third type of graphic interface, the selection list, includes multiple preprinted responses to a specific question. It allows the clinician entering clinical assessments into an electronic H&P to document information by selecting one or more of the items on the list. For example, selection lists prove extremely effective in helping physicians indicate which one of the four levels of risk of presenting illness applies to a patient. This design is not appropriate for sections of the record, such as the ROS, that require a documented response (eg, positive or negative) to *each* listed element.

Part 3 of this book will demonstrate that graphic interfaces are extremely useful and efficient for the following sections of the H&P:

- Past medical history
- Family history
- Social history
- ROS
- Physical examination (normal findings)
- Elements of medical decision making (including data reviewed, data requested, complexity of data, and risks of illness, diagnostic tests, and treatments)
- Nature of the presenting problem

Narrative Interface

The *narrative interface* consists of a blank space for the entry of free text for documenting more complex clinical information. Designers of EHR systems must recognize that physicians require a *narrative* approach for obtaining (and for documenting) the thorough and in-depth descriptive information required for significant medical history information, recording specific abnormal physical examination findings, and describing the medical decision making involved in the diagnostic process. This type of interface allows documentation to reflect the way physicians are taught to obtain a medical history, delving, layer-by-layer, into the details of the course of a patient's illness. Obtaining an effective HPI, for example, uses a sophisticated evaluation process. The patient's response to an initial question or set of questions directs the content of the physician's next set of questions, and those responses direct selection of the next group of inquiries. The process continues until the physician can securely identify a reasonable differential diagnosis. This approach elicits responses that are unique to each patient and to each encounter, and this individualized information is optimally documented using a descriptive narrative. The restricted yes-no or linear vocabulary of the graphic interface would limit the quality and extent of information that can be recorded; therefore, it "is not suited to 'tell a story' of each patient's unique medical history or to adequately describe the nuances that distinguish each patient's abnormal physical exam findings."[3]

The narrative interface offers the optimal design for compliant and efficient documentation of the following sections of the H&P:

- HPI
- Details concerning positive responses to inquiries in the ROS (these discussions should function like "mini" HPIs.)
- Positive findings of the physical examination
- Descriptive details and qualifying remarks for the "impressions" and "plans" sections in the medical decision making portion of the medical record

Options for Data Input by Medical Personnel and Patients

The Documentation Guidelines provide that "the ROS and PFSH [personal, family, and social history] may be recorded by ancillary staff or on a form completed by the patient."[2(p6)] Therefore, it is unnecessary for physicians to personally obtain and enter all preliminary medical history information into the medical record to satisfy compliance specifications. However, the guidelines require that physicians review this information, ask their patients about positive responses, record these details, and apply the responses appropriately to patient care. In the world of paper records, mobilizing patients and medical staff to obtain and record appropriate portions of the medical history has significantly increased efficiency while maintaining compliance and enhancing medical quality. Designs for EHR software should, in a similar manner, provide the capability for patients to record their own responses for the PFSH and ROS by direct or indirect entry into the electronic H&P.

Options for the Medical Record Format

The term *format* refers to the medium used for collecting and storing medical record information. Writing, transcribing (or dictating), and electronic data entry and storage are conventionally considered the three potential formats. It remains important to differentiate between the data entry and the data storage components of medical records. By focusing attention on EHRs, the electronic format for data storage and retrieval has already been selected. However, when evaluating data entry options for clinical information, it will be important to consider the relative strengths and weaknesses of each of the three common formats, plus the potential advantages of hybrid alternatives. Hybrid approaches can combine several of the three formats to maximize their strengths and minimize their weaknesses. Providing a full range of options for documenting the electronic H&P allows each physician to select the data entry format that matches his or her practice patterns and personal preferences.

SUMMARY

The earliest designers of electronic systems did not have an understanding of the relationship among compliance, the medical diagnostic process, and quality care. They also lacked a compliant model in paper medical records to guide their efforts.

On the other hand, although medical students receive training for performing a comprehensive H&P, the only tools they are taught to use—a pen and a blank sheet of paper—are highly inefficient, and they are insufficient to help physicians function effectively in today's real practice environment. As a result, to complete their care in the time available under current economic constraints, almost all physicians have been forced to compromise the provision and/or documentation of comprehensive care in favor of speed.

To meet the needs of the health care system and of practicing physicians, designs of EHRs must facilitate *all* of these features: appropriately comprehensive care, the diagnostic process, compliance, and maximal efficiency. Attaining this result requires that medical practices and vendors have access to a model for identifying the strengths and weaknesses of various EHR data entry designs and for reassessing design and functionality capabilities desired for future electronic systems. A conceptual toolkit is required to analyze the effect of various design options on quality care, usability, and efficiency. This analysis includes consideration of *interface* designs, *data entry personnel* options, and data entry *format* opportunities. Combining these building blocks in an optimal manner will allow creation of designs that meet the needs for effective H&P components and avoid unacceptable compliance problems.

References

1. US Department of Health and Human Services. Improper Fiscal Year 2001 Medicare Fee-for-Service Payments (A-17-01-02002). http://oig.hhs.gov/oas/reports/cms/a0102002.pdf. Accessed January 15, 2008.

2. American Medical Association. Evaluation and Management Services Guidelines. In: *Current Procedural Terminology CPT®*. Chicago, IL: American Medical Association; 2007:1-7.

3. Levinson SR. Model for analyzing medical records. In: *Practical E/M: Documentation and Coding Solutions for Quality Patient Care*. Chicago, IL: AMA Press; 2005:63-73.

4. American Medical Association, Health Care Financing Administration. *Documentation Guidelines for Evaluation and Management Services*. Chicago, IL: AMA Press; 1997.

chapter 7

The Source of Electronic H&P Design Issues

Most physicians' challenges in using electronic health records (EHRs) arise when working with the electronic history and physical examination (H&P) record at the point of care. This chapter investigates the underlying factors that can cause these problems by adversely affecting software designs. Identifying the source of H&P issues should provide the knowledge and incentive to approach enhancements of electronic H&P design and functionality with the same level of energy and creativity already being applied to data storage, retrieval, and exchange features of EHRs.

Defining Functionality

The term *functionality* is commonly used when referring to features of software programs. The Web site http://usinfo.state.gov/products/pubs/intelprp/glossary.htm describes *functionality* as "[t]hat aspect of design that makes a product work better for its intended purpose, as opposed to making the product look better or to identifying its commercial source."

REIMBURSEMENT POLICIES AND PATIENT CARE

Careful analysis reveals that one of the major challenges physicians face when using electronic H&P records parallels the greatest obstacle they encounter when using paper records: attempting to achieve high levels of care, thorough documentation, and E/M coding compliance within the time constraints imposed by payment limitations under the Resource-Based Relative Value System (RBRVS) for physician reimbursement. For example, Current Procedural Terminology (CPT®) descriptors call for physicians to spend "typically" 60 minutes for a level 5 initial visit (CPT code 99205) and 45 minutes for a level 4 initial visit (CPT code 99204).[1(pp9-10)] However, current Medicare and insurer (managed care) payment conversion factors (Medicare conversion is now about $37.00 per relative value unit, or RVU[2]) provide insufficient funds to cover medical practice overhead costs for this amount of medically appropriate physician time.

Calculating Time-Based Reimbursement

Although medical practice overhead costs vary based on factors ranging from specialty to geographic location to size of practice, current expenses far exceed the amounts actually paid under the RBRVS system for practice expense

continued

plus liability insurance costs. For example, examination of the 2008 RVUs assigned to CPT code 99205, a service that the *CPT* manual designates as warranting 1 hour of care, reveals that *practice expense value plus the liability expense value* totals 1.93 RVUs.[2] At the current national Medicare conversion rate, practices receive overhead reimbursement of only about $74 for this complex evaluation and management (E/M) service (currently scheduled to be reduced to less then $67 on July 1, 2008). In some "high-risk" medical specialties (eg, obstetrics and neurosurgery), this level of payment is insufficient to cover the premium for liability insurance alone. For most practices, an accounting of expenses will reveal true hourly costs that may be as much as three to four times the amount that Medicare and insurers currently pay (ie, real practice expense costs of $200 to $300 per hour, even higher in high-cost locations).

Appendix B (pp.340-342) provides three sets of computations that medical practices can use to calculate approximate values for their own:

i.   Gross practice overhead cost per physician per hour

ii. Overhead cost per physician per hour for provision of medical care alone (excluding income, and its associated expenses, generated by ancillary personnel and ancillary services)

iii. Percentage of actual overhead expense being provided by Medicare and insurers, combined with the amount of time this reduced funding actually allows for commonly performed outpatient E/M services.

To maintain the economic viability of their medical practices, physicians have little choice except to devote less time to each patient visit than CPT® designates as "typical." If, for purposes of this simple example, physicians were to spend only 30 minutes per level 5 visit instead of 60 minutes, the practice would receive overhead reimbursement of approximately $142 during that hour, which is an improvement but still inadequate to meet the current overhead and liability insurance expenses of most medical practices. Only when the length of a level 5 visit is reduced to 20 or even 15 minutes will the hourly overhead reimbursement meet the economic requirements for most medical practices. However, this limitation of time spent caring for patients creates a significant conflict between quality care and documentation and coding compliance on the one hand and efficiency (ie, speed of a visit) on the other.*

Reaching a resolution for this conflict requires consideration of two concepts that apply to providing E/M care with the assistance of an EHR. First, well-designed EHRs should help physicians maximize their efficiency while maintaining the principles of quality care and documentation compliance. Second, physicians, insurers, and government agencies must all understand that there is a limit to how quickly physicians can see patients and continue to maintain *high-quality* E/M care, provide *appropriate* counseling to patients about their health issues, and complete *meaningful* documentation of those visits. It is important to note that the speed limit seems to have been reached. Any further decrease in the time that physicians have available for each patient visit owing to further reductions in reimbursement (and/or increases

---

* In markets in which medical practices have the highest overhead expenses, the level of payment for overhead with the current RBRVS conversion factor is even farther below the cost of the practice expense resources. As a consequence, a preponderance of physicians in those locations have become unable to see patients for required Medicare payment rates or contracted insurer payment rates. The result has been a significant limitation of patient access to quality medical care.

in practice expense costs) may reasonably be expected to lead to decreases in quality care, patient safety, patient access, and cost-effectiveness.

As noted, achieving appropriate levels of medical care and compliant documentation in the time currently available can be facilitated by sophisticated medical record tools, which is a powerful reason for physicians to seek well-designed EHRs. However, as discussed in Chapter 5, there is currently significant evidence that certain H&P designs intended to increase documentation speed have done so at the expense of individualized care and compliant documentation and coding. Medical practices must be diligent in avoiding systems that have made such trade-offs. They must insist that software companies ensure that their H&P tools do not facilitate increased speed at the expense of high-level, compliant patient care and the diagnostic process on which it is based.

IDENTIFYING THE COMMON CAUSES OF DATA ENTRY DESIGN PROBLEMS

Careful examination of the compliance and quality issues created by current EHR efforts at increasing efficiency reveals that at the heart of the H&P problems are two fundamental data entry assumptions intrinsic to most existing EHR systems: (1) the physician personally must directly enter all clinical information into the software, and (2) these data must be entered into the patient's record during the patient visit. Designers acting on these assumptions significantly limits the range of options that can be made available in H&P components. The consequences of designs that impose these restrictions have included compromised quality of graphic interfaces, limited (until recently) effectiveness and compliance capabilities of narrative interfaces, inability to use alternative data entry personnel, and reduction of the range of formats available for data entry.

Assigning the physician to be the sole person responsible for entering clinical information into the electronic H&P record has created numerous issues for physicians at the point of care, including the following:

■ Many physicians do not type well enough to enter free-text narrative information efficiently into the software.

■ For good patient relations, most physicians prefer to maintain eye contact with their patients during the care process, rather than sharing their attention with a keyboard and a computer screen that is commonly placed, like a barrier, between the physician and the patient.

■ Similarly, most patients want their physician's attention during the care process to feel a sense of personal connection and concern rather than a sense of being a data input resource.

■ Attempting to type meaningful and individualized narrative descriptions into a computer while providing patient care is neither user-friendly nor time efficient for most physicians.

Physicians in practice have found a comfortable routine for working with patients and documenting the care provided. In planning for transition to EHRs, it will be advantageous to offer a variety of successful tools that match physicians' preferences instead of compelling changes that might increase documentation time and/or disturb patient care patterns.

The requirement that all data entry be synchronous with the time of the visit precludes use of the potentially valuable alternative of delayed data entry, which allows physicians to avoid typing by recording their findings and conclusions on a data transfer medium (eg, writing on paper or dictating on a recording device at the time of the visit—an image of the paper and/or the dictation file would be uploaded directly into the computer or given to professional transcriptionists who enter the physician's notes into the patient's electronic record file). Additional data entry options are also becoming available with software that permits physicians' direct entry into devices that translate the information indirectly into the electronic H&P record with only minimal delay.

Time Trial for Physician Typing Medical Information

As a relatively fast physician typist, I performed a time trial for a system requiring the physician to enter all documentation into an EHR at the time of a visit. All data from a real medical chart with an efficient paper system were typed into electronic screens designed to identically match the sections of the paper record. This task included checking boxes for graphic interface areas and typing word-for-word the descriptive free-text narrative.

The time spent during the actual patient encounter and documentation on an efficient paper form for this 99205 patient visit required 15 minutes. The visit was made more efficient through the use of a structured questionnaire that the patient completed to provide screening information for the past, family, and social history (PFSH) and review of systems (ROS). The 15 minutes included the physician personally obtaining the history of the present illness (HPI) and details of positive ROS responses, examining the patient, counseling the patient, writing prescriptions, and documenting in the medical record.

By comparison, copying all data for accurate keyboard entry, including typing narrative text plus point-and-click for marking check boxes, required more than 15 minutes and did not include any patient interaction. Additional time would have been required if the preliminary PFSH and ROS responses had to be obtained by the physician by interviewing the patient (rather than having the patient fill out a form).

Physicians are accustomed to a variety of modalities for documenting their care effectively and efficiently. For many physicians, systems requiring direct keyboard entry have created significant usability issues and resistance to purchasing or using EHR systems. To overcome this problem, software system developers introduced a number of alternatives designed to reduce the amount of typing and the number of mouse clicks needed for documentation of E/M visits. However, these alternatives also have the potential to introduce new obstacles to accurate and individualized documentation and serious concerns for E/M compliance. Examining the stages of this progression should help analyze these issues and point the way toward continuing design evolution that can meet the needs of physicians and software developers.

THE EVOLUTION OF H&P DESIGN AND FUNCTIONALITY

Keyboard and Mouse-Click Entry

During the mid- to late 1990s, most electronic systems offered physicians only two options for data entry of narrative information: typing on the computer keyboard for direct narrative entry or "point and click" with a mouse to build pseudonarrative descriptions from "pick lists," which are drop-down menus of individual words and phrases. Both of these options proved laborious, and drop-down menus introduced the additional problem of offering a severely limited vocabulary and a limited set of documentation options. This lack of precise descriptive capabilities may, at times, prove frustrating because it can interfere with physicians' ability to record details that accurately describe each patient's history and examination findings.

Pre-entered Documentation

Since the late 1990s and early in the 21st century, many designs have included preloaded templates for documenting graphic sections of the H&P record and preloaded macros for the narrative sections. *Graphic templates* can be efficient and compliant, provided that they do not contain boxes that are already checked (so-called documentation by exception) and that data entry screens do not include a "global" box that, when checked, automatically checks all the other boxes in a predetermined manner (eg, checking all the physical examination elements as normal).

Narrative macros, designed by vendors or customized by physicians themselves, are intended to speed the process of documenting the narrative sections of the H&P record. Macros contain generic text that can be brought forward (ie, using computers' capabilities to copy and paste an existing file) into portions of the medical record in lieu of individualized *narrative descriptions* documented at the point of care. Even though the physician can modify the preloaded information, the use of macros almost invariably results in the creation of "cloned" documentation and the potential for significant compliance and quality issues, as discussed in Chapter 5. Advocates of generic narrative macros contend that physicians can modify the text as needed to accurately depict a valid picture of a patient's history or examination. Although this modification may be possible, it would require more time to accurately modify pre-entered text than to write or dictate an individualized narrative H&P report. Of greater concern, the use of macros requires physicians to presuppose a patient's diagnosis (usually on the basis of nothing more than the patient's chief complaint) to select an applicable macro for the HPI. This selection process, requiring a presumptive diagnosis to derive a generic medical history, reverses the highly valued medical diagnostic process in which physicians use the medical history to derive the differential diagnosis.

Templates vs Macros

Some vendors and physicians have applied the term *template* to describe preloaded generic narrative descriptions. For clarity, *Practical EHR* uses the term *macro* to refer to a preloaded narrative, reflecting the terminology used for preloaded text in word processors; and the term *template* to describe a structured graphic interface design.

Reintroduction of Free-Text Narratives

On a positive note for physicians and their EHR goals, during the last several years, a significant number of EHR systems have reintroduced the option of free-text entry into several of the narrative sections of their medical records.

Specifically, these EHRs provide the option for physicians to dictate abnormal examination findings, the HPI, and, occasionally, details of positive findings in the ROS. The dictated information is transcribed into the appropriate section of the electronic H&P record through the use of voice recognition software, which functions synchronously with dictation, or by sending the audio file electronically to a transcriptionist, who enters the information into the software within a reasonably short time frame.

This development is a progressive and constructive step and a dramatic reversal of the previously noted restrictive data entry design assumptions, allowing some portion of the data entry to be asynchronous and performed by a professional entry person rather than by the physician. It also opens a doorway to a wide range of potential hybrid data entry approaches that can increase usability and flexibility of the software. These tools should be capable of optimizing efficiency while promoting the documentation of high-quality, patient-specific clinical information and preserving E/M compliance.

One of the remaining barriers, however, is that most software systems that have introduced this dictation design have also retained the option for physicians to use problematic documentation tools, such as pre-entered macros and pick lists. A primary theme for *Practical EHR* is that the electronic H&P must avoid any design or functionality that might promote, guide, or allow physician actions and documentation capable of interfering with optimal medical care and/or compliance. At this point, the general design issues that violate these principles, thereby causing concerns for physicians and coders, are examined in greater detail.

COPY AND PASTE FUNCTIONALITY

Computers have the ability to duplicate significant blocks of information from one file to another. Because patients' return appointments often deal with issues related to previous visits and their past histories tend to be relatively stable, some EHRs have introduced the functionality of copying the information from a patient's previous visit and pasting it into a current visit. Physicians are then supposed to use the old information as a starting point and update changes in the patient's history, examination findings, and/or medical decision making.

Some software designs have carried this functionality to the extreme of having "standardized" canned H&P reports for each of the common medical problems the physician encounters. These macros generally take the form of a traditional, dictated H&P report. The physician is instructed to identify a patient's primary symptom or probable diagnosis (usually derived from an assessment of the chief complaint) and then choose the macro appropriate for this problem from a stored repository of macros. The selected macro is then copied and pasted into the patient's record, with instructions for the physician to enter variations found during the patient encounter.

From a compliance perspective, this approach creates cloned records. They are word-for-word identical, with the exception of a minimal number of changes. Another physician or a compliance auditor who reviews such records is unable to determine if the medical history was truly reviewed, the body areas were reexamined, or any significant decision making occurred. In its May 2007 final report, "Recommended Requirements for Enhancing Data Quality in Electronic Health Records Systems," the Office of the National

Coordinator for Health Information Technology highlighted the severity of compliance danger and even the risk of fraud, by indicating that

> "[T]he use of defaults, templates, copying, and others [tools that enable a provider to be more efficient when documenting an encounter] . . . can also open the EHR-S [EHR systems] up to fraud or abuse. . . . specific warnings regarding the use of these tools by different payers may be a consideration. However, having an audit version of the EHR that shows the tools used and the individuals who used them can enable retroactive detection of patterns of abuse or fraud."[3]

From a quality of care perspective, such automated documentation tends to discourage physicians from adhering to one of the primary directives of their training, approaching each patient and each visit with an open perspective and allowing the medical history and examination findings to lead to the proper diagnoses. Although the software's documentation is prewritten as if the physician performed comprehensive care, the copy-and-paste approach reinforces problem-focused care and not comprehensive care as intended, by allowing a clinician to attend solely to the presenting problem; while the automated macro defaults all other components as if a normal history and/or normal examination were also performed. It tends to focus the physician's attention on the single issue of a patient's chief complaint and creates barriers to finding other symptoms or findings that may either be contributing to or unrelated to the initial presenting problem. In summary, copy-and-paste functionality interferes with the diagnostic process rather than reinforces it.

From a compliance perspective, the use of automated entry of clinical information conflicts with the requirements for proper documentation. Since the physician has neither dictated nor typed any of the canned information that is preloaded (by the software) into a record, the physician has not actually documented this data. The software through the computer has. Combining this reality with one of the fundamental principles cited by the Centers for Medicare & Medicaid Services (CMS), "[i]f care was not documented in the medical record, it was not done,"[11] leads to the conclusion that portions of the record that have automated entry have not been adequately documented by the physician. Therefore, no care can be credited in an audit of these sections. In summary, *automation is not documentation.*

The same compliance and quality issues will be echoed in the subsequent discussions of documentation by exception for the graphic user interface and the use of macros as a documentation tool for the narrative interface.

GRAPHIC USER INTERFACE ISSUES

Overview of the Graphic User Interface

The graphic user interface is a type of design that permits rapid selection of straightforward responses to pre-entered structured information, such as the check box design illustrated in Figure 7.1. This type of interface can provide the electronic H&P with highly efficient tools for obtaining and documenting information, when it is applied in sections of the medical record for which it is appropriate to use straightforward questions (or descriptions) and succinct answers. During a patient's initial visit, the information obtained in the graphic interface sections of the medical record (ie, PFSH, ROS, and normal examination findings) allows physicians to piece together the picture of each patient's overall health status at the time of the visit. They

FIGURE 7.1

A Hypothetical Graphic Interface for the Family History. The yes-no boxes allow rapid documentation. There are also areas adjacent to the boxes for entering free-text narrative details for positive responses.

Family History	Yes	No	
Heart problems or murmurs	☐	☐	
Allergy	☐	☐	
Diabetes	☐	☐	
Cancer	☐	☐	
Bleeding disorder	☐	☐	
Anesthesia problems	☐	☐	

accurately identify all history and examination elements that are normal, provide details of previously established abnormalities, and help to identify new concerns that the physician must address in detail. When properly completed, well-designed graphic interface templates for the patient's PFSH and ROS should provide a clear picture of the patient's current overall health status. It should metaphorically present the physician with the cover of a jigsaw puzzle box, showing how the patient "looked" before he or she became ill, with highlights surrounding all the body areas (and conditions) that need to be explored in detail during the present encounter.

During the medical history portion of an established patient visit, even though physicians are permitted to use the same graphic user interface to repeat the list of inquiries from an initial visit, they are not required to do so. Instead, physicians are permitted (according to the Documentation Guidelines) to "review and update the previous information,"[4(p6)] an alternative that takes less time for the patient and the physician while providing valuable information about the patient's present health. This option provides the physician with the medical equivalent of referring back to the picture on the cover of the puzzle box from the previous visit and ask the patient whether there have been any changes or additions to this picture. For the other portions of an established patient visit, physicians continue to use the other graphic interface tools that assist in documentation of physical examination findings and medical decision making.

Figure 7.1 illustrates a check-box and short answer type of graphic interface that might appear on the screen for the family history component of the medical history. Compliant graphic interface functionality requires the active entry of a *yes* or *no* response to each question about a possible illness in the family. This requirement for *active* entry attests that the physician actually asked the questions and recorded the patient's responses. In later chapters, a variety of options will be considered that allow the patients to use this same type of interface to enter their family history data directly into their own electronic file.

Potential Problems With EHR Graphic User Interface Design and Functionality

Problems can arise when an EHR system's graphic user interface design introduces documentation shortcuts in an effort to further shorten the brief time that physicians need to enter information into these templates. Some of the noncompliant documentation practices caused by such efforts include the following:

1. Documentation by exception, type 1

    In this variation, the graphic section's design would have only one check-box next to each illness (instead of the two check-boxes for *Yes* and *No* illustrated in Figure 7.1). The header for the section would state, "All responses negative except for those checked." The automated label *implies* that the physician has, in fact, asked about each of the illnesses and obtained a negative response. However, an empty box is not documentation. In the extreme, when the entire section remains unchecked, it is impossible to ascertain whether the physician asked all questions and obtained negative responses, asked only some of the questions, or overlooked the entire section. Such uncertainty affects not only compliance but also quality care and even liability. For another physician seeing the patient or even for an attorney reviewing the chart, this design cannot ensure that the questions were asked and answered.

    > Assessment: Although this documentation approach may seem reasonable to the person entering information at the time of care, the documentation becomes unclear and unreliable when reviewed at a later date, particularly by a third party such as another physician, an auditor, or an attorney. When reviewers encounter a preponderance of uncompleted check-boxes in case after case (as often occurs with this approach), they conclude that the documentation has been electronically automated, with no confirmation that all the questions were asked. In summary, the *absence of documentation is not the equivalent of documentation.*

2. Documentation by exception, type 2

    This graphic user interface documentation shortcut is encountered fairly frequently in a variety of software designs. The most common design appears identical to that shown in Figure 7.1, with the addition of an action button or check-box labeled *All negative*. When the physician clicks this button, the software automatically checks all the boxes in the *No* column (or in the *Normal* column for the graphic user interface portion of the physical examination section). The physician is then supposed to manually document all exceptions to *no* responses, clicking each *Yes* box for a positive response (and each *Abnormal* box for abnormal findings in the examination section) and reclicking a checked *No* box to make it blank if the question had not been asked (or if a specific physical examination element had not been performed). The problem is that automated checking of the boxes does not provide certain or reliable *documentation* that each question was asked or each examination element completed. Without a requirement for separate documentation of each individual check-box, there can be no verification that the documentation reflects the care provided rather than the software's ability to provide automatic documentation.

    > Assessment: Once again, although this documentation approach may seem reasonable to the person entering information at the time of care, the documentation becomes unclear and unreliable when reviewed at a later date by a third party. When reviewers encounter a similar pattern of *No* check-boxes in the history section or a similar pattern of *Normal*

check-boxes in the examination section in case after case (as often occurs with this approach), they conclude that the documentation has been electronically automated, with no confirmation that all questions were asked or all body areas examined.

3. Documentation by exception, type 3

    This is a variation of type 2, which automatically loads each section with all *No* (or *Normal*) boxes checked. Although this variation is not generally encountered in most popular software, the programming would be similar to that of type 2, without using the additional "action" button. The assessment for type 3 is also identical to that for type 2.

The general problem for all three categories of documentation by exception used with the graphic user interface is that they contain substance (ie, preloaded clinical information) in addition to structure. Effective templates should have only preloaded structure, and their functionality should require active entry (checking individual boxes) to document the clinical substance. This principle reflects the guidance provided in the report on antifraud model requirements, issued by RTI International in January 2007 at the request of the Office of the National Coordinator for Health Information Technology.[5] This review suggests that templates may be used in EHRs "if the intent is simply to provide common terminology or phraseology."[5] That is, the report advises that to ensure compliant documentation, any preloaded terminology must not indicate clinical care was actually performed until the physician actively checks a box to attest that a specific element of care occurred.

All documentation by exception approaches have the potential to create cloned medical records, which were discussed in Chapter 5. This problem becomes apparent when nearly every one of a physician's medical records not only includes a complete PFSH and ROS and/or a comprehensive examination (whether or not this extent of care is medically indicated by the nature of the presenting problem [NPP]), but also has all responses marked as *Negative* (or *Normal*), except for questions or examination elements specifically related to the present illness.

Furthermore, accurately recording a complete PFSH, ROS, and examination when using a graphic form with pre-entered responses as *No* or *Normal* actually requires more physician time than completing a compliant blank template. It generally requires far more effort to find and change preloaded *Normal* responses to *Abnormal* or to blanks (to indicate not asked or not performed) than to simply start with a clean slate. This observation may be a contributory factor to what coders commonly find when reviewing records created through the use of documentation by exception, which is that nearly every visit for every patient reports all *No* responses for the graphic sections of the history report. Similarly, nearly every visit also reports all *Normal* responses for the graphic sections of the physical examination, except for elements relating to the affected body area. Therefore, this electronic preprogramming frequently creates the appearance that physicians perform problem-focused care but the computer documents comprehensive care. As a result, this functionality creates concern about overcoding and even potentially fraudulent documentation.

NARRATIVE INTERFACE ISSUES

Overview of the Narrative Interface

Physicians exercise the highest levels of their semiology (assessment of signs and symptoms) skills through the portions of the H&P that call for documentation with a narrative interface. These are the sections of the medical record in which physicians chronicle the distinct and in-depth features of each patient's medical history, abnormal examination findings, differential diagnosis, and treatment protocol:

- Medical history: A narrative "tells the story" of the patient's illness and its background.
  - HPI
  - Details of positive responses in the PFSH
  - Details of positive responses in the ROS
- Physical examination: The narrative "paints a verbal picture" of the abnormal findings.
- Clinical impressions: The narrative "creates a logic tree" describing the physician's rationale for the differential diagnosis (ie, the probable diagnoses and potential alternatives).
- Treatment recommendations: The narrative "designs a blueprint" for current and future care that fits that patient's particular medical and personal profile.

The objective of obtaining a detailed and accurate medical history is to find the unique course of each patient's illness and capture this information accurately as a patient-specific narrative in the electronic H&P. As shown in Table 3.1, the *Bates' Guide to Physical Examination and History Taking*[6] reference text describes this documentation as "a chronological description of the development of the patient's present illness from the first sign and/or symptom or from the previous encounter to the present. It includes the following seven elements: location, quality, severity, timing (including duration), context, modifying factors, associated signs and symptoms."[6(pp3-4)] It should be apparent that the timeline of each patient's illness has specific features that differ from those of most other patients. Obtaining and recording this diagnostically important information requires the use of a narrative interface to record free text.

Compliance as a Codification of the Quality-Care Process

The definition of HPI in the Documentation Guidelines[4] clearly parallels the quality-based explanation in the clinical medicine reference source *Bates' Guide to the Physical Examination and History Taking*.[6] It emphasizes the chronological description of the development of the illness and includes the same eight elements, albeit with the Documentation Guidelines describing "duration" as separate from "timing."

Figure 7.2 illustrates a sample free-text narrative interface that could be used for the HPI section of an electronic H&P. It includes a compliance-based documentation prompt to inform physicians of the extent of care appropriate for the nature of each patient's presenting problem(s).

Figure **7.2**

Suggested Narrative Interface for the History of the Present Illness (HPI) in an Initial Outpatient Visit. The form includes an area for free-text entry (by typing, dictation, or other alternatives), plus documentation prompts to provide compliance-based guidance relating levels of care provided to medical necessity. The prompts also include a reminder of the need for a chronological description and a list of the eight HPI elements that contribute to this narrative.

Present Illness	Chronology with: 1. one to three elements (level 2) 2. four to eight elements; OR status of 3 chronic or inactive conditions (level 3, 4, or 5)
	(1) duration (2) timing (3) severity; (4) location (5) quality (6) context (7) modifying factors (8) associated signs and symptoms

Potential Problems With EHR Narrative Interface Design and Functionality

When using EHRs, most physicians find the option of typing narrative descriptions at the point of care to be significantly more time-consuming than writing or dictating the clinical information. As a result of this common challenge, software designers introduced a number of alternatives to free-text entry that still sustained the concepts of the physician directly entering the data at the time of the visit. However, problems can arise when an EHR system substitutes graphic user interface design shortcuts into narrative interface sections. Some of the noncompliant practices include the following:

Design Issue 1: Use of Short-Answer Graphic User Interface to Create the HPI

This type of design typically presents a list of the eight elements of an HPI described in the *CPT* manual, and it directs the physician to provide short descriptions for some of these elements. This approach not only precludes the use of full narrative documentation, it discourages the physician from obtaining a true medical history (ie, a chronological description of the course of the patient's illness) because it does not provide a practical mechanism to easily capture the details of the time course of an illness even if the physician were to elicit them. Instead, physicians simply ask questions related to the eight elements, and the resultant documentation reveals only a snapshot of the patient's symptoms on the day of the visit, without insight into the event-by-event course of the illness. This loss of information and of a thorough HPI provides insufficient information about the patient's illness and, therefore, handicaps the physician's ability to fully follow the diagnostic process, which requires knowledge of variable features to distinguish one patient's diagnosis from that of another patient who may have an otherwise similar complaint.

FIGURE 7.3

Example of a Type of Short-Answer Graphic Interface Used for the History of the Present Illness Instead of a Free-Text Narrative. All sample physician entries are shown in italics.

History of Present Illness	
Chief complaint	*Chest pain*
Location	*Chest*
Quality	*Dull*
Severity	*Mild to Moderate*
Timing	*Intermittent*
Duration	*9 weeks*
Context	
Modifying factors	
Associated signs and symptoms	*No shortness of breath*

Figure 7.3 illustrates the limited amount and quality of information recorded in this *graphic* type of HPI. Although its structure elicits features of the patient's illness on the date of the visit, it precludes the recommended approach to the HPI, which follows the time course of a patient's illness and asks about the appropriate elements of the HPI during each significant event that occurs during that time course. This example demonstrates that even though a physician may document four or more elements of the HPI, an auditor could not consider the HPI to be "extended," because it lacks a chronological description of the course of the illness, as required by CPT compliance standards. It also lacks sufficiently detailed descriptive information about the course of the illness to permit a physician to develop a meaningful and complete differential diagnosis.

Design Issue 2: Use of Generic Macros to Create a HPI

In this approach to documenting the HPI, the physician must select from among a collection of generic macros, which are nonspecific medical histories that have previously been created and loaded into the software for future access. Each macro is usually based on a different chief complaint. Some EHR companies provide a series of preexisting macros, while others encourage physicians to develop their own personalized versions. The underlying concept in the construction of these macros parallels that used for the alternative short-answer graphic-type interface. Each macro usually consists of fill-in-the-blank information related to the *CPT* manual's eight elements of the HPI, with nonspecific connecting language to make it seem as though the physician obtained a true narrated medical history.

Figure 7.4 shows a sample generic macro that physicians might develop for a patient complaining of chest pain. Only the information in bold is original data entered, which was prompted by the cues shown in italics. A review of multiple patient records easily reveals that these pseudonarratives all have identical language except for the few words

Example of a Generic Macro Used for the History of the Present Illness (HPI) Instead of a Free-Text Narrative. This example illustrates a macro for chest pain, using the same example as in Figure 7.3. The macro uses the same premise of creating an HPI by asking questions about the 8 elements. The preloaded macro appears in normal font. The physician's entries are shown in **bold**. For illustration purposes, the cues that guided the physician about which history elements to enter into the macro are shown in parentheses and italics; these cues would not appear in the final record.

History of Present Illness

The patient arrives with a chief complaint of chest pain. The pain is located in the **chest** (*location*) area and feels **dull** (*quality*) to the patient. The patient reports that the severity of the pain is **mild to moderate** (*severity*). The symptom's onset was **9 weeks** (*duration*) ago. Episodes occur **intermittently** (timing), with the following background information: **none** (*context*). Factors affecting the pain include **none** (*modifying factors*), and the patient reports the following associated signs and symptoms: **no shortness of breath**.

---

that are changed in each chart, resulting in cloned documentation. In addition, by definition, it is not possible to predesign a macro that can create a true medical history. It is the process of obtaining a patient's history that must generate the medical record, not vice versa. Because the time course and sequence, severity, and interrelationship of events of an illness are unique to each patient and these details cannot be generalized or known in advance, it is not possible for pre-entered information to depict "a chronological description of the development of the patient's present illness."[1(p3)]

Software vendors do not claim that the purpose of the macro approach is to improve patient care, but rather that it is to reduce the time for documentation. However, the time normally required to write or dictate a true HPI is actually very small. Therefore, the preponderance of time saved intended with this approach must come at the expense of obtaining an effective history, which is, therefore, at the expense of patient care. As discussed previously, instead of helping a physician obtain a true medical history that tracks the course of events from the onset, pre-entered macros guide physicians to obtain and record only a snapshot of the patient's status on the date of the visit. Consequently, this documentation device fails to meet CPT compliance standards. It also fails to tell the patient's entire medical story, generally precluding the discovery of contributory factors and secondary illnesses that may only have affected the patient earlier in the course of the illness, prior to the date of the visit. Yet, all of these details and contributions are required for physicians to develop a reliable differential diagnosis. The macro approach discourages physicians from asking the questions that will elicit a real medical history because it fails to guide or encourage documentation of chronological information. The physician would have to add any such clinical information separately, as free text. Although it is acceptable to add such free text to a macro to create a true history, if this were the designers' intent, there would be no need for the macro. Using a macro in addition to free text would, in fact, tend to add time to the encounter rather than make it more efficient.

Design Issue 3: Use of Problem-Focused Algorithm Macros for the HPI

Instead of focusing on the eight elements of the HPI, this variation of the macro uses a narrow, targeted approach to the patient's history, based on determining whether a patient has a specific problem or warrants a specific intervention. As in the approach described in design issue 2, the physician chooses a macro based on the patient's chief complaint. The algorithm in the macro usually asks a predetermined set of specific questions. These are not open-ended inquiries, and the macro does not include questions about the course of the illness or the eight HPI elements. For example, to evaluate a pediatric patient with a presenting complaint of recurrent tonsillitis (or frequent sore throats), the physician might use a preloaded HPI macro that concentrates solely on the questions commonly used to determine whether the patient has sufficient frequency and duration of episodes to warrant recommending possible tonsillectomy. Little attention is directed to whether the presumed diagnosis is valid, whether past responses to treatment confirm the probable diagnosis, or whether there might be correctable associated illnesses or predisposing circumstances contributing to the patient's problems. Figure 7.5 illustrates a preloaded macro that a physician might use when evaluating a patient with this chief complaint.

FIGURE 7.5

Example of a Preloaded Algorithm-Type of Interface Used for the History of Present Illness of a Pediatric Patient with a Chief Complaint of Recurrent Tonsillitis. All sample physician entries are underlined and in bold type.

History of Present Illness

The patient arrives with a chief complaint of recurrent tonsillitis. The episodes occur **3-4** times per year. They have been occurring during the last **4** years. The patient misses approximately **2-3** days of school with each of these episodes. Treatments have included **antibiotics**.

Impression: **Recurrent tonsillitis**   Recommendation: **Tonsillectomy**

In addition to the compliance issue that the documentation lacks a chronological description of the illness, this sample record illustrates the clinical concerns raised by using a presumptive diagnosis or a chief complaint to generate a patient's history. The limited number and range of questions in the algorithm leave only a finite range of possibilities for the physician. In this example, there are two choices available: the patient has sufficient clinical indications for surgery or the patient does not. However, there is insufficient information in the HPI to determine whether the patient in fact has recurrent episodes of bacterial tonsillitis. This same limited amount of information could also support a diagnosis of viral upper respiratory infection that the patient and/or another physician could have mislabeled as "tonsillitis." In addition, the limitations of the algorithm suggest that no further questions are required. Yet, further inquiry into the patient's home environment might reveal significant exposure to cigarette smoke, or asking about associated symptoms could suggest chronic acid reflux pharyngitis. Treatment for such predisposing factors could provide the opportunity to resolve the patient's problems without surgical intervention. Other questions could yield responses that might suggest significant underlying disease contributing to the infections, such as immune deficiency or leukemia.

Potential Impact of Pre-entered Macros on Quality

A physician who was pleased with the increased speed of care and documentation achieved by using the tonsillitis algorithm in Figure 7.5 was asked four questions that would reasonably have been answered through the use of a full narrative history:

■ Who confirmed the diagnosis of bacterial tonsillitis and how?

■ What was the medical history of the episodes that supported such a diagnosis?

■ Was there smoke exposure at home, the elimination of which could have changed the course of the patient's illness without surgery?

■ Did the patient have reflux symptoms, the treatment of which could have altered the course of the patient's illness without surgery?

The physician replied, "Oh, you're talking about a quality of medical care that no longer exists."

This assessment summarizes the concerns for quality that can result from suboptimal EHR documentation approaches. It conveys that this physician believes he has insufficient time to provide anything more than problem-focused care, which is less than the level of care warranted, according to CPT standards, by the nature of this presenting problem. By using this limited algorithm, the physician delegated the diagnostic process to the computer.

In contrast, the goal for design of the HPI section should be to facilitate the physician's use of the full potential of the comprehensive medical history and the diagnostic process. Physicians should consider any designs that have the potential to discourage or compromise this effort to be unacceptable.

Design Issue 4: Use of Generic Macros to Document a Physical Examination

In some systems, physicians are allowed or encouraged to create macros that automatically report a normal comprehensive physical examination for their specialty. This report will read like an original dictated examination. The text automatically attests that the physician has performed a comprehensive examination with all normal findings, and it appears this way, with every word identical, on every visit for every patient. The physician is theoretically supposed to "undocument" the macro, inserting abnormal findings and deleting all portions of the examination that were not performed. However, this method creates significant challenges and numerous compliance problems.

Undocumenting is inefficient, and it is counterintuitive to the way physicians are trained to document care in medical records. Many medical problems do not warrant a comprehensive examination, but physicians can easily fail to delete descriptions of one or more body areas they did not examine. As a result, the software program commonly reports a comprehensive examination for every visit, regardless of medical necessity and, in many cases, regardless of whether the care was provided. Physicians also frequently fail to modify descriptions of findings that are inaccurate or incomplete in the context of a given patient (eg, the following record [Figure 7.6] provides a detailed description dictated by a physician about the unique abnormal findings in a patient's right ear; however, the physician neglected to change the macro for the left ear, which read "same as right"). These problems can result in imprecise or inaccurate records, which is what EHRs are intended to eliminate because inaccurate records can lead to medical errors.

FIGURE 7.6

Sample Record Adapted from a Real Patient Record in Which a Macro Was Used.
The record confirms the use of a macro because all text in standard print was preloaded, and the software printed all changes to documentation in bold text. Underlining indicates areas where the physician should have modified the pre-entered text but did not; the information is incompatible with the remaining documentation, is present without any medical indication to perform that portion of the examination, or is inappropriate for this generally healthy 8-year-old patient.

Physical Examination

Constitution: Height: <u>5 ft 9 in</u>. Weight <u>180 lb</u>
   General appearance: well developed; well nourished; easily responsive to visual, verbal, and <u>tactile stimulation</u>; <u>oriented x 4</u>; no apparent deformities; well groomed; cooperative; appears healthy; well-coordinated gait
   Ability to communicate: normal

Head, face, salivary glands, and temporomandibular joint
   Inspection of head and face: Normal contour and symmetry. No masses, lesions, or significant scars observed
   Palpation/percussion of face: <u>No tenderness, deformity, or instability</u>
   Palpation of parotid and submaxillary glands: Normal
   Facial mobility: Normal
   Temporomandibular joints: Normal

Eyes: Conjunctivae without redness, lids normal. <u>No arcus senilis visible</u>. Pupils round, equal, and reactive to light. Gaze appears conjugate in all positions; no evident nystagmus

Ear, nose, mouth and throat
   Pinnas: Normal
   External nose: Normal
   Otoscopic examination
      Right ear: External auditory canal normal. Tympanic membrane **red, injected, brownish yellow, meniscus level behind the tympanic membrane**.
      Left ear: <u>same as the right</u>
   Nasal interior: Septum **deviated** to the right 2+ (1–4 scale)
      Turbinates and middle meati: Inferior turbinates **hypertrophied** +3. Middle turbinates normal. Middle meati normal. Nasal airway **obstructed** on the right side estimated 30%. **Rhinorrhea:** bilateral, moderate, mucoid, yellow
      Mucosa: **Pale, congested;** no nasal polyps
      Lips, teeth, and gums: <u>Normal</u>.
      Base of tongue, pharyngeal walls, vallecula and pyriform sinuses: <u>Normal</u>
      Nasopharynx examination: The adenoids are **inflamed and swollen, hypertrophied with over 50% obstruction** of the posterior nasal airway. The posterior choanae are normal.

Neck and thyroid
   Neck: Symmetrical; no masses; trachea midline; <u>normal laryngeal crepitation</u>
   Thyroid: Normal size, no masses

Lymph nodes
   <u>Normal neck lymph nodes</u>

Skin
   Palpation of scalp and inspection of hair on scalp, eyebrows, <u>face, chest, and extremities normal</u>

Neurologic
   Higher integrative functions: Normal orientation, <u>memory</u>, attention span and <u>concentration</u>, language, and <u>fund of knowledge</u>

Psychiatric The patient is awake and alert. <u>Oriented x 4</u> . <u>The judgment and insight of the patient are normal</u>.

---

continued

> Comments: In this record, when the physician dictated "hypertrophied," the software automatically attached "+3" as the default degree of severity. Also, although the medical history and the impressions sections of this record (not shown) documented severe dental abnormality as a reason for the visit, the examination report shows the default setting that the teeth are "normal." There are other significant areas of inappropriate documentation unrelated to the head and neck examination: (1) Eight-year-old children do not have hair on the face, chest, and extremities, as documented in the skin section. (2) They are not evaluated for arcus senilis (seen only in elderly patients). (3) There is no reason to assess the child's memory, fund of knowledge, judgment, and insight; it is doubtful that the physician would have done so, even though this assessment is included in the neurologic examination section.

Even when a physician is motivated to thoroughly undocument all nonexamined body areas and meticulously modify all areas with positive findings, the process is time-consuming and far less efficient than other compliant documentation alternatives. Furthermore, every unaltered portion of the macro still reads word-for-word the same as the corresponding portion of every other medical record. This is automated, or cloned, documentation, which does not provide the ability to differentiate between care that was provided and information that was entered automatically. In a compliance audit, the reviewer can only give credit for the examination of the body areas for which documentation was changed from the standard macro because it is clear that these areas were examined. Figure 7.6 illustrates an actual EHR physical examination report created from a macro and used by an otolaryngologist.

The macro approach to examination documentation is compromised because the pre-entered narrative descriptions verify only that the computer has a preloaded macro. This amazingly documented comprehensive examination is for a young child whose only complaint in the medical history was poor dental alignment. Yet, the preprinted comprehensive examination, which possibly appears the same, word-for-word in each of this physician's records, proclaims that the teeth are normal. In addition, it demonstrates (in bold) original documentation in only two areas of the head and neck: the right ear and the inside of the nose. (The nasopharynx examination cannot be performed on a patient of this age other than with a fiberoptic telescope, so this part of the original report came from that evaluation). This type of *pseudodocumentation* cannot certify that the physician actually performed all the elements documented for this physical examination or for the almost-identically documented examinations in the records of all the physician's other patients. As illustrated, this design approach almost always results in cloned documentation, which was discussed in detail in Chapter 5.

SUMMARY OF PROBLEMS WITH THE USE OF MACROS

None of the various macro alternatives illustrated offers documentation capable of certifying that the physician performed all elements of a history and/or physical examination, even though documentation is generated as if comprehensive care has been performed in every case. In addition, in many encounters, there are no medical indications to examine all of the body areas reported because some of them are not relevant to the patient's medical problems. Not only does the inclusion of non-medically necessary services seem inappropriate, but it is impossible for an auditor to ascertain whether these identically documented services were actually performed.

Compliance Issues With Macros

The compliance concerns created by the use of such macros derives from the fact that they are predisposed to the creation of cloned documentation, which generally fails review for compliance and medical necessity, as detailed in Chapter 5. This type of documentation could subject the physician to charges of false claims owing to systematic overcoding and lack of appropriate medical necessity.

Medicare Carrier Director's Assessment of Cloned Documentation

Robert A. Pelaia, an attorney, a certified coder, and director of compliance at the University of Florida College of Medicine, Gainesville, reported and commented on medical record documentation guidance that had recently been issued by the medical director of First Coast Options, Inc, the Medicare Part B carrier for Florida and Connecticut. The Carrier Director advised

"Documentation is considered cloned when each entry in the medical record for a patient is worded exactly alike or similar to the previous entries. Cloning also occurs when medical documentation is exactly the same from patient to patient. . . . Cloned documentation does not meet medical necessity requirements for coverage of services rendered due to the lack of specific, individual information. All documentation in the medical record must be specific to the patient and her/his situation at the time of the encounter. Cloning of documentation is considered a misrepresentation of the medical necessity requirement for coverage of services. Identification of this type of documentation will lead to denial of services for lack of medical necessity and recoupments of all overpayments made."[7]

Pelaia added further caution to this analysis, noting "Specifically, it may seem obvious, but providers must ensure that what is being represented in the medical record actually took place and is not something the provider normally does but may not have done for that particular patient."[7] The danger of macros is that they have a high potential to create cloned documentation, and cloned documentation has the potential to report comprehensive care identically and repeatedly in every case. As a result, there is no way for a reviewer, another physician, or even the physician himself or herself to know whether the reported care was actually provided. Unfortunately, these designs provide the capability, even if not intended, for a physician to perform problem-focused care and report detailed and comprehensive levels of care.

Quality Care Issues With Macros

There are multiple reasons that the macro approaches illustrated interfere with quality care. First, the graphic user interface macro and narrative macro options interfere with a physician's ability to obtain a true *history* of the patient's present illness. Although a good medical history should record the entire course of a patient's illness, from onset until the date of the visit,[6(chap 1)] it is not possible to preprogram such a chronological description into the text of a macro because the time course of every patient's illness differs from the time course of every other patient's illness. Because an HPI macro does not provide a means for physicians to document a true history, there is a strong incentive not to inquire about the time course of their patients' illnesses. However, eliciting only the information concerning the status of the *CPT* manual's eight elements of the HPI on the date of the visit provides physicians with insufficient clinical information. As illustrated in Figures 7.3, 7.4, and 7.6, these alternatives restrict the physician's inquiries to such an extent that they record nothing more than a *snapshot* of the patient's signs and symptoms on the date of the visit, with the possible additional notation of a date when the problem(s) began. Nevertheless, there is no guidance to help physicians learn what transpired during the period between the onset of symptoms and the date of the visit. Without a true medical history, the physician loses the most important diagnostic tool in his or her armamentarium.

The information obtained and recorded using such macros is usually inadequate for a physician to detect additional features or unrelated problems that may occur during the course of a patient's illness. It is also generally insufficient to enable a physician to make a secure differential diagnosis, reliably figure out the probable cause or genesis of the patient's problem, and identify the best treatment plan. Instead, deprived of the power of a rigorous medical history, the physician may default to batteries of laboratory tests and/or sophisticated radiographic studies in an effort to make a diagnosis. When, as often occurs, the test results are negative, the physician is left with nothing more to give the patient than a ruled out diagnosis, such as "you haven't had a heart attack." Although this is good news, it does not provide an acceptable explanation of the problem to the physician or the patient, and it may result in delayed diagnosis and treatment.

When EHRs Include Options for True Narrative and Macros

Many EHR systems now include the option for free-text entry by typing or dictating a report. However, many of these enhanced systems also continue to include preloaded macros as well, and their software vendors continue to advocate that physicians use and complete these macros for their HPIs, because they are "faster." On the other hand, the same vendors do not promise or contend that the macros provide compliant documentation and coding or that they promote quality care.

It is reasonable to assume that the primary rationale for developing these various types of pseudonarrative macros was to increase the speed of documentation because typing free text is potentially slow and laborious and may interfere with physicians' communications with their patients. On the other hand, the speed of free-text narrative documentation is not a significant issue for physicians familiar with medical records that provide data input by modalities other than typing. For physicians who prefer to dictate their narrative reports when working with conventional records, dictating an HPI may require an additional 30 seconds beyond the time required to obtain the history. For physicians who prefer to write their narrative reports, documenting an HPI requires no additional time because they can write in the chart while eliciting the history from the patient.

Fortunately, current technologies can allow efficient documentation of free text using information capture by writing or by dictation, as well as by typing. Physicians should be able to select whichever data entry modality best suits their personal preference. When coupled with a guidelines-based design for the narrative sections of the electronic H&P, these capabilities each have the potential to provide speedy documentation while also ensuring compliance, increasing usability, and promoting good care.

The Electronic Rubber Stamp

Analyzing a computer-generated medical history (or physical examination) created with the use of a macro can be a challenge, primarily because it is clothed in the aura of EHR respectability. However, the challenge can be readily eliminated by stripping away the aura and viewing the use of macros as the electronic equivalent of a *rubber stamp* that a physician would imprint on a blank piece of paper to create the HPI for every visit of every similar patient.

Despite the fact that the stamped document would provide four or five blank spaces in the precomposed paragraph for the physician to enter a few brief phrases about symptoms and a laboratory test result, the compliance problems are readily apparent. For compliance purposes, coders and auditors know that only the uniquely entered verbiage represents valid documentation and provides meaningful information about the patient. Also, physicians understand that the stamped history provides too little meaningful information to convey what is truly wrong with the patient. Finally, medical educators would recognize that such an abbreviated approach fails to allow physicians to apply the medical diagnostic process, which is essential for finding the source of a patient's medical problems.

Impact of Macros on the Diagnostic Process

A primary principle guiding care is that a high-quality medical history leads the physician to derive an accurate differential diagnosis. When using macros, the exact opposite applies: the EHR requires the physician to select which macro to load solely on the basis of the chief complaint, and this macro then drives the questions the physician asks. In other words, instead of the history leading to an informed diagnosis, a presumptive *unsupported* diagnosis dictates the medical history.

The consequences of replacing a true narrative interface resonate through all of the critical components of the H&P. Owing to their inability to document an individualized medical history, examination findings, "rule out" diagnoses, and/or alternative management options, these systems might dissuade physicians from making such individualized assessments. Quality is compromised when every patient seems to fit into one of a limited number of categories and when the unique features of each patient and each episode of illness are overlooked, including the evolution of a disease process over time as it is affected by outside factors and medications and its own natural history. Training tells physicians that their patients are their best teachers, but gaining the benefit of the insights they provide requires that physicians investigate each patient's history, examination findings, and diagnostic studies in depth. It is often even more important to find and address the differences among patients with similar clinical manifestations than it is to recognize their similarities. The ability to detect these patient-specific features is what years of training and experience teach physicians. This critical thinking and ability to synthesize medical clues is the basis of the art of medicine. This art cannot be programmed into a computer, but what can be programmed are designs that allow software to accurately capture the elements of this diagnostic process.

Graduation

Thomas Koenig, MD, Associate Dean for Student Affairs, Johns Hopkins School of Medicine, delivered the keynote address at the 2007 convocation ceremony. In his conclusion, he reminded the students to "[g]ive thanks to the best teachers of all—our patients. They teach us better than any text book ever could."

It is the responsibility of physicians to perform an effective H&P to give patients the opportunity to impart this wisdom.

INCREASING SPEED IS NOT THE SAME AS ACHIEVING EFFICIENCY

Practical EHR differentiates between the concepts of "efficiency" and "speed." Design and functionality tools that increase "efficiency" should allow physicians to perform the same high quality of care and meaningful documentation in a reduced amount of time. For example, the graphic check-box tools for documenting past medical history, family history, social history, and review of systems that appear on the initial visit forms, as illustrated in Appendix F, promote increased efficiency. They allow physicians to pre-enter standard questions rather than writing or dictating these same questions during every new patient encounter. The questions are the same, the patient responses are recorded individually for each new patient, compliance is maintained, and the amount of physician time for documentation is significantly reduced, particularly when the patients answer the questions by marking the check-boxes.

Design and functionality tools that increase "speed" (without achieving efficiency) may reduce physician time, but they do so at the expense of introducing a significant potential for compromising high-quality care, meaningful documentation, and/or compliance. "Speed tools" mobilize software capabilities for copying and pasting previously-entered documentation from prior visits, for preloading check-box forms with normal responses, and for copying and pasting canned generic macros that enter near-identical descriptive information for patients with similar chief complaints. All of these techniques tend to create "cloned" documentation, which produces nearly word-for-word identical charts in case after case after case. In the vast majority of medical records created in this fashion, the only modifications the physician makes to the standard macro are in the portions of the H&P that refer to the present illness. There is rarely, if ever, any documentation of abnormalities in aspects of the medical history or physical examination that are unrelated to the HPI. This contrasts significantly with medical records that do not employ macros or prefilled template check-boxes, in which some degree of individual differences and variations from "normal" are the rule, rather than a rare exception. As a consequence, reviews of "cloned" medical records give the impression that the physician has performed problem-focused care, and the remaining standard text gives the *appearance* of comprehensive care, without visit-specific documentation to confirm that such care was performed.

Ironically, when handicapped by having to use "speed tools," physicians attempting to record *individualized* patient information, accurately and with full detail, actually require significantly more time than they need for documenting a free-text narrative. As a result, designs that provide "speed" but not "efficiency" are at the core of many of the electronic H&P concerns voiced by physicians who are committed to performing and accurately documenting care that reflects the diagnostic process. They are frustrated and unhappy when they find that "speed tools" paradoxically increase the time they need to accurately document their care. This consequence may lead to decreased productivity and ultimately to implementation failure.

"Speed tools" confront physicians with two unacceptable choices: working at rapid speed to create cloned records or requiring unacceptably increased time in order to record individualized (and compliant) patient information. In contrast, Part 3 of this book explores designs that provide true "efficiency," increasing documentation speed while maintaining and promoting physicians' quality and compliance needs for the electronic H&P.

E/M COMPLIANCE AND THE NEED TO ADDRESS MEDICAL NECESSITY

During the early years of EHRs, most EHR companies seemed entirely unaware of the E/M system and the importance of E/M compliance for medical documentation. More recently, most companies have made efforts to incorporate compliant E/M documentation and coding functionality as an integral component of the electronic H&P, creating their own integrated coding engines or incorporating coding software built by independent developers. Unfortunately, these efforts have largely been unsuccessful. Most EHR companies seem to acknowledge their deficiencies in achieving compliance because they commonly claim that their software only provides guidance, and they formally assign the responsibility for correct documentation and coding to the physicians' judgment.

The fundamental stumbling block for software coding engines is that they almost uniformly fail to integrate the concept of medical necessity into their documentation and coding functionality. Yet, all of the authoritative publications on E/M documentation and coding emphasize that medical necessity is an essential component in achieving compliance. In particular, the *Medicare Claims Processing Manual,* published by the CMS, advises that "[m]edical necessity of a service is the overarching criterion for payment in addition to the individual requirements of a CPT code."[8] This policy echoes the government's general policy on necessity, which appears in Social Security Law: "Medicare will not pay for services that are not medically necessary."[9]

The *CPT* E/M documentation and coding system includes the contributory factor NPP as its measure of medical necessity. This is shown in the definitions of NPP, which consider the natural course and prognosis of medical conditions in the absence of medical intervention, including risks of morbidity without treatment, the risks of mortality without treatment, and the probability of prolonged functional impairment without treatment.[1(pp3-4)] These factors support medical necessity for the different levels of E/M service. In addition, Appendix C of the *CPT* manual provides clinical examples of patients with medical conditions having various levels of medical necessity that correlate with the E/M descriptors for NPP. Furthermore, every type of E/M service that considers the three key components also includes a level for the NPP. The *CPT* manual repeatedly emphasize the importance of medical necessity in determining appropriate levels of care (ie, the proper E/M code). It advises that "Clinical examples . . . are provided to assist physicians in understanding the meaning of the descriptors and *selecting the correct code* [italics added]."[1(p5)4] Appendix C reiterates this relationship, stating "The Clinical Examples, when used with the E/M descriptors ... provide a comprehensive and powerful tool for physicians to report the services provided to their patients."[1(p450)] Because these services are reported by submission of E/M codes for medically appropriate (ie, medically necessary) levels of care, the clinical examples illustrate the association of an illness's severity and relative risk (ie, the NPP) with appropriate levels of care.

The publication, *Documentation Guidelines*[4] reiterates the CPT emphasis on the importance of medical necessity and the NPP. Concerning the medical history component of E/M, it states "The extent of history of present illness, review of systems and past, family and/or social history that is obtained and documented is dependent upon clinical judgment and the *nature of the presenting problem(s)* [italics added]."[4(p5)] It provides a similar correlation for the physical examination component of E/M, stating "The type ... and content of examination are selected by the examining physician and are based upon clinical judgment, the patient's history, and *the nature of the presenting problem(s)* [italics added]."[4(p10)]

Demonstrating the parallel between compliance principles and quality care practices, the *Bates' Guide to Physical Examination and History Taking*, in its section explaining the concept of clinical reasoning, instructs physicians to "make hypotheses about the *nature of the patient's problem* [italics added]."[6(p785)] The *Bates' Guide* reports that gaining this insight involves the physician applying knowledge and experience to weigh the patient's most critical complaints and findings, match these against the possible and probable conditions that might produce these complaints, and consider whether the "worst case scenario" for these symptoms could possibly be the cause the patient's problems.[6(pp785-786)] This description summarizes the complex synthesis and interplay of numerous factors that physicians must bring together to derive proper diagnosis and treatment. It provides a clinical equivalent of the CPT descriptors for the NPP and their reflection in the CPT clinical examples.

The message from all three of these authoritative sources highlights the significance of medical necessity in medical care and in correct documentation and coding. The importance of considering the NPP is summarized in *Practical E/M* with the principle that "[a] critical insight to coordinating coding and documentation with medical necessity and appropriate quality care is to include NPP as a mandatory fourth factor."[10(p39)] This realization leads us to the insight that it is the failure of EHRs to incorporate this essential E/M component into their H&P designs and coding engines is one of the significant factors that has precluded them from achieving physicians' goal of compliant documentation and coding.

Interrelationship Among Medical Necessity, Compliance, and the Standard of Care

The CPT clinical examples make a powerful statement about the relationship between E/M compliance and quality care. These examples were developed by physicians' medical specialty societies and approved by CPT committees of the American Medical Association to indicate the level of care that is medically indicated for patients with different severities of illness (ie, NPP). They therefore establish an approved *standard of care* that is warranted for patients with such illness severity.

Thus, when Appendix C provides examples of patients who have very severe illness and, therefore, appropriately deserve level 5 care,[1(pp452,455-456,458,462-463,464-465)] it indicates that the medical *standard of care* for this severity of illness warrants, per the E/M descriptors, a *comprehensive* history, a *comprehensive* physical examination, and medical decision making of *high complexity*. EHR software that does not guide physicians to consider medical necessity during patient care fails to assist them in performing and documenting appropriate levels of care. Failure to consider the NPP can lead to overcoding (submission of claims at higher levels of care than warranted by medical necessity) or undercoding (submission of claims at lower levels of care than warranted by medical necessity). It can also result in provision of lower levels of care than medically indicated, as demonstrated in the following examples.

Example 1: Patient Warranting High Levels of Care Based on Medical Necessity

The first clinical example in *CPT* Appendix C for code 99205 states "Initial office visit for a patient with disseminated lupus erythematous with kidney disease, edema, purpura, and scarring lesions on the extremities plus cardiac symptoms."[1(p452)] Three specialty societies—dermatology, general surgery, and internal medicine—confirmed that this patient warrants level 5 care (which correlates with CPT's descriptor for an NPP level of "moderate to high" or "high"). Submission of E/M code 99204 for a patient with this severity of illness would represent undercoding. In addition, it would represent underdocumentation and care below accepted standards if the physician were to provide and document only level 3 care (99203) for this patient (ie, a detailed history, detailed examination, and/or medical decision making of low complexity).

In contrast, effective electronic H&P functionality would guide the physician to identify and document the NPP for this patient as high, warranting level 5 care. It would then provide documentation prompts to guide the physician to perform and document the *medically indicated* degree of history, physical examination, and medical decision making warranted for this patient's illness.

Example 2: Patient Warranting Low Levels of Care Based on Medical Necessity

Conversely, the CPT's first clinical example for code 99212 presents an "Office visit for an 11-year-old, established patient, seen in follow-up for mild comedonal acne of the cheeks on topical desquamating agents."[1(p453)] Three specialty societies—dermatology, family medicine, and pediatrics—confirmed that this patient warrants level 2 care (which correlates with an NPP level of "self-limited or minor"). The CPT descriptors for established patient visits state that two of the three key components must support this level of care, including a problem-focused history, problem-focused examination, and/or straightforward medical decision making. Submission of a level 3 or higher code for a patient with this level of NPP would be overcoding based on medical necessity, regardless of the levels of the key components performed and documented.

The NPP establishes the *maximum* and appropriate level of care (and E/M code) considered *medically necessary*. Even in cases in which the documentation might include more than a problem-focused history, a problem-focused examination, and/or straightforward medical decision making, consideration of the NPP as a "mandatory fourth factor" helps physicians recognize the medical necessity of this patient's illness to be "minor," thereby establishing that the appropriate upper limit of the code for care to be submitted should be 99212.

Integrating Medical Necessity Principles for Quality and Compliance

Properly integrating consideration of the NPP into an EHR's H&P interface design and E/M coding functionality (which generally depends on a separate but linked software coding engine) will allow the software to guide physicians to identify medically necessary and medically appropriate levels of care. This will help ensure that physicians can always identify the appropriate levels of care to provide, particularly for patients with severe illness, by establishing the amount of history, examination, and medical decision making that are *medically indicated* and warranted by the standard of care. It also ensures E/M compliance by establishing an upper limit for code submission based on *medical necessity,* thereby eliminating overcoding.

It is clear that physicians cannot provide quality care if they fail to meet the standard of care that is recognized by their own specialty societies. Performing the appropriate extent (level) of history, examination, and medical decision making gives physicians the best opportunity to identify all appropriate diagnoses and treatment options. The EHR coding engines that fail to consider medical necessity fail to ensure that physicians using those systems can provide this opportunity for every patient and every visit. Chapter 13 presents effective design solutions for bringing consideration of the NPP into physicians' normal workflow and care processes.

Current national health care policy calls for the adoption of EHRs to promote quality care, not to permit systems that can foster levels of care that are below recognized standards. However, EHR systems that lack the functionality to consider medical necessity are unable to guide appropriate amounts of history, examination, and medical decision making to meet these standards. In addition, two of physicians' goals in purchasing an EHR system are creating higher quality medical H&P records and elimination of the E/M coding challenge. Systems that fail to incorporate medical necessity into their coding engine functionality and their H&P interface designs lack the tools to fulfill these needs.

SUMMARY

Analysis of current EHRs reveals a high prevalence of design features in critical components of the H&P record that, when used by physicians as intended, can lead to problems in quality care, usability, and E/M compliance. A significant number of these issues result from designs that seek to increase speed of care and documentation, but may do so in a manner that potentially compromises quality of care and compliance. These problematic features include preprinted lists of information that presume that the *absence of documentation* indicates "negative" history responses or "normal" exam findings, and they also include the insertion of *automated information* in lieu of true documentation. This latter type of problem can arise from functionality that allows copying and pasting of information from previous visits or different patients, from graphic user interface designs that can prepopulate data fields, and from narrative interface designs that rely on pre-entered generic descriptions (macros). Additional concerns are also derived from the failure of current software systems to incorporate functionality capable of addressing the critical issue of medical necessity.

Physicians require the design and functionality of EHR software to fulfill all of their requirements for an effective H&P record. To accomplish this, EHRs must promote the positive features of quality, compliance, usability, efficiency, productivity, and data integrity. In addition, these sophisticated systems need to provide safeguards against designs that could lead to improper use and/or suboptimal results.

In October of 2007, the American Health Information Management Association (AHIMA) passed a resolution recognizing the importance of ensuring that these compliance and quality concepts are integrated into EHR designs. The resolution advises:

> "Whereas, the healthcare industry is in transition to electronic health records (EHRs) and EHRs need to yield quality documentation and data in order to support patient care, health information exchange, quality management, compliance and other secondary uses of data;
>
> Whereas, EHR systems are an important tool and provide a significant opportunity to improve documentation and patient care when properly designed and used;
>
> Whereas, EHR systems may contain design features and functions that can potentially contribute to suboptimal quality of healthcare data and documentation;
>
> Therefore, be it
>
> Resolved, That AHIMA advocates that organizations developing or implementing EHR systems take steps to ensure that the functionality of their EHR system supports quality care, valid documentation, and data integrity;[12]
>
> Resolved, That AHIMA advocates that HIM professionals, particularly those with expertise in data capture methods, compliance, and data quality management, actively participate in EHR system selection, design and development, implementation, and maintenance;
>
> Resolved, That AHIMA advocates that organizations implementing EHR systems ensure that process analysis and improvement is performed in order to enhance documentation and avoid inaccurate, incomplete, inappropriate, or non-compliant documentation;
>
> Resolved, That AHIMA advocates that HIM professionals collaborate with clinician users of the EHR, including training, to ensure that the best quality of data and documentation is maintained for patient care, quality management, compliance, health information exchange; and secondary use purposes; and
>
> Resolved, That HIM professionals actively participate and contribute to organizations that develop standards for the EHR to ensure that data and documentation in the EHR meets the needs of healthcare organizations.

References

1. American Medical Association. *Current Procedural Terminology (CPT®)*. Chicago, IL: American Medical Association; 2007.

2. Smith S, ed. *Medicare RBRVS 2008. The Physicians' Guide.* Chicago, IL: American Medical Association; 2008.

3. Office of the National Coordinator for Health Information Technology, US Department of Health and Human Services. Recommended Requirements for Enhancing Data Quality in Electronic Health Record Systems: Final Report.

May 2007:46-47. www.rti.org/pubs/enhancing_data_quality_in_ ehrs.pdf. Accessed June 15, 2007.

4. American Medical Association, Health Care Financing Administration. *Documentation Guidelines for Evaluation and Management Services.* Chicago, IL:1997.

5. RTI International Anti-Fraud Model Requirements, http://ehrantifrauddev. rti.org/Home/tabid/36/Default.aspx. Accessed January 20, 2007.

6. Bickley LS, Szilagyi PG. *Bates' Guide to Physical Examination and History Taking.* 8th ed. Philadelphia, PA: Lippincott Williams & Wilkins; 2004.

7. Pelaia RA. Medical record entry timeliness; what is reasonable? *Coding Edge.* September 2007:21.

8. Centers for Medicare & Medicaid Services. Selection of level of evaluation and management service. In: *Medicare Claims Processing Manual.* Chapter 12:-section 30.6.1. http://new.cms.hhs.gov/manuals/downloads/clm104c12.pdf. Accessed June 15, 2007.

9. Social Security Online. Compilation of the Social Security laws. 1862(a)(1)(a). www.socialsecurity.gov/OP_Home/ssact/title18/1862.htm#act-1862-a. Accessed June 15, 2007.

10. Levinson SR. Features of the E/M coding system and the *Documentation Guidelines.* In: *Practical E/M: Documentation and Coding Solutions for Quality Patient Care.* Chicago, IL: AMA Press; 2005:39.

11. Center for Medicare & Medicaid Services Carriers' Manual, Chapter 7: Overpayments: Physician Liability; section 7103.1(I).

12. American Health Information Management Association (AHIMA). Resolution on Quality Data and Documentation in the EHR. 2007-08 House of Delegates, October 7, 2007; Philadelphia, PA. Available at: http://library.ahima.org/ xpedio/idcplg?cookieLogin=1&portal=gomain. Accessed 24 January, 2008.

chapter 8

Data Entry Design Issues: The Medical History Component

The realization that physicians can use the medical record to facilitate the diagnostic process provides a powerful lens for examining the effects of various design and functionality options on patient care for each component of the electronic H&P record. Although there are hundreds of different software systems available, each with its own variations of screen layout and data entry designs, the present task is to analyze the types of data entry features that, when used as instructed, may interfere with physicians' efforts for optimal care, effective documentation, and compliant coding. Conversely, as will be explored in Part 3, the creation of H&P designs that prioritize support of the diagnostic process will help promote quality care and ease of use.

The issues identified and discussed in this chapter and in Chapter 9 are representative of the problems that can occur with a variety of existing data entry designs; they are not, however, intended to provide a comprehensive list of all possible design and functionality issues. The goal is to illustrate how physicians and administrators can (and should) analyze the various H&P sections of electronic health records (EHRs), enabling them to detect problems and have them remedied by the system's software design team. Ideally, these modifications should take place—and be verified—before a practice implements a new system and, preferably, before making a final commitment to purchase EHR software.

POTENTIAL SIDE EFFECTS OF INCREASING SPEED OF DOCUMENTATION

As noted previously, most software systems commonly require increased time at the front end to record individualized clinical information. This characteristic places a greater burden on physicians when they are assigned the task of data entry, but physicians cannot afford to invest more time than they already expend while using a familiar and effective paper documentation system. Therefore, software designers have frequently devoted considerable effort to mobilizing the abilities of computers to use and reuse standardized or preexisting documentation during subsequent encounters. However, this approach to documentation can generate a number of significant problems. Although these designs seek to increase documentation speed, they commonly fail to guard against potential negative consequences for the physician-patient interaction, the application of the medical diagnostic process, and compliant documentation and coding.

This chapter evaluates the possible difficulties created by commonly encountered designs in each section and subsection of the medical history component of evaluation and management (E/M) services. Analysis can be streamlined by reviewing these design approaches in terms of two categories that include different elements of physicians' goals for medical records:

- The first category, *quality and compliance*, addresses physicians' demand for the electronic H&P to facilitate the interrelated elements of quality care, E/M compliance, usability, and data integrity. Because the E/M system is a codification of the medical diagnostic process, these four components are naturally interrelated. An EHR structure that follows the diagnostic process and guides compliance should facilitate quality and data integrity through individualized documentation. It should also increase usability because of its compatibility with physicians' optimal patient care workflow.

- The second category, *efficiency*, analyzes the ability of the electronic H&P to allow rapid documentation while guarding against designs that also tend to speed up the care process to a degree that may negatively affect one or more of the elements of quality, compliance, usability, and data integrity.

Physicians' final EHR need, *productivity*, depends on the successful fulfillment of all the other elements that occur in both of the aforementioned categories.

Prioritizing Physicians' Requirements

Our goal is for EHR designs and functionality to satisfy all six of these medical practice requirements (quality care, compliance, usability, efficiency, data integrity, and productivity). Although some current systems focus primarily on speed of documentation, *Practical EHR* mandates that quality, usability, compliance, and data integrity have the highest priority. Efficiency can be maximized only to the extent that it does not interfere with optimal results for these critical factors.

OVERVIEW OF THE MEDICAL HISTORY COMPONENT

Early in their medical education, nearly all physicians encounter the truism that a good medical history is the foundation of accurate diagnosis and quality care. Most have heard the aphorism "with a good medical history, a physician can make the correct diagnosis 95% of the time before he or she even picks up a stethoscope." However, it is in this section of the H&P that physicians often encounter their greatest challenge in achieving a balance between efficiency and quality and compliance. During an initial patient visit, software designs that require physicians to personally ask and document all appropriate questions required for a clinically comprehensive medical history demand an inordinate amount of physician time. Other designs that provide documentation shortcuts may, as previously discussed, lead to "cloned" documentation that negatively affects compliance and the quality of information.

Speakers at health information technology conferences, articles in information technology journals, and presentations by EHR vendors sometimes discuss the potential for physician offices to make electronic versions of medical history forms available for patients to complete. These solutions include the options of patients entering much of their own medical history (specifically, the chief complaint; past medical, family, and social history [PFSH], and review of systems [ROS] elements) into the EHR by using an electronic kiosk in the waiting room or logging on to the physician's Web site to complete the forms from home or another site. These elegant data entry alternatives have the potential to fully satisfy efficiency and quality and compliance criteria. Using the patient as the data entry operator (DEO) reduces to zero the physician's time for asking routine questions and documenting responses. With a properly designed graphic user interface, plus controls to ensure physician review and addition of pertinent details to positive responses, this creative approach promises to capture and make available meaningful clinical information in a compliant and physician-friendly package.

Although this ability to permit patient documentation directly into the EHR seems to be an ideal solution for an ideal world, few medical offices have implemented this approach. It faces numerous obstacles, including increased costs for equipment and personnel (to instruct and assist patients in using the hardware) for the medical practice, compounded by the real-world obstacles that not all patients are computer literate, not all patients are Internet literate, and not all patients want to invest their personal time at home for completing medical forms. Even in the best of circumstances, this hardware-dependent approach to using the "patient as DEO" offers a solution for only a small percentage of patients. Until this option becomes widely available, acceptable to a significant majority of patients, and much less costly, software developers and designers need to identify a more effective alternative than requiring the physician to ask these questions and be the DEO.

CHIEF COMPLAINT AND PFSH (INITIAL VISIT)

Although the time-honored approach to obtaining a medical history began by physicians asking a patient about the chief complaint (the primary reason for the visit) and the history of present illness (HPI), practicing physicians who use paper records now often use structured patient questionnaires that allow patients to document the other portions of the medical history before seeing the physician. This paper design approach matches the electronic option, discussed above, of patient pre-entry of the chief complaint, PFSH, and ROS via kiosk or Internet.

Benefit of Initiating the Medical History With the PFSH and ROS

Traditionally, medical students are taught to begin the medical history by investigating the chief complaint and present illness. The consequence of using this approach, however, is the natural tendency to view obtaining the PFSH and ROS as being peripheral or as an interruption to taking care of the patient's presenting medical problem. With this order of history taking, physicians tend to move through this clinical background information quickly so they can proceed to the examination, diagnosis, and treatment of the patient's chief complaint.

---

continued

In contrast, by using an "intelligent medical record" in the paper format, physicians can become accustomed to reviewing every new patient's completed PFSH and ROS forms before entering the examination room. After greeting the patient, the next step is to interview the patient to obtain details of positive responses in this background information before investigating the HPI. This order of evaluating medical histories provides a reasonable understanding of the patients' general health, including active medical problems and treatments, before turning attention to the symptoms for which the patient scheduled their visit. This approach, which requires far less time than personally obtaining the PFSH and ROS, automatically orients the physician toward a holistic perspective, first considering the patient as a whole and then assessing the present illness.

Experience shows this to be a more comprehensive and logical approach to patient care. It helps physicians to better understand their patients' health concerns and to appreciate their current complaints in the context of their overall health, family health, and social setting. It also increases the likelihood of detecting other unsuspected health problems and issues that call for preventive counseling. Most important, this sequence of the medical history orients physicians to taking care of a "patient who has a lung problem," rather than the problem-focused approach of "treating a sick lung."

Efficiency Concerns

When an EHR requires that a physician personally obtain and document the chief complaint, PFSH, and ROS, there is a significant loss of physician time. Because the Documentation Guidelines specify that "[t]he ROS and/or PFSH may be recorded by ancillary staff or on a form completed by the patient,"[1(p6)] most practices using paper medical records have outsourced obtaining and documenting these portions of the medical history directly to the patient, particularly during initial visits and consultations. When an EHR's design returns this task to the physician, it creates a significant loss of efficiency, particularly in comparison with paper records.

PFSH Quality and Compliance Concerns

Most electronic screens for the PFSH wisely provide a graphic interface screen for data entry, with *Yes* and *No* check-boxes for the person recording information to indicate whether the patient does or does not have a particular illness, social issue, or family medical history. Figure 6.1 illustrated an example of this design, including check-boxes and an adjacent text box to record explanations of positive responses.

These designs present two potential problem areas. First, very frequently, they fail to *require* the person entering the data (whether it is the physician, member of the clinical staff, or the patient) to provide details of each positive response. In addition, some designs fail to offer the option of entering explanatory data, presenting the check-boxes but not a means of documenting narrative details (such systems would look similar to Figure 6.1 but would lack the associated boxes for free-text entry). This design defect not only fails to meet documentation compliance requirements, but it also significantly impacts completeness of the clinical data and the quality of care. Physicians should investigate the details of patients' positive responses. Although it is important, for example, to recognize that a patient has a diagnosis of "diabetes," this information should trigger a number of additional questions to reveal greater depth and detail, such as the following:

- Do you have type I or type II diabetes?
- How long have you had diabetes?
- How do you manage it?
- Is it under control?
- Have you had any problems with your eyes, kidneys, or feet?
- How often do you see the physician who treats your diabetes?

The potential negative impact of this design limitation on the quality of care is compounded by the fact that, realistically, the inability to successfully record these details of the medical history also discourages physicians from asking these additional questions. Furthermore, even if physicians have asked the questions, inability to properly document the responses means that the information is not carried forward to the next visit or the next practitioner. Over time, the loss of this level of detail promulgates and reinforces problem-focused care.

The second consideration in design problems in the PFSH section relates to E/M compliance. The Documentation Guidelines require that, when the PFSH and/or ROS are recorded by staff or by a patient, "To document that the physician reviewed the information, there must be a notation supplementing or confirming the information recorded by others."[1(p6)] My interpretation of this guideline is that it calls for explanatory documentation of positive responses, which requires a narrative (ie, free-text) interface, and an electronic signature specific to this section of the H&P record for the physician to attest that he or she has reviewed the negative responses.

REVIEW OF SYSTEMS (INITIAL VISIT)

A well-designed ROS questionnaire has the potential to provide a remarkable amount of important information about a patient's health. Effectively phrased questions inquiring about signs and symptoms among the 14 recognized organ systems may reveal a variety of potentially significant medical issues, including some that the patient may not otherwise recognize as relevant.

The ROS as a Bridge to Comprehensive Care

The introduction of a complete ROS into every initial-visit medical records greatly increases a physician's ability to identify patients who have symptoms of potential illnesses that warrant higher levels of care, including problems related to that physician's particular specialty, as well as unrelated issues warranting care from specialists in other fields.

In my own field of otolaryngology, it became common to find that patients with a simple complaint, such as ear wax, could present completed ROS forms that suggested additional problems ranging from chronic sinusitis to life-threatening obstructive sleep apnea. At other times, the ROS might reveal symptoms suggesting thyroid illness, asthma, or acute myocardial infarction. For example, a patient whose ROS form indicated "recent weight loss" replied, when asked how much weight she had lost, "40 pounds in the last 4 months." With further interviewing, she stated that the loss had occurred without her

---

continued

trying to lose weight, and subsequent questions suggested mild gastrointestinal symptoms. Consultation was requested from a gastroenterologist who found stage I lymphoma of the intestine, which had an excellent prognosis for cure owing to early diagnosis.

The message in this story is that having patients complete an effective ROS survey (and PFSH review) provides sufficient information, with almost no investment of physicians' time, to change from a problem-focused history to a comprehensive one. This transformation can help physicians detect symptoms suggesting a broad range of significant health problems, such as asthma, chronic obstructive pulmonary disease, congestive heart failure, myocardial infarction, gastric ulcer, diabetes, thyroid problems, and cerebral aneurysm.

Efficiency Problems

As with the PFSH, electronic designs that require physicians to ask all questions of the ROS and document the patient's responses, rather than delegating the documentation of responses to the initial screening questions to patients and staff, result in a significant loss of efficiency.

Quality and Compliance Problems

Similar to the designs for PFSH data entry, most EHRs provide a graphic interface screen for data entry of the initial responses to questions in the ROS. This design usually includes appropriate *Yes* and *No* check-boxes that document whether the patient is experiencing specific signs or symptoms. (A sample of this design is shown in Figure 12.5.) Although this design helps physicians to fulfill compliance standards for inquiring into the number of systems appropriate for a comprehensive ROS, it also presents the same two issues in documentation requirements that raised potential concerns for the PFSH section.

As suggested by the Documentation Guidelines, physicians should electronically sign this section to verify their review of information obtained and documented by others.[1(p6)] In addition, just as for the PFSH, physicians must *supplement* the screening information by investigating and documenting the details of all positive responses.[1(p6)] Although brief descriptions are generally sufficient to provide meaningful additional information in the various PFSH subsections, positive responses in the ROS should usually be explored in greater depth, similar to the diagnostic approach used to evaluate the presenting symptoms in the HPI. Physicians need to inquire about the chronological course of the symptom and investigate the elements of the HPI (duration, timing, severity, location, quality, context, modifying factors, and associated signs and symptoms) that are appropriate to each circumstance. As discussed in the following section on the HPI, the only design option that is capable of meeting these compliance and quality standards is a narrative interface that permits documentation of free text. For example, when a patient's ROS indicates a positive response to the question about "chest pain," it is incumbent on the physician to investigate this symptom in greater depth, just as if it were the patient's presenting complaint. This will include asking a series of questions and documenting the patient's responses to trace the history of this symptom from its onset until the time of the visit, allowing the physician to determine whether this is a stable controlled problem under physician care, a new problem calling for appropriate evaluation in the near future, or an urgent problem requiring immediate medical attention.

The Case of the Overlooked Chest Pain

When auditors review medical records for compliance, one of the most alarming documentation lapses they can encounter occurs when a physician fails to review or address positive ROS responses documented by a patient or staff member. For example, a patient checks the *Yes* box for chest pain, and the physician initials the page (to attest to having reviewed the information), yet no details were documented about the chest pain in any part of the medical record, including the "impressions" section of the chart.

It is chilling to imagine the possibility of the patient having a myocardial infarction shortly after the visit and to think of the physician's indefensible position when the patient's attorney sends a subpoena for the medical records. The records will document that the patient advised the physician of the chest pain and that the physician failed to acknowledge or address that complaint.

One of a physician's primary responsibilities is to determine when a symptom may be dangerous, life threatening, or an indication of a serious underlying condition or illness. The EHR should provide tools to aid in this process, not tools that allow it to be bypassed.

Some electronic ROS designs create an immediate compliance problem by having only a check-box-type of graphic user interface without a narrative section for the physician to add critical supplemental details. Furthermore, systems that do provide an option for narrative entry may fail to include a safety feature requiring physicians to address all positive responses, potentially allowing physicians to proceed without providing the requisite medical detail. Just as described for the PFSH, designs that lack the option for physicians to document critical medical history details for the ROS may even discourage physicians from obtaining this information because they would be unable to record it. The lack of a narrative interface component for the ROS, therefore, not only challenges physicians' ability to achieve E/M compliance, but it may also lead to less effective care and/or the potential for problems with medical liability.

"Counting" the Chest Pain

At the October 2006, Medical Group Management Association's annual meeting, a number of EHRs from a variety of excellent vendors were available for review. Although the ROS section of many systems provided a reasonable graphic user interface section to allow documentation of patients' *Yes* or *No* responses to questions about a variety of signs and symptoms, several had no free-text capability for this part of the H&P.

When representatives demonstrating systems with such limitations were asked "What does your system do if I check the *Yes* box for chest pain?" puzzled looks and a variety of perplexed reactions were the usual responses. One sales person simply replied "We count it," referring to the software's E/M code calculator having the ability to count check-boxes in the H&P sections of the chart and to use these "counts" to suggest an E/M code.

While an effective coding engine is a desirable EHR feature, this representative's response overlooks physicians' primary concern, which is the patient's health and well-being. This system had no entry mechanism in the ROS section to enable a physician to describe, for example, when the patient's chest pain began, how severe it was, and whether the patient had previously visited a physician because of this problem. Although the software was able to count organ systems, it was unable to allow a physician to document the patient's medically indicated evaluation. Although it could measure the *quantitative* elements of E/M compliance, it failed to facilitate the *qualitative* aspects of E/M and the medical diagnostic process.

PFSH AND ROS (ESTABLISHED PATIENT VISIT)

It is also clinically important to reassess patients' medical history during follow-up visits because significant illnesses or symptoms may have developed since the last visit. Although neither physicians nor patients want to repeat the entire inventory of medical history questions that were completed on the initial visit, the Documentation Guidelines recommend a valuable approach to eliciting PFSH and ROS information during follow-up visits that is highly efficient and clinically valuable: The physician is permitted to review and update the previous information, which is documented by:

- "describing any new ROS and/or PFSH information or noting there has been no change in the information; and
- noting the date and location of the earlier ROS and/or PFSH"[1(p6)]

Applying this approach facilitates the discovery of invaluable clinical information ranging from changes in medications to recent new diagnoses, hospitalizations, operations, and the onset of new health symptoms. These insights may prove pivotal in managing existing problems or finding new ones. Even the knowledge that the patient's general health remains stable makes a valuable contribution. Just as with initial patient visits, obtaining a comprehensive medical history at the beginning of follow-up visits triggers the medical diagnostic process and provides the best opportunity for providing quality care.

Comprehensive History in Follow-up Visits: A Bonus of E/M Compliance

Although medical school training emphasizes the value of a comprehensive history during every initial visit, most physicians report that there is little or no instruction in the extent of the medical history that ideally should be obtained during follow-up visits. Moreover, there is no presentation of a formal structure for reviewing the PFSH and/or ROS during subsequent care. The *Bates' Guide*[2] also includes no such discussion.

As an alternative to repeating a complete PFSH and ROS survey during each follow-up visit, the inclusion of PFSH and ROS updates as integral elements of outpatient established visits and of ROS updates during inpatient subsequent care visits seems to be an innovation of the Documentation Guidelines. Formally including questions to elicit this update during every follow-up visit frequently reveals surprising and sometimes critically important clinical information that facilitates quality care, just as it does during initial visits. The following is an example:

A patient had an appointment to review results of a sinus computed tomography scan, with a discussion about surgery to treat the problem that had remained unresponsive to medical therapy. The physician usually would have reexamined the patient and then discussed and potentially scheduled surgery, but the requirement on newly adopted compliant E/M forms for updating the PFSH and ROS prompted first asking whether the patient had experienced any nonsinus medical issues or symptoms since the last visit (3 weeks earlier). The patient responded: "Oh yes, 2 weeks ago I had an angioplasty, and now I'm taking Coumadin." This information clearly modified the care sequence and process, leading to planning and support with the patient's cardiologist before, during, and after the successful operation. It helped increase patient safety and avoid potential medical error and it, thereby, saved the patient and physician from potentially trying moments in the operating room.[3]

In the inpatient setting, where patients are seen by physicians on a daily basis, E/M compliance calls for an update of the ROS, although it does not require an update of the PFSH. Inquiring each day about symptoms unrelated to the patient's primary illness gives the opportunity for detecting potential problems at their earliest stages, when corrective action can lead to rapid resolution and prevent major complications. It takes only a few seconds after greeting a patient to ask, eg, "Have you had any new symptoms since yesterday, such as chest pain, shortness of breath, or pain in your calves?" Yet, a positive response may permit identification of the beginnings of a heart, lung, or venous clotting problem before it becomes a serious threat to the patient.

Quality and Compliance Problems

The most commonly encountered compliance issue in this portion of the electronic H&P for established patient visits results from using noncompliant copy and paste functionality to increase the speed of documentation. Recognizing that it is time-consuming and inefficient for physicians and patients to repeat a complete list of pertinent medical history questions on every visit, some software systems use this documentation shortcut in an effort to fulfill E/M requirements for the medical history. Instead of providing a narrative interface to enable documentation of an update of the PFSH and ROS, the systems using this tool can copy and paste, word-for-word, the entire PFSH and ROS from the initial patient visit directly into every subsequent visit. Even if the physician is given the opportunity to update the copied information, doing so would require repeating all of the questions from the initial visit, an approach already identified as being unsatisfactory.

Although instantaneously fast, this copy-and-paste approach suffers from lack of compliance, from failure to enter meaningful (ie, current) data, and, most important, from not satisfying quality care standards. From the compliance perspective, this approach creates cloned medical records. It is apparent that the *work* of the history was not actually performed on the date of the visit, it was simply copied. Cloned documents are inadequate to support medical necessity because they refer to the patient's status on a previous date. Finally, when audited, this approach risks a determination of "false claims," because it includes submitting codes based on care performed during previous visits rather than the current one.

From a quality perspective, the physician needs to be concerned with the patient's health status on the date of the visit and how it evolved from the date of the last visit. For example, it is not relevant to the current visit that the patient did not have chest pain at the previous visit, 3 months ago. What is medically relevant and critical is to know whether the patient has had chest pain during the 3 months since the previous visit.

The copy-and-paste approach also may create medical liability issues. When the medical record reports a normal ROS that is merely copied from a previous visit, it represents that the physician performed a complete inquiry into the patient's signs and symptoms on the day of the visit. However, if a serious health issue subsequently develops and the physician had not actually updated the PFSH and ROS, this noncompliant functionality could place the physician at risk.

Many EHRs fail to provide the compliant alternative of a narrative interface section that prompts the physician to update the PFSH and ROS since the previous visit. This is a simple design solution, and the narrative interface is the most appropriate approach because the range of potential patient responses is vast, and updates in the ROS section call for free-text narrative of any positive responses to document a true history of the events.

History of Present Illness

Knowing how to obtain a comprehensive HPI is a cornerstone of quality patient care. Physicians love to share their stories of making the right diagnosis for a patient with an unusual illness or with uncommon manifestations of a more common disease. These heroic tales invariably hinge on the patient volunteering a critical piece of information during a well-timed, open-ended question or the physician resorting to a "magic question," a focused inquiry that has the ability to elicit a specific response that will confirm or rule out a potential diagnosis.

Obtaining an effective history requires a combination of open-ended questions, designed to elicit the patient's interpretation of the signs and symptoms, and more directed and specific questions, focused on verbally narrowing the list of possible diagnoses. This combination of questioning starts with asking the patient to describe how the symptoms began, followed by tracing the course of events over time, from the onset to the present, obtaining specific details to describe what happened during each significant turn in the illness. This process is described in essentially the same way in the *Current Procedural Terminology* (*CPT*®),[4] in the Documentation Guidelines,[1] and in the *Bates' Guide*.[2] All three references describe the HPI as a "chronological description"[4(p2)] or a "chronological account"[2(p4)] of the course of the illness from the first sign and/or symptom to the present. They also all state that this descriptive account additionally includes the eight clarifying elements or attributes of a symptom (location, quality, severity, duration, timing, context, modifying factors, and associated signs and symptoms). The *Bates' Guide* explains that the role of these eight attributes is, for all symptoms, "to fully understand their essential characteristics."[2(p27)] A well-documented history will usually include a number of significant episodes, and the HPI will include some of the eight elements that are pertinent for each episode.

It is critical to design the HPI interface in a way that guides physicians to obtain and document the medical history in this manner. It should first facilitate a chronologically based description of the symptoms affecting the patient and then guide inclusion of appropriate details related to the eight clarifying elements. The most usable and intuitive design to accomplish these needs is the narrative interface, combined with documentation prompts to provide physicians with a list of the eight elements of the HPI and to emphasize the requirement for a chronological description. Physicians elicit patients' stories as sequential narratives, which are unique to each patient. Physicians are accustomed to documenting this type of history information as a free-text description, just as the patient tells it. Physicians currently writing their records on paper commonly document this narrative as they are obtaining it, and those who prefer dictation are advised to dictate the history at the conclusion of the patient's visit.

Efficiency Problems

Chapter 7 pointed out the fact that many physicians would face a significant efficiency challenge and has voiced considerable resistance to EHR adoption, if required to type individualized free-text descriptive narratives, such as the HPI, directly into the electronic H&P. The prevalence of this problem likely accounts for one of the primary reasons that EHR designers created alternative means of recording the HPI. Figures 7.3 and 7.4 illustrate two of the more common design alternatives to a straightforward narrative interface. The first demonstrates a short-answer style of graphic interface, and the second illustrates a pre-entered generic macro. Both are built solely on the eight elements of the HPI listed in CPT codes and the Documentation Guidelines. Unfortunately, along with increased speed of documentation, this approach predisposes to an associated decrease in the time physicians devote to obtaining a true HPI. A second and less obvious consequence of these solutions is that this approach alters the nature of the history obtained.

The designs of both of these alternatives focus solely on the eight elements of the HPI to the exclusion of the core medical history requirement for a "chronological description of the development of the patient's present illness."[4(p2)] Instead, by not providing for the documentation of a patient's actual medical *history*, these types of designs guide physicians to obtain a snapshot that reveals only the patient's symptoms on the date of the visit. In cases that include the element of duration, the record will state the time of onset (eg, "symptoms began 6 months ago") and then proceed with the snapshot of symptoms on the date of the visit, neglecting to obtain or document a description of the course of historical events that has transpired between the date of onset and the date of the visit. On the other hand, if a physician were to attempt to document a true medical history using the preset designs in Figure 7.3 or 7.4, it would be inefficient and time-consuming, if not impossible, to properly enter a chronological description of the course of an illness.

The Inefficiency of Macros

During the 2006 Medical Group Management Association annual meeting, data entry designs for HPI in the current generation of EHRs were available for review. Only a minority of these systems completely failed to provide an option for free-text data entry, while most offered one or two options for physicians to record narrative information. However, even for designs capable of recording a narrative history by typing and/or dictating, the demonstration staff members always emphasized the benefit of reduced time for documenting the HPI by loading and modifying pre-entered macros.

In his effort to demonstrate how quickly a physician could document an HPI using a generic macro, one of the salesmen asked me to describe the HPI of a patient with chest pain. After expertly uploading his EHR system's chest pain macro onto the computer screen, he readied his mouse to complete the few blanks spaces in the macro by pointing and clicking on brief descriptions of duration and severity from drop-down pick-lists, I began my description of a patient presenting with chest pain: "Seven weeks ago, the patient was in an auto accident and suffered a steering wheel injury to the mid-chest and rib cage. As a result, he experienced some bilateral chest pain with deep inspiration, which was worse on the left side. He was seen in the emergency room the next day, where X-rays were negative for rib fracture. These symptoms gradually improved over the next two weeks. Two weeks after the accident, while jogging on a treadmill at the gym, he had an episode of feeling short of breath and felt some mild discomfort in the left neck and jaw. This resolved after resting for about ten minutes and. . . ." "STOP!" interrupted the vendor. "I can't do it this way. I'll put away the macro and just type as you speak, but you'll have to speak much more slowly."

The salesman explained that it was much slower to enter data by typing out the free text, but he then assured me "it will go much faster once you learn to

continued

change how you take a history, so that you can use macros." This statement underscores one of the central issues physicians must confront when presented with the option of using macros as substitutes for narrative free text. The goal of EHR design should be to fit the way physicians obtain a high-quality H&P; it should not require them to abandon the proven diagnostic process in order to accommodate inadequate and noncompliant software designs.

Quality and Compliance Problems

Designs that do not facilitate or allow physicians to obtain and document a chronological description of a patient's illness not only fail to satisfy the definition of an HPI in CPT codes and the Documentation Guidelines, but they also interfere with physicians' ability to obtain and record a true medical HPI. In an audit following strict interpretation of the Documentation Guidelines, absence of a valid HPI might result in the reviewer reducing the code level significantly or entirely disallowing an E/M service because of a physician's failure to document a *history* of the present illness.

Quality care concerns with this approach compound the compliance issue. Because the medical history is physicians' most powerful diagnostic tool, decreasing its scope and effectiveness necessarily limits their insight into patients' medical problems and physicians' ability to develop a complete and accurate differential diagnosis. Reducing this capability compromises the overall quality of patient care. HPI design solutions are needed that can maximize documentation efficiency without requiring a trade-off of compromised compliance and scope of care; Chapter 12 presents alternative medical history design approaches that facilitate compliance, quality care, and efficiency.

Implications of Loss of a Chronological Description for the HPI

A travel metaphor illustrates the problems that can result from obtaining a "history" that lacks a chronology. For example, asking about a friend's recent trip and omitting the chronological elements might elicit the following information: "I left home 3 weeks ago. I just returned and came to see you. I've brought you some gifts and have photos of some mountains and lakes. My back is aching a bit, I broke my glasses, and I met two really interesting college students who were also traveling abroad." While it might seem that some travel information was shared, descriptions of what happened between the friend's leaving and her visit today were left out, including where she visited and how long she stayed in each destination, and what she did at each location. We know she took a trip, but she has conveyed very little meaningful information about the details.

Similarly, asking a patient about chest pain by following the guidance of an HPI template such as shown in Figures 7.3 and 7.4 discourages a physician from obtaining a true medical history and using the conventional diagnostic process. Those sample designs might, for example, allow the physician to overlook diagnostically important details about each symptomatic episode the patient experienced. Investigating the interim episodes might enable a physician to learn critical information that could change the impression of illness severity and/or modify the differential diagnosis. For example, this additional information might reveal that the patient had sustained trauma to the chest or experienced episodes with symptoms that would lead a prudent physician to consider gastroesophageal reflex as the cause for the pain symptoms. These designs also make it difficult to appropriately document details that do not fit into macros.

The Impact of Coding Software Limitations on Designs for the Medical History Record

Chapter 7 detailed concerns about the functionality of E/M coding software that fails to consider medical necessity, relying solely on the three key components of E/M to determine E/M code levels. In addition, coding software functionality that concentrates only on the *objective* elements of the CPT codes and Documentation Guidelines and fails to incorporate the overriding *subjective* considerations of the E/M guidelines can lead to consequences that are more subtle than those related to the nature of the presenting problem, but can also have more far-reaching consequences than just an impact on compliance.

The discussion of design limitations of the HPI interface illustrates the extent of this problem. Software designers are not physicians. They cannot be expected to appreciate that the overriding consideration for an HPI is obtaining and documenting a true medical history (chronological description of the course of the patient's illness), not just a compilation of the eight elements (which, when used properly, should help to characterize each of the significant episodes during the course of that illness). Most coding engines incorporate only the HPI values they can easily count: the eight elements. It is possible, but more challenging, to incorporate the subjective element of chronology, and most existing programs have, unfortunately, failed to do so. Because many interface designs have been constructed to provide the data these coding engines need to capture, the elements left out of the coding software are often consequently excluded from the H&P screens.

The failure of EHRs to incorporate medical history record designs that meet physicians' optimal workflow extends beyond the HPI. Similar issues occur for the PFSH and ROS sections, in which software that correctly prompts physicians to inquire about diseases and symptoms may fail to incorporate the associated requirement for physicians to elicit and document medical details about all positive responses. Chapter 9 describes similar challenges that imperfect coding software functionality can create for interface designs of the physical examination, medical decision making, and medical necessity.

There are significant secondary problems generated by coding engines with functionality that fails to incorporate the subjective elements of E/M care. Such deficiencies are commonly reflected in interface designs for the electronic H&P where they can result in systems that are incompatible with physicians' normal workflow and ability to carry out all components of the diagnostic process. Failure to recognize the necessity of maintaining and facilitating physicians' workflow and the entire diagnostic process is at the core of EHR issues that challenge usability, compliance, quality care standards, efficiency, and data integrity. As a fundamental principle, software designs should not change or disrupt physicians' normal workflow for achieving optimal patient care; rather, the designs should reinforce and facilitate this process.

Software and the Science and Art of Medicine

A major focus of the coding software in EHRs has been to measure the *objective* components of the quality care process. This functionality capably evaluates the science of medicine, including counting the number of tests performed, the number of body areas examined, the number of elements of

continued

the HPI reviewed, and the number of diagnoses selected. It is far more difficult, if not impossible, to measure the elements of care that contribute to the art of medicine, ie, the subjective components of the quality care process. These elements encompass the *complexity* of the data, the *illustrative* description of abnormal examination findings, the *historical* sequence and relationship of events in a high-quality medical history, and the *individual assessment* of severities and probabilities in determining a sophisticated differential diagnosis.

One cannot truly "quantify" Da Vinci's *Mona Lisa* or place on it a "measurable" value, to compare its magnitude against the "value" of Michelangelo's frescoes on the ceiling of the Sistine Chapel or Beethoven's Ninth Symphony. This lack of objective assessment enhances the value of these artistic accomplishments; it certainly does not give reason to overlook them. Similarly, even though they are not readily quantified, it is necessary for software designs to maintain and nourish the subjective portions of the electronic H&P, not to discourage or interfere with their performance.

Physicians have the ability to place a relative value on the subjective elements of the H&P. Coding engines must, therefore, have the ability to accept and value such input, and software designers must incorporate this functionality into the interface of each appropriate component of the H&P record.

SUMMARY

The medical history has a pivotal role in helping physicians effectively evaluate patients' conditions and provide appropriate levels of medical care. Accomplishing this goal requires the design and functionality of the EHR to meet a number of major objectives. The obvious requirement is that physicians must be able to document the care they provide accurately and efficiently. The design must also work intuitively for physicians— easy to use while caring for patients and ensure E/M compliance— because physicians rely on their records to guide appropriate care and documentation to satisfy coding requirements. Finally, because physicians rely on their records as an integral part of the patient care process, the quality of the care they provide is a reflection of the quality of the medical record tools they use. Designs that are unable to record certain types of information will discourage physicians from obtaining that information, and this may negatively impact diagnosis and treatment. Therefore, electronic H&P designs must use appropriate interfaces for each section of the record to assist physicians in providing the appropriate type and amount of care.

In many cases, the source of H&P design problems derives from non-compliant E/M coding software, which either neglects to consider some of the critical elements of compliance (eg, the levels of risk and the nature of the presenting problems) and/or fails to match physicians' optimal workflow. These shortcomings can lead to suboptimal interface designs that may interfere with a systems' usability and may negatively impact physicians' ability to provide optimal patient care and compliant documentation. Therefore, medical practices must carefully analyze the electronic H&P designs and the E/M coding functions of every EHR they consider. Any compliance or usability problems that exist should be successfully addressed before finalizing a decision to bring that EHR into their practice.

References

1.   American Medical Association, Health Care Financing Administration. *Documentation Guidelines for Evaluation and Management Services.* Chicago, IL: American Medical Association; 1997.

2.   Bickley LS, Szilagyi PG. *Bates' Guide to Physical Examination and History Taking.* 8th ed. Philadelphia, PA: Lippincott Williams & Wilkins; 2004.

3.   Levinson SR. Quality of care and the role of the medical record. *Practical E/M: Documentation and Coding Solutions for Quality Patient Care.* Chicago, IL: AMA Press; 2005:3-8.

4.   American Medical Association. *Current Procedural Terminology* (*CPT*®). Chicago, IL: American Medical Association; 2007.

chapter 9

Data Entry Design Issues: Examination, Medical Decision Making, and Nature of the Presenting Problem

In the medical diagnostic process, physicians generally formulate a preliminary differential diagnosis and a preliminary assessment of the severity of a patient's illness during the course of obtaining a comprehensive medical history. As more information is gathered, this initial evaluation becomes further refined, and physicians select increasingly precise questions until establishing a working diagnosis, a set of alternative diagnoses, and a reasonable appraisal of the nature of the presenting problem (NPP; degree of risks associated with the illness).

The *Bates' Guide*[1] emphasizes this interweaving of diagnostic reasoning into the medical history as an advanced medical skill, advising medical students that "[b]ecause assessment takes place in the clinician's mind, the process of clinical reasoning often seems inaccessible and even mysterious to the beginning student.... ***As you gain experience, your thinking process will begin at the outset of the patient encounter, not at the end*** [emphasis added]."[1(p784)]

Similarly, Guidance in the *Current Procedural Terminology* (*CPT*®) manual's Clinical Examples Section (Appendix C) on evaluation and management (E/M) compliance encourages the determination of the severity of a patient's problems during the early stages of a visit; and cautioning that only after having identified the medically indicated level of care that "[t]he three components (history, examination, and medical decision making) must be met and documented in the medical record to report a particular level of service."[1(p450)]

The approach of *Practical EHR* to solving the E/M compliance challenge builds on this relationship between physicians' accustomed diagnostic methods and the *CPT* manual's instructions for providing and documenting the levels of care warranted by the NPP. Therefore, *Practical EHR* recommends that at the conclusion of reviewing (and documenting) the patient's *comprehensive* medical history, physicians should consciously determine a preliminary assessment of the NPP and identify the associated level of care they deem appropriate for this severity of illness. The design of the medical record itself should include a section that provides secure guidance in this choice, based on the *CPT* manual's E/M descriptors and clinical examples. Defining the medically indicated level of care in this manner ensures that subsequent coding and documentation will meet criteria for medical necessity. The medical record should provide additional guidance based on *CPT*'s E/M guidelines to alert physicians to describe the extent of examination and medical decision making (MDM) warranted by the NPP. At this time, it seems that none of the current electronic health record (EHR) systems available include this functionality on the basis of medical necessity. However, the following analysis of potential issues in the examination, MDM, and NPP sections takes into consideration not only existing design issues, but also designs that may arise when this functionality becomes available, we hope in response to physician demand.

One of physicians' requisite goals for EHRs is complete assurance of E/M compliance as an integral component of patient care. One of the fundamental requirements for achieving this goal is that documentation performed using EHR software must satisfy two fundamental compliance principles that are derived from the Center for Medicare & Medicaid Services (CMS) payment rules:

- Medicare will not pay for services that are not *medically necessary* [emphasis added].*2
- If care is not documented in the medical record, *it was not done* [emphasis added].*3

Auditors and coders enforce these standards whenever they review physician charts. The *Practical EHR* method addresses both of these issues because the converse of these rules is also true: (1) Medicare will pay for services that are medically necessary, and (2) when care is documented, the record attests that the care was performed. Therefore, compliance standards dictate that EHRs provide physicians with the ability to *document* medical necessity as a mandatory component of every patient visit. In addition, the design of the electronic history and physical examination (H&P) record needs to allow physicians to record all elements of E/M services, including all elements involved in MDM and the NPP.

ANALYZING THE PHYSICAL EXAMINATION COMPONENT

Experienced physicians are able to perform a comprehensive physical examination, appropriate for their specialty, remarkably quickly. Never are physicians heard complaining that it requires too much time to complete the examination. The primary challenge is designing an EHR interface that enables physicians to document the normal and abnormal findings with efficiency and compliance. Doing so requires the right combination of an optimal graphic interface (to indicate whether an examined area is "normal" or "abnormal") plus a narrative interface to document individual details of all abnormal findings. An additional design enhancement is the inclusion of documentation prompts that remind physicians of the extent of examination that is warranted by the NPP.

---

*This concept is derived from the CMS Carrier Manual, Part 3 (Claims Process), which states "the following are examples of situations in which the physician is liable for refunding an overpayment (section 7103.1). . . . physician does not submit documentation to substantiate that he performed services billed to program where there is question as to whether they were actually performed" (Section 7103.1(I))

Clinical Example of NPP Related Guidance

Physicians commonly evaluate patients for a recent onset of abdominal pain, which may or may not be associated with other gastrointestinal symptoms such as nausea or reduced appetite. This presents a reasonable example of how physicians would evaluate an otherwise healthy, established patient to determine the appropriate level of service and NPP, and then use this information to guide the performance and documentation of the medically indicated level of care.

If the physician's initial clinical impression following the completion of a comprehensive medical history indicates that the patient has a probable diagnosis of acute appendicitis, the next step would be to identify the appropriate NPP and level of care for this severity of illness. The EHR can provide a documentation prompt that informs and provides physicians with such information (as illustrated in Figure 13.1) because physicians should not have to memorize these details. The physician can use this prompt to identify that appendicitis would correlate with a *moderate to high* NPP and level 4 care that matches appropriately with *CPT*'s clinical examples in Appendix C.

Similarly when the physician proceeds to the physical examination, the EHR's documentation prompt for this component should eliminate the need for physicians to memorize compliance guidelines with a reminder that the identified level 4 care warrants a *detailed* examination (illustrated in Figure 14.2), and that physicians are required to provide and document at least 12 of the exam elements included under the 1997 Documentation Guidelines.

In the MDM portion of the electronic H&P, prompts should likewise be made available to indicate that this level of care warrants a *moderate* complexity decision making and that this is achieved by documentating the appropriate number of diagnoses or treatment options (three in this example) and levels of risk (moderate in this example) indicated to support this level of care. Finally, the software should provide for documentation of the *moderate to high* severity of the NPP.

Efficiency Problems

In the physical examination section, the problem commonly found is that software designs that increase documentation speed may have adverse effects on compliance and patient care. One of the most common features for increasing data entry speed is "documentation by exception," a software tool whose problems were discussed in detail in Chapter 7. In an effort to automate documentation of the examination, this design almost invariably leads to "cloned" documentation. Although this approach is fast, it creates a significant compliance problem because it is highly inefficient for physicians to "undocument" the software's pre-entered generic information. As a result, physicians make frequent documentation errors or leave most of the macro or template unchanged, even when there are portions of the examination they did not perform or that are not medically indicated for the patient's medical problem.

To remedy these problems, there are a number of design features whose inclusion can optimize documentation efficiency while also providing an approach that is compliant and easy for physicians to use. Including a graphic interface with dual check-boxes, based on the 1997 Documentation Guidelines[4] examination criteria (and not prefilled with check marks), allows physicians to indicate rapidly the elements of the examination they performed and whether the findings were normal or abnormal. An additional enhancement to this graphic component would be the inclusion in the template of a brief explanation of what the physician means when indicating that findings are normal (an example of this feature is shown in Figure 14.1). This added information increases efficiency because checking a box that includes this information requires less time than using the narrative interface section to fulfill the Documentation Guidelines requirement of recording "relevant negative findings of the examination of the affected or symptomatic body area(s) or organ system(s)."[4(p11)] The third positive design element for this component of the H&P is the use of a narrative interface to report "specific abnormal findings."[4(p11)] Entering free text to describe the *specific* findings for each individual patient, as advised by the Documentation Guidelines, is faster and more accurate than selecting generic phrases from pick lists. Software that includes these three design features will increase the speed at which physicians can perform compliant, individualized documentation of the physical examination component.

Quality and Compliance Problems

The EHR systems that use documentation by exception, using a graphic or narrative appearance to automatically enter preloaded normal findings for a comprehensive examination findings, anticipate that clinicians will go through the tedious effort required to change all normal descriptions for findings that are abnormal and to erase all elements that were not examined. Experience shows that carrying out such changes would actually require more time and effort than using compliant tools to document the care accurately using blank, compliant graphic and narrative designs. As a result, physicians using such systems are incentivized to address only the examination areas related to the patient's presenting illness and leave all other pre-entered normal findings unchanged. These designs, therefore, inherently have the potential to create charts that appear cloned and the ability to provide documentation for care that was not actually provided. Such circumstances could lead to serious compliance issues, including allegations of *false claims*. This functionality also presents the potential danger of placing a physician in an indefensible position in a medical liability action in which he or she could be accused of failure to diagnose an obvious abnormality because the chart attests (by default) that the examination of the body area in question was normal (even though the physician did not examine this area).

Another design issue for the examination section is that some EHR systems provide only a check-box–type of graphic interface that allows documentation of the body areas examined and whether they are normal. They fail to provide a narrative interface for physicians to enter detailed individualized descriptions of specific abnormal and pertinent normal findings.

Still other EHRs may provide a narrative interface but continue to offer the alternative of entering a more generic description through the use of a limited-vocabulary pick list. The pick-list option may seem convenient, but it should be removed from the design because of its potential problems. This approach to recording an examination invariably provides generalized terminology, which is usually insufficient to fulfill the Documentation Guidelines requirement for recording abnormal findings that are *specific* to each individual patient. Such generalized language fails to paint a descriptive picture of the precise findings for a patient. For example, simply clicking the mouse on a drop-down list to enter the generic term *rales* to describe a patient's lung sounds is insufficient to distinguish one patient's findings from those of any other patient with similar abnormal findings. When the patient returns 1 month later, this nondescript portrayal of the findings will not provide sufficient information for a physician to assess whether the status of the lung abnormality is stable, improved, or worsening. To enhance quality care, physicians should document in-depth findings, such as "2+ inspiratory rales on deep inspiration, right upper lobe." This brief but effective assessment is easily and quickly entered using free text, whereas the same task would be cumbersome and imprecise using a pick list. In addition to enhancing care and patient management, high-quality narrative descriptions offer a degree of liability protection by providing clinical evidence that supports making particular medical decisions and evidence for not making other decisions.

In summary, design needs for the physical examination section begin with elimination of all design features that present the potential for interfering with physicians' ability to provide and document care in an optimal manner. Instead, this component of the H&P requires an appropriate combination of graphic and narrative interface elements to satisfy the need for efficient documentation of normal findings and individualized documentation of abnormal findings that enables physicians to meet medical requirements for quality and compliance.

ANALYZING MDM

After completing the physical examination, physicians may further refine the list of possible diagnoses and the assessment of the severity of the patient's medical problem. They then review (and document) the results of all available medical data, including laboratory and radiology test results, documents from other physicians, and any other medical information pertinent to the patient. Following this step, physicians usually will have completed their diagnostic process and proceed to document their clinical impressions, which should be in the form of a differential diagnosis, and their recommendations for further evaluation and/or treatment. This step marks the conclusion of the traditionally documented H&P.

However, the E/M system includes several additional subcomponents of the MDM component that must be addressed for complete documentation. These extra elements include the complexity of data reviewed or ordered and assessment of the levels of three types of risk: (1) associated with the presenting problem(s), (2) associated with diagnostic tests ordered, and (3) associated with possible management options.[5(p6)] Although physicians generally appreciate these supplemental features at a subconscious level during their care process, they have, in general, not been taught to document them, nor have they been provided satisfactory tools with which to do so.

Failure to include documentation of these additional elements is one of four reasons that MDM has proven to be the most challenging of the three key components of the E/M system for physicians and EHR designers. There are three additional MDM factors that contribute challenges to compliant design and documentation. First, because there has not been a guideline for MDM published in the Documentation Guidelines, some of the CPT descriptors for this section remain *qualitative* rather than quantitative, evidenced by the use of terms such as the *number* of diagnoses, the *number* of treatment options, the *amount* of data ordered, and the *amount* of data reviewed. A second problem is that physicians customarily document treatment plans together with the data they are ordering, even though these are considered separate MDM subcomponents for compliance purposes. Finally, MDM calls for a computation comparing the levels of two of the three subcomponents of MDM, and this calculation commonly proves to be inconvenient and even burdensome during the provision of patient care.

Subsection 1: Data Reviewed and Data Ordered

It is most convenient to provide the *data reviewed* subcomponent as the first portion of MDM because physicians customarily look at existing data after completing the examination and before reaching their final conclusions for diagnoses and treatments. This section lends itself to a number of reasonable design options. Although templates allow for "fill-in-the-blank" functionality for laboratory test results, such as blood cell counts and serum chemistry results, this section also calls for a capability for entry of some free text. This ability is needed to accommodate entry of the physician's own analysis of radiology images, electrocardiograms, reports from consultants, summary information from reviewing outside records, and other diagnostic materials.

The *data ordered* subsection is a component of the "plans" section, which physicians commonly document after listing their clinical impressions (diagnoses). The design of this section lends itself to some form of graphic interface for selecting commonly ordered tests and diagnostic procedures, which may be in the form a drop-down menu or check boxes with a preset list of diagnostic studies. This section also requires some capacity for the entry of free text to accommodate entry of unusual tests or to specify details of a common test. For example, the graphic interface readily accommodates selection of a "Brain CT [computed tomography] scan with contrast." However, an attached narrative entry section is warranted for the physician to specify a request such as "with fine cuts in the left temporal lobe."

Quality and Compliance Problems in the Subsection for Data
Quality documentation is rather straightforward for this component of the electronic H&P record. The software design simply needs sufficient flexibility, including the option to enter free text, to permit an accurate recording of data results, on the one hand, and the details of data ordered, on the other.

The compliance perspective for the data subcomponents requires additional attention. In most current EHR software, an integrated coding engine is able to count the number of data reviewed and the number ordered. However, this same software does not usually provide an interface that allows physicians to document assessment of the *complexity* of the data reviewed and ordered. In the event of an audit, absence of this documentation leaves the interpretation of data complexity to the discretion of a reviewer, and, in some cases, this could result in inappropriate downcoding.

A second concern relates to failure of systems to provide separate documentation for data ordered and management options. This is a common concern in paper-based records, and current EHRs duplicate this problem. Physicians are generally trained to first list their impressions and then record their plans, which include treatments and diagnostic tests they plan to order. However, the E/M coding system considers the number of treatment options separately from the amount of data ordered. Lumping them together has the potential to cause compliance errors and prevent coding engines from distinguishing them as separate subcomponents. To avoid this problem, providing separate fields for each of these categories is preferable.

Subsection 2: Number of Diagnoses and/or Number of Treatment Options

When physicians document their clinical impressions, they usually list the most probable diagnoses first, but it is appropriate to include all probable and a reasonable number of possible diagnoses. For each diagnosis, this documentation may also include a description of its relative probability and/or its relative severity.

Physicians usually enter a straightforward list of treatments they will be recommending, but this section also provides for recording treatment alternatives that have been considered or that might be considered pending the outcome of test results and/or treatment success.

Quality and Compliance Problems in the Subsection for Diagnoses

In the diagnosis (impressions) section, design efforts are frequently encountered that are intended to increase the speed of data entry or the ease of mining data but that have overlooked negative consequences for compliance and patient care. In many systems, rather than presenting a narrative interface for free-text entry, designers provide a drop-down menu that has been preloaded with International Classification of Diseases, Ninth Revision, Clinical Modification (ICD-9-CM) codes that list diagnoses appropriate for a particular specialty or field of practice. In EHRs that include practice management capability, this functionality may also simultaneously post the diagnosis codes in the practice management system to complete that portion of charge entry function.

Although this approach allows rapid entry of diagnosis codes, it also has limitations that can negatively impact E/M compliance and quality considerations. In systems that include charge entry, the rules for completing claim forms (CMS 1500) prohibit the submission of "rule-out" diagnoses. However, this restriction contradicts the mandates of E/M and quality documentation, both of which encourage documenting a complete differential diagnosis, including rule-out diagnoses, to accurately record the physician's analysis and interpretation of all possible causes for the patient's symptoms.

Even in software that does not link the diagnoses section to charge entry, the pick-list approach allows only documentation of the diagnosis code information on the preset list. It does not allow physicians to elaborate on their impressions by adding descriptive adjectives to reflect the medical analysis and thought process. Adjectives are required to indicate severity of the illness. For example, "life-threatening" obstructive sleep apnea has far different implications for risk, the NPP, and urgency of treatment than "mild" obstructive sleep apnea. Adjectives also explain and convey an in-depth sense of physicians' impressions of the probability of each diagnosis included in the differential list, with the descriptions such as "probable," "possible," "unlikely," and rule out. The solution to this problem is that this section of MDM must provide a narrative interface so that physicians may accurately record their thought processes instead of simply listing codes to be used for billing purposes.

Physicians also need the option to include free-text information when listing diagnoses to be able to describe many important illness features that are not included in a list of ICD-9-CM codes. These factors include, for example, emphasizing the particular manifestations of an illness that require attention, listing the possible causes of the problem, describing an abnormal laboratory test result for which a diagnosis has not been established, and considering social and family concerns. Having this descriptive information available is essential during follow-up visits, immediately orienting the physician (or any other physician seeing the patient) to the original assessment, probabilities, and most significant concerns. As an additional benefit, having the ability to identify rule-out diagnoses also fulfills compliance requirements to document "the number of possible diagnoses and/or treatment options that must be considered."[5(p6)]

Weed Weighs in on the Importance of the Problem List

Lawrence Weed, MD, placed a spotlight on the "diagnoses" subcomponent of the H&P section of the medical record in 1968, when he introduced his concept of the problem-oriented medical record. His writings emphasize the importance of documenting a problem list with a structure and logic that provide future assistance and guidance in optimally managing each patient on an individual basis. His use of descriptive language that shows the relationship between different diagnoses underscores the need for *free-text* data entry in this subsection. He provides the following example:

> "Problem #1. ASHD [arteriosclerotic heart disease] with heart failure
> Problem #2. Supraventricular tachycardia—2° to Problem #1"[6(p28)]

This documentation of the relationship between two separate diagnoses illustrates the importance of providing physicians with a narrative interface for listing their diagnoses. It would be impossible to record this physician's impression of the relationship between the two diagnoses by using a software design that provides only a drop-down menu of diagnosis codes.

Weed's medical record insights summarize the quality care benefits of a descriptive narration in this portion of the medical record, advising that "It's not sufficient to just know what was done. It's a very incomplete record if we don't know why it was done."[7] This philosophy encourages physicians to go beyond just recording clinical impressions to include documentation of the medical diagnostic process itself. The problem list must have the ability to present a multi-faceted story of the physician's assessments, interpretations, and reasoning.

Quality and Compliance Problems in the Subsection for Treatment Options

Similar problems can arise in the management options subsection if data entry design fails to provide for free-text entry of descriptive information. Compliance calls for documenting "the number of management options that must be considered,"[5(p7)] but if the software provides only selection of treatments from a drop-down menu, physicians cannot describe alternative options or indicate the reasons for selecting one option in preference to another. Free text also permits physicians to enter a blueprint for future care, listing optional treatments that would be most appropriate in response to specific test results or appropriate secondary choices if a patient's condition fails to respond to the primary treatment. Finally, finding and selecting multiple treatment items from one or more pick lists is often less efficient than using free-text entry, particularly with the variety of medical therapies now available.

Medical Liability Concerns

In the diagnoses and treatment options sections of the MDM part of the H&P record, there are potential medical liability implications from data entry designs that lack a narrative interface. These systems limit or eliminate physicians' ability to list all reasonable alternative diagnoses, to describe consideration of various treatment options, and to briefly explain the reasoning for choices recommended or discouraged. The lack of free text further prevents documentation of discussions with patients related to illness severity and complexity, interrelationships among diagnoses, and contributory social or dietary factors. Documentation of such information can powerfully assist a physician accused of malpractice; its absence can prove detrimental. Finally, recording only the primary management option selected could reduce physicians' ability to defend against litigation that claims lack of informed consent (which legally requires physicians to discuss all reasonable treatment options with their patients).

Subsection 3: Risks of Significant Complications, Morbidity, and/or Mortality

Although the *CPT* manual makes no distinction in importance or requirements between the levels of risk and the other two MDM subcomponents, conventional training in E/M compliance usually addresses this subsection of MDM differently. Whereas experts commonly advise physicians of the importance of documenting the data reviewed and ordered and their diagnoses and management options, they commonly do not provide a similar recommendation to document their assessment of the three levels of risk. Perhaps overlooking the need to document these elements of MDM reflects the fact that, as with the complexity of data reviewed, physicians have generally not been taught to document these elements during medical school.

Compliance Problems in the Subsection for Risks

The lack of documentation of the three categories of risk leaves physicians' documentation and coding subject to uncertainty and potential exposure in the event of a compliance audit. Years after caring for a patient, an auditor unfamiliar with the case may review the chart and judge that the risk was low, resulting in potentially significant downcoding. On the other hand, when this information is entered into the medical record, the documentation confirms the physician's clinical assessment at the time of the visit. As noted earlier about the power of documenting all E/M elements, "When it was documented, it was done." Having this documentation in the medical record prevents reviewers from imposing their own interpretation of risk, compelling them to follow the physician's legitimate interpretation.

Although the code-calculating engines included with many EHRs give physicians the option of selecting a level of risk to calculate an E/M code, none of the software systems I have reviewed to date have offered a mechanism for documenting the three levels of risk in the actual H&P record. Because auditors have no access to the code selection software, which may or may not retain input elements for each visit, they will review only the H&P recorded by the physician. Systems that lack the ability to document this critical MDM subcomponent fail to provide complete MDM documentation and, therefore, place physicians at compliance risk.

ANALYZING THE NPP

Consideration of the severity of illness is an integral part of the medical diagnostic process that all physicians should apply in quality patient care. Physicians following this method gauge the severity of illness from the earliest phase of obtaining the medical history. This assessment continues in parallel with refinement of the differential diagnosis throughout the remainder of the encounter, including examination, review of diagnostic test information, and compilation of probable diagnoses and optimal treatment options. Assessing the risk of morbidity, risk of mortality, and threat of loss of significant physiologic function (ie, the NPP) helps physicians determine the appropriate level of care and the relative urgency of diagnostic and therapeutic intervention.

The NPP also occupies a central guidance role in the entire E/M process because of the important role of medical necessity in determining appropriate levels of care. Even though the NPP has not been categorized as one of CPT's three "key components" for E/M services, the organization of the CPT code descriptors in effect elevates NPP to a mandatory fourth factor by including a value of the NPP with every E/M service that uses the key components to determine the level of care. The *CPT* manual also devotes an entire section of the book to clinical examples that illustrate the NPP.[8] This section infers that the NPP assumes an *overarching* role in determining appropriate levels of E/M care and documentation. As noted above, its introduction instructs that after a physician determines an appropriate level of care based on the clinical examples, "the three key components...must be met and documented in the medical record to report a particular level of service."[8(p450)] In other words, just as CMS assigns to medical necessity an overarching role in payment criteria,[9] the *CPT* manual directs that the NPP determines the level of care warranted and the extent of history, physical examination, and MDM appropriate to fulfill the criteria for that level of care.

Quality and Compliance Problems in the Subsection for the NPP

As with the absence of documentation capability for the three levels of risk, failure of an EHR design to provide physicians with the means to document the NPP in the H&P record exposes physicians to problems in the event of an E/M compliance audit. Lack of documentation of the NPP leaves the measure of medical necessity to the judgment of an auditor instead of properly assigning this evaluation to the judgment of the physician who evaluated the patient's condition at the time of care.

On the other hand, when a system allows physicians to confirm the medical necessity of care by *documenting* the level of the NPP as a component of the H&P, an auditor must acknowledge and respect the physician's selection.* As an additional benefit, a system that provides physicians with the information

---

*The auditor's acknowledgement of the NPP requires, of course, that the NPP level that the physician has documented is reasonable and appropriate for the severity of the patient's illness, ie, it must be compatible with the types of patients included in the *CPT* manual's clinical examples as warranting the selected level of care.

and guidance needed to formally assess the level of NPP throughout the care process will facilitate their accomplishment of compliant documentation and coding as a natural consequence of providing appropriate (ie, medically indicated) levels of care. At the conclusion of each visit, physicians will have successfully performed and documented all components of care necessary for E/M compliance, including fulfillment of medical necessity requirements. This approach also fulfills physicians' medical record goal of having the E/M *problem* disappear. It is not possible for medical records that lack the capability to include NPP documentation and guidance to meet this goal.

CODING SOFTWARE COMPLIANCE LIMITATIONS

Many EHRs have incorporated a coding engine designed to provide automated E/M code calculations. Some software vendors create their own coding engines, whereas others license coding software from other developers. These systems usually include a caveat stating that whereas the coding engine is "suggesting" code levels, the ultimate responsibility for all coding decisions resides with the physician.

Most current coding engines contain intrinsic design problems that arise from deficiencies in one or more of the following general categories.

- Consideration of medical necessity in code assessment, including requiring input of documentation of the level of the NPP
- Documentation of the level of the NPP
- Documentation of subjective elements of the E/M system
  - Medical history details of positive responses in the past history, family history, and social history and review of systems
  - Chronological description aspect of the history of present illness
  - Detailed description of the abnormal findings in the physical examination
  - Specific documentation of subjective MDM components: (1) complexity of data, (2) risk of presenting problem, (3) risk of diagnostic procedures, and (4) risk of treatment options
- Inclusion of only approved, compliant auditing tools for coding functionality

Consideration of Medical Necessity: the NPP

Practical EHR has emphasized that medical necessity is an essential element of compliant care and documentation. It also provides the key to physician understanding of how to seamlessly integrate compliant documentation into their normal workflow. The EHR coding engines that fail to incorporate physician-guidance consideration of the NPP into E/M code determination lack the capacity for reliable coding compliance. To ensure reliable coding functionality, a coding engine must include consideration of medical necessity in code determination for all types of service (eg, outpatient visits and consultations, hospital inpatient visits and consultations, emergency department services, and nursing home visits) that consider the three key components. Optimal coding engine functionality should also include two additional features. First, it should require the EHR's design for the

H&P to include an interface that requires physicians to document their clinical assessment of the NPP during various stages of the patient encounter. In addition, the coding engine should have the ability to actively send compliance guidance to physicians, helping them ensure provision and documentation of appropriate levels of care on the basis of medical necessity.

Consideration of Subjective Elements of the E/M System

Quality care involves the science and the art of medicine. Because the E/M system is a codification of the quality medical care process, to be successful, a coding engine must incorporate both objective *and* subjective elements of documentation. Chapter 8 explored the consequences of coding engines that fail to consider the subjective aspects of medical history, including the history of the present illness and positive responses in the past, family, and social history and review of systems. It showed how this shortcoming could not only impair compliance, but also have a negative influence on physicians' ability to provide essential portions of patient care. For compliance purposes, it is equally important that coding engines not only are able to accept input related to the subjective elements of the physical examination and MDM, but also that they require H&P interface designs to include features that compel physicians to document them.

Consideration of Noncompliant Auditing Tools

Since its inception, the E/M coding system has presented auditors and physicians with challenges in the interpretation of many of the compliance rules. Following the introduction of the Documentation Guidelines to provide objective measures for the medical history and the physical examination, the most prominent remaining challenges have resided with the subjective components of MDM and NPP. In the mid-1990s, some shortcuts were advanced using formulas that attempted to convert the challenging subjective components of the MDM (which, as noted, physicians were failing to include in their documentation) into quasi-objective measures. These shortcuts were adopted by certain clinical tools that are currently available. The assumptions that underscored the shortcuts in converting subjective measures into quasi-objective measures lead to noncompliant coding determinations that contradict the results of audits performed based on the principles of CPT coding and Documentation Guidelines.

Overview Assessment of a Prevalent Currently Available Audit Tool

One of the currently available audit tools used in certain systems tends to credit too much complexity of MDM to "new problems" that are of relatively minor severity (eg, assigning *moderate complexity* of MDM for simple new problems, such as an insect bite or a sprained ankle) and too little severity for established problems with a high probability of morbidity or mortality (eg, recurrence of lymphoma). Furthermore, systems that use this tool give no attention to the NPP and medical necessity.

A number of coding engines use this tool for their assessment of MDM. This functionality permits a coding engine to derive an MDM level from some of the recorded objective MDM information to compensate for EHR systems that lack the ability to document physicians' subjective impressions. However, the levels of MDM derived in this manner are unreliable because they are frequently incompatible with evaluations performed using CPT-compliant E/M review tools.

The Coding Conundrum of Software That Lacks Full Compliance Features

The interplay between coding engine functionality and EHR interface design can create insurmountable challenges for physicians seeking a successful E/M compliance solution. Coding engines that fail to consider all of the subjective elements of the E/M system (eg, the chronological component of the history of present illness) may influence the creation of interface designs that lack the ability to document these subjective elements. Similarly, interface designs that do not allow physicians to document certain subjective elements of the E/M system (eg, the three levels of risk) can disrupt coding functionality. These problems are compounded by systems with interface designs *and* coding engine functionality that overlook the role of medical necessity in coding compliance.

Resolving this conundrum requires insistence by medical practices that to be considered for possible purchase, any EHR system must provide a coding engine and interface designs that include all elements needed for E/M compliance, use only compliant tools and functionality, include consideration of medical necessity, and work together cohesively to provide physician guidance and ensure compliant documentation and coding.

SUMMARY

Medical practices have the right to expect that a sophisticated EHR will guide and ensure E/M compliance as an integral component of the medical care process. These systems should also facilitate creation of high-quality patient records capable of helping physicians provide optimal care for their patients. In the physical examination and MDM sections of the electronic H&P, ensuring compliance requires elimination from the EHR of any interface designs that present pre-entered clinical information, such as documentation by exception or macros for normal examination findings.

Achieving compliance also requires systems to provide a free-text narrative interface section for indicating diagnoses and treatment options. This type of interface is needed to provide physicians with the ability to document rule-out diagnoses, relative severity of an illness or symptom, relative probability of an uncertain diagnosis, and consideration of features of an illness that are inadequately explained by ICD-9-CM codes and descriptions. Another design feature that can facilitate compliance is the separation of data ordered and treatment options into individual sections of the record, rather than lumping them into a section labeled "Plans." Significantly, software designs must also include sections for documentation of commonly overlooked MDM elements for complexity of data, risk of presenting problems, risk of diagnostic studies, and risk of management options. These uncommonly documented elements must be included to confirm compliant levels of MDM in the event of an audit.

The indispensable feature that affects both care and compliance that is absent from nearly all currently available EHRs is consideration of the NPP, which is the E/M system's measure of medical necessity. Failing to document the NPP risks repeated downcoding for "lack of medical necessity" in an E/M audit. Even more important, NPP functionality should provide guidance for identifying the *medically indicated* levels of care and the appropriate levels of history, examination, and MDM based on medical necessity. Consideration of the NPP throughout a patient visit provides the true key to helping physicians integrate E/M documentation and coding into their medical care process and making the E/M challenge disappear.

References

1.   Bickley LS, Szilagyi PG. *Bates' Guide to Physical Examination and History Taking.* 8th ed. Philadelphia, PA: Lippincott Williams & Wilkins; 2004.

2.   Social Security Law, section 1862(1)(a). www.ssa.gov/OP_Home/ssact/title18/1862.htm. Accessed May 12, 2007.

3.   Centers for Medicare & Medicaid Services. Part 3—Claims Process. In: *Medicare Claims Processing Manual.* Section 7103.1(I). www.cms.hhs.gov/Manuals/PBM/itemdetail.asp?filterType=none&filterByDID=99&sortByDID=1&sortOrder=ascending&itemID=CMS021921&intNumPerPage=10. Accessed May 12, 2007.

4.   American Medical Association, Health Care Financing Administration. *Documentation Guidelines for Evaluation and Management Services.* Chicago, IL: American Medical Association; 1997.

5.   American Medical Association. *Current Procedural Terminology (CPT®).* Chicago, IL: American Medical Association; 2007.

6.   Weed LL. *Medical Records, Medical Education, and Patient Care.* Cleveland, OH: Press of Case Western Reserve University; 1969:28.

7.   Versel N. Dr. Weed's software cure. Digital HealthCare & Productivity.com. June 7, 2007. www.health-itworld.com/emag/070104/289.html?page:int=-1. Accessed August 10, 2007.

8.   American Medical Association. Appendix C. In: *Current Procedural Terminology (CPT®).* Chicago, IL: American Medical Association; 2007:450-467.

9.   Centers for Medicare & Medicaid Services. Selection of level of evaluation and management service. In: *Medicare Claims Processing Manual.* Chapter 12, section 30.6.1. http://new.cms.hhs.gov/manuals/downloads/clm104c12.pdf. Accessed May 12, 2007.

Reenvisioning the Electronic H&P

This section takes a fresh look at building the electronic history and physical examination (H&P) record from the ground up. It examines a variety of available design and functionality options that can be combined to fulfil physicians' requirements for documenting the H&P, while also avoiding the potential problems identified in Part 2 and permitting flexible solutions capable of accommodating individual physician differences and preferences. EHR vendors are capable of incorporating these types of solutions, and physicians can anticipate that they will do so as medical practices demand these features as prerequisites for purchasing EHR systems.

chapter 10

Design and Functionality Criteria for H&P Success

Practical EHR seeks to facilitate the development of EHR (electronic health record) systems designs for the history and physical examination (H&P) component that work easily and intuitively for physicians at the point of care. These systems should include design and functionality features that inherently address all requirements physicians have for their H&Ps. For many years, physicians have trained using the medical diagnostic process as their approach to patient care. Therefore, EHRs that incorporate this process into the foundation for their H&P design should prove usable and effective for most physicians. For convenience, records meeting these criteria are referred to as "intelligent" electronic records (IERs).

The various participants in the health care system envision different goals for implementing EHRs in every physician's office and for establishing a national health information network that allows sharing of medical information among patients, their physicians, testing facilities, and information processing centers. Insurers, of course, look forward to the predicted financial savings, which should increase their profitability. (Ash and Bates[1] state that 90% of the financial savings from electronic records accrue to payers, while physicians bear the costs of purchasing, operating, and maintaining these systems.) Legislators and health policy professionals expect that EHRs will provide data and insights that can direct the development of future health policy tools and protocols to increase medical care quality and patient safety.[2] They anticipate that these benefits also have the potential to create significant savings for Medicare and Medicaid and in overall health care spending.

Achieving these admirable goals must start with medical records that work for physicians, facilitating quality care one patient at a time and recording patient data that are *individualized* and meaningful. This objective also requires that standards for the electronic H&P eliminate designs that create automated, or cloned, H&P documentation, which results in medical charts that contain similar (or nearly identical) information for each of a patient's visits and similar documentation for all patients with related symptoms or diagnoses. The H&P compiled using such preprogrammed tools leads to records with unreliable clinical data, which is of little or no value to understanding of disease, treatments, and optimal care. As noted in Chapter 2, "The best [HIT (health information technology)] system in the world can't be effective without good content."[3] Identifying the design principles that promote meaningful content is the focus of Part 3 of this book.

Physicians must set the standards for their medical records. They must be leaders in identifying the features that facilitate optimal care and in rejecting features that might obstruct it. *Practical EHR* advocates the following guiding principle for EHR quality:

> The EHR is a sophisticated tool whose design and functionality must be directed to helping physicians practice the best patient care possible. The EHR must supplement physicians' knowledge and judgment, not supplant them through automatic insertion of programmed clinical information and/or automated decisions regarding patient care.

OVERVIEW OF PART 3

This part of the book begins by bringing together a review of physicians' requirements for the electronic H&P requirements. These are presented to launch the dialogue and the design effort in a positive direction toward achievable goals. Because physicians' concerns with the electronic H&P have been identified as a primary cause of the "electronic chasm," EHR companies need to bring the same degree of innovation to electronic H&P design and functionality that they are already generating for clinical decision support, interoperability, health information exchange, and the potential uses for excellent clinical information once it has been recorded.

Chapter 11 identifies a variety of design tools that can help meet physicians' standards. The remaining portions of Part 3 explore how designers might apply these tools appropriately for each component of the electronic H&P record to create an IER. These approaches are suggested to promote analysis of the potential advantages and disadvantages of each available option. Because physicians have their own personal preferences and styles for performing and documenting the H&P, the goal of this book is not to promote one specific approach or solution as ideal. Rather, physicians should be able to choose from among a number of alternatives, all of which meet their the goals for compliance and quality. Each physician can then select design the designs that are best suited to his or her personal preferences. It is hoped that each EHR system will incorporate multiple options into their systems to afford maximum flexibility and choices for users of their programs. Creating physician awareness of and demand for designs that enhance the patient care process should provide an impetus to developers to include these performance-enhancing technologies in their systems and create blueprints for integrating these improvements into EHR design.

GOALS FOR THE ELECTRONIC H&P

The medical record establishes a solid foundation for a physician's ongoing care of patients. It is the knowledge warehouse accessed during every visit, documenting the longitudinal health history of every patient encounter, phone call, laboratory result, and written correspondence. The H&P component is not only the central repository for patients' clinical information, but it is also the embodiment of the process used to evaluate and treat patients. Physicians refer to the road map laid out by the H&P as they care for patients so that the nature and extent of that care also reflect the medical record that guides them.

Physicians first learn how to provide medical care through the structure of a comprehensive H&P, which they memorize and meticulously write out free hand during each patient encounter in the early years in medical school. By following this structured approach, physicians learn and imprint the methodology of the medical diagnostic process. However, once these skills are acquired, there is no further educational benefit to the inefficient process of manually writing the structure of the H&P (ie, the medical history questions and the descriptions of areas examined) during every patient visit. Yet, physicians continue to require and rely on the presence of this structure as an integral part of the record, not only for compliance, but even more important, to create meaningful documentation and to support the diagnostic process. Therefore, a record that provides the H&P structure while allowing physicians to fill in all patient responses, examination findings, and decision making is not only reasonable and efficient, but also assists in promoting optimal workflow for physicians.

In its preface, *Practical E/M* proposed that physicians should anticipate achieving four major goals when employing compliant E/M methodology combined with intelligent medical record designs, even for records stored in a paper format[4(p x)]:

- Equal or increased quality of patient care
- Equal or improved efficiency (time spent)
- E/M-compliant and "audit-proof" documentation and coding
- Equal or increased levels of productivity, ie, compliant E/M code levels should actually increase (unless a physician is systematically overcoding)

Physicians using this approach with effective H&P tools have commonly reported that in addition to meeting these four goals, they have achieved additional secondary benefits, including reduction or elimination of after-hours time for completing patient charts, reduced concern about the risk of financially damaging compliance audits, and increased enjoyment of the patient care process.[4(p x)]

Physicians believe that they have a right to expect EHR systems to equal or exceed those positive results achieved with paper-based documents. In addition, when this approach is translated to an electronic format, physicians should expect three extra benefits. The first two are intrinsic features of EHRs that satisfy two primary goals of medical practices: (1) immediate medical record access at all times and (2) elimination of the cost of managing a paper record system. The third advantage is "error proofing," which is another special capability that only EHRs can bring to clinical documentation. This concept requires software developers to incorporate intelligent guidance into their designs to ensure that physicians follow their own protocols for compliance and quality. Such features may include, for example, the following:

- Monitoring electronic signatures
- Guaranteeing documentation of a comprehensive medical history during every visit
- Ensuring narrative documentation of details about positive responses to inquiries about the past, family, and social history (PFSH) and review of systems (ROS)
- Ensuring narrative documentation of details about examination findings reported as abnormal in the graphic user interface portion
- Ensuring appropriate extent of examination and complexity of medical decision making (MDM) to fulfill the medically indicated levels of care based on the nature of the presenting problem (NPP)
- Requiring documentation of the severity of the NPP

In Chapter 11, "error proofing" is included as one of the essential tools for constructing an effective electronic H&P.

GOALS FOR DESIGN

The H&P has multiple component parts, and each section calls for its own specialized designs and tools to achieve maximum effectiveness for physicians during patient care. The Preface identified six standards that medical records should meet in any medical record format. These requirements provide the criteria for evaluation of the effectiveness of possible design options for each section of the H&P record.

It is interesting that when an H&P is designed to meet the criteria for being usable, compliant, and efficient, it usually also achieves the other three standards: facilitating quality care, ensuring the integrity of the clinical data, and promoting appropriate productivity.

Usability and Flexibility

Usability provides an appropriate starting point for defining how the electronic H&P record should function. Many current systems ask physicians to adopt new ways of obtaining a medical history, documenting clinical impressions, or entering data into the record. What physicians want and should demand are systems that fit the way they are taught to practice. They do not want to change optimal patient care workflow to fit the demands or restrictions of software.

Using E/M compliance, which codifies the diagnostic process as a foundation for constructing the H&P, recreates the method physicians have learned as the basis for clinical care. In addition, it provides efficient tools, which allow physicians to accomplish compliant levels of care within a realistic and reasonable time frame. Even for physicians whose current paper records

---

Like Riding a Bicycle

I experienced this type of dramatic reintroduction of the comprehensive H&P and the medical diagnostic process in 1995. During my own medical training, I maintained the structure of a comprehensive H&P throughout medical school and 5 years of residency training. However, when I entered private practice and faced the (economic) reality of needing to see 4 to 6 patients per hour, I was forced to adopt a more problem-focused approach. The structure for this more-limited H&P reduced the extent of the background medical history and led to documenting fewer alternative diagnoses and treatment options into the chart. Incredibly, this conversion from comprehensive to problem-focused care and documentation occurred without any real understanding or insight on my part. I simply made the change to my care and my record that was required to adapt to the changing circumstances without assessing what I had lost or its effect on the level of care I was providing to my patients.

I practiced with this more restricted approach for many years. Yet, when I introduced E/M-compliant medical record tools that allowed me to see the same number of patients per hour while once again providing appropriately comprehensive care, there was no challenge or learning period. This was just a return to using the comprehensive care medical record of my training. It was just as if someone had asked me to ride a bicycle for the first time in 20 years—no learning curve was needed.

present issues for E/M compliance, reintroducing the familiar H&P model and diagnostic process will not present a significant usability challenge, and it requires only a brief learning period.

EHR systems also need to build in sufficient flexibility to meet individual physician preferences within this optimal framework. Although some physicians are comfortable entering data at the point of care, others prefer attending solely to the patient during the visit and recording information afterwards. Many physicians prefer to dictate documentation, others prefer writing, and some prefer interacting with patients while typing on a keyboard and working with a mouse. In fact, each section of the record offers multiple reasonable data entry possibilities. When systems make them available, many physicians likely will choose to use a variety of modalities, with one approach for certain portions of the record and a different approach for other sections.

The key to designing a usable electronic H&P record is to have it fit physicians' optimal practice habits and style like a well-made leather glove would fit a hand. Although the structure of the glove provides the required coverage, it must be flexible enough to fit different people, with hands of different shapes, who use them to perform different functions. Physicians cannot be required to mold practice patterns to fit a rigidly designed H&P record, particularly if it fails to provide effective design, functionality, and/or data entry options. Instead, H&P record designs need to be flexible enough to fit the optimal needs of all physicians.

E/M Compliance

The positive effects of medical records constructed to ensure compliant E/M documentation and coding go beyond the obvious benefit of protection against significant financial loss after a medical record audit by Medicare or insurers. These records also guide performance of medically indicated levels of care, thereby promoting quality performance. Providing levels of care based on physicians' standards for medical necessity also allows practices to submit claims for higher levels of care when clinically appropriate, thereby appropriately increasing productivity. An added benefit of records that document levels of care appropriate for the severity of each patient's condition is that they provide an extra degree of protection if a medicolegal review occurs. Defense attorneys and physician expert witnesses agree that well-documented medical records usually present physicians' most effective defense.

Creating medical record designs capable of promoting and ensuring compliance has presented a major challenge since the introduction of the E/M coding system in 1992. The absence of a recognized medical record model ensuring E/M compliance before 2005 has likely contributed to the difficulties software designers have encountered in creating the electronic H&P record. This task has been compounded by the need for designs that encourage optimal efficiency while ensuring compliance. At this time, however, it is possible to adapt the method and design principles of the *Practical E/M* approach in EHRs to ensure that E/M coding compliance is an intrinsic feature of every patient encounter.

Several fundamental design elements must be incorporated into the structure of the electronic H&P to meet this standard. The first priority is to provide for documentation of all components of E/M services, including the following portions of E/M that most records overlook:

- Complexity of data reviewed
- Risk of presenting problem(s)
- Risk of diagnostic procedures
- Risk of management options
- NPP
- All elements needed for complete documentation of time-based visits

When a medical chart documents all E/M components, it attests that all care was performed as described, including assessment of medical necessity (the NPP). As long as the documentation is reasonable and appropriate to the patient's illness, a reviewer cannot superimpose his or her own opinion of these E/M components but must respect the physician's judgment (ie, when care has been documented, it has been done). As a result, because in this method the actual level of care, documentation, and code submitted are selected and performed based on the NPP, such records fully document the appropiate level of care provided and coded, including medical necessity, which make them "audit protected."

In this approach, graphic design elements, such as check box templates for PFSH, ROS, and physical examination, must provide both a rigid structure to meet compliance needs and maximum flexibility to allow physician customization. The basic structure must include all the elements defined by the Documentation Guidelines[5] for a comprehensive H&P to allow the appropriate levels of documentation in cases of suitable severity. Within that framework, physicians need the flexibility to determine the details of which history questions to ask and which additional examination elements to include.

In accordance with the diagnostic process, the H&P record design should also provide for a comprehensive medical history during every visit. For initial patient visits, this includes a complete PFSH and a complete ROS, in addition to documentation of the patient's chief complaint and an extended history of the present illness. For achieving a comprehensive

---

Combining Rigid Structure With Flexible Details and Customization

The ROS offers a good illustration of how designing an H&P to fulfill compliance and quality requirements can also allow physicians to have the record reflect their own specialty and personal preferences. The *Current Procedural Terminology* (*CPT*®) manual[6] and Documentation Guidelines[5] describe 14 organ systems that may be reviewed to find signs and symptoms the patient has at the time of the visit or may have had in the past. The Documentation Guidelines also state that to provide a *complete* ROS, which is indicated for patients with a moderate to high or high NPP, "at least 10 organ systems must be reviewed."[5] Therefore, ensuring compliant care and documentation for patients warranting the highest level of care indicates that the basic structure for the ROS must include one or more questions for at least 10 of the 14 defined organ systems. However, meeting these basic requirements is just a starting point, ensuring that the electronic H&P has the capacity for compliant documentation for all levels of care. Designs must

continued

also provide physicians with the flexibility to include more than 10 organ systems and to include the full range of signs and symptoms about which they inquire. Physicians should be encouraged to enhance their ROS design by listing as many questions as they believe appropriate for quality care.

Practical EHR recommends that in designing the various components of the electronic H&P record, compliance should provide a starting platform on which each physician can build a quality-based superstructure that meets the highest standards of his or her specialty and personal values.

history during visits with established patients, the H&P design can replace the complete background survey used in initial visits with sections for documenting an update of the PFSH and ROS[5(p6)](ie, noting whether the patient has experienced any change in the subcomponents since the preceding visit). From a quality perspective, this approach gives physicians an opportunity for optimal care, making sure that the patient does not have new medical problems in addition to the presenting complaint. For optimal compliance, obtaining a comprehensive history contributes essential information that physicians require to make an accurate assessment of the NPP, which allows determination of the appropriate extent of care and documentation.

Another enhancement for compliance success is the inclusion of "documentation prompts" in the design. These tools are able to replace the conventional E/M compliance approach, which involves complex coding paradigms and calculations at the end of a visit, with guidance during the patient visit to facilitate medically indicated care and documentation. These prompts integrate the qualitative E/M descriptions from the *CPT* manual[6] with quantitative measures from the Documentation Guidelines.[5] They help physicians meet compliance standards by guiding care and documentation based on the physician's own determination to facilitate medical necessity, not on "care for coding's sake." These prompts bring physicians the precise criteria approved by medical societies for defining the extent of history, examination, and decision making warranted to meet CPT standards for medically indicated problem-focused, expanded problem-focused, detailed, and comprehensive levels of care. The prompts are specific to each type of visit reflecting the fact that the E/M guidelines differ for each type of service. Incorporating prompts into the electronic H&P design eliminates the need for physicians to memorize or look up E/M compliance requirements. More important, by integrating documentation and coding into the process of providing care, this approach makes the E/M problem go away!

Efficiency

The demands for parameters of efficient documentation, and even for "efficient" care, are not the product of medical education, quality standards, or CPT guidelines. Rather, they are the consequence of cost-saving efforts of payers to get more care for progressively less payment, creating ever-increasing economic pressure on physicians to complete their patients' E/M visits in reduced amounts of time. Nevertheless, EHR developers face the reality of facilitating care and documentation within the same time frame physicians customarily use when using writing or dictating their records. For most physicians, this means seeing between four and six patients per hour, with variations based on specialty and severity of illness for the "average" patient in each practice.

The Impact of Reduced Payment on Time Devoted to Caring for Patients

Because Medicare and most insurer payments are based on the Resource-Based Relative Value System (RBRVS), reductions in the conversion factor (or a stable conversion factor in the present environment of steadily increasing overhead costs) put ever-increasing cost pressure on all medical services, including procedures and cognitive (ie, E/M) care. Although physicians can consider reducing preparation time for procedures, they quite reasonably understand that it is not safe to operate faster and faster. Yet, when it comes to E/M services, which also rely on having enough time to provide quality care, insurers and policy makers presume that physicians can and should work faster and faster. This is an unreasonable assumption. Insurers and policy makers also champion the philosophy that quality care leads to the most cost-effective care. Yet, they fail to appreciate that *quality care is not a speedy process.*

The negative impact of reduced payments on quality of E/M care is easily illustrated. The E/M descriptors for level five initial-visit care (CPT code 99205, which is appropriate for the most severely ill patients) offer the following guideline: "Physicians typically spend 60 minutes face-to-face with the patient and/or family."[6] In today's medical environment, this guideline likely sounds totally unrealistic to physicians and patients alike. The inconsistency between guidelines and the real world derives from the fact that RBRVS values practice expense costs (including liability insurance) for code 99205 at 1.94 relative value units (RVUs). However, today's Medicare conversion factor of $37.34 per RVU (which has been relatively unchanged for more than 20 years) provides overhead payment of merely $72.44 for the visit. This level of reimbursement covers only about 25% or less of physicians' current true cost of overhead for 60 minutes of practice time. In other words, CPT guidelines advise that code 99205 warrants 60 minutes of care, but payers are paying for only about 15 minutes or less. Policy makers must come to the realization that the severe underpayment, caused by the failure of the conversion factor in reflecting the true cost of resources, imperils medical quality far beyond the potential benefits of EHRs.

The most effective approach for optimizing documentation efficiency while maintaining the quality care process will result from selecting the most appropriate data entry tools for each section of the electronic H&P. This includes identifying the best graphic or narrative interface, most suitable data entry person, and fastest format(s) for data entry. Because there are significant differences among physicians for the techniques they find most comfortable for entering data, EHR software should ideally offer multiple options, providing the most efficient means for physicians who prefer to write, dictate, or to enter data directly into the computer. With these options, physicians will have the opportunity to choose different formats for each component of the record. While encouraging maximum creativity and flexibility for efficient data entry designs, *Practical EHR* applies the following primary axiom to guide this development:

> Design elements intended to promote rapid entry of clinical information must also ensure compliant documentation and maintain the medical diagnostic process.

> **Setting the Limits of Efficiency (Have we hit the speed of light for speedy care?)**
>
> In physics, the speed of light is the ultimate barrier; it sets a maximum limit for how fast any object or particle can move. In medicine, efficiency is composed of two elements: the speed of documentation and the speed of providing patient care. The documentation tools presented in Parts 2 and 3 of *Practical EHR* are the product of 12 years of continual improvements and refinements, evolving through questions and suggestions from many physicians and confirmed as efficient and compliant by physicians and coders. These tools and techniques appear to have reached their maximum possible speed while adhering to the primary axiom of maintaining compliance and quality.
>
> (These tools help physicians spend most of their time during each visit performing the appropriate level of care and talking with patients; documentation of that care requires little additional time. If there were an EHR capable of reading physicians' minds and translating their thoughts into data, the combined care and documentation process could not occur much faster without sacrificing the care process itself.)
>
> Critically, physicians attest that they have already reached, or even exceeded, their maximum speed for providing quality care. Most practicing physicians complain that economic constriction does not allow them to spend enough time with patients to achieve the best quality of care. Patients also complain that physicians are too rushed and have insufficient time to answer questions and explain problems. In other words, the evidence is overwhelming that the equivalent of the speed of light for medical care efficiency has already been reached. It is predictable that further reductions in reimbursement (and/or failure to keep pace with inflation of medical practice costs) will cause health care to implode, impeding access to care, lowering quality, and increasing the overall cost of health care (a process described in *Practical E/M* as "Medicaidization"[4(p255)]). This financial environment creates a de facto rationing of access and rationing of medical quality.
>
> It should be the responsibility of physicians and organized medicine to evaluate this thesis and confirm that the limits to which Medicare and insurers should be permitted to push their drive for reducing payments (relative to costs) for physician services have been reached. The three pillars of the medical profession—quality care, patient advocacy, and medical ethics—should confirm the absolute limit beyond which inadequate payments harm patients. It is hoped that focusing attention on these consequences will mobilize support from patients, politicians, and health policy experts for a conversion factor sufficient to realistically meet today's cost of providing quality care.

Facilitating Quality Care

Health information technology proponents (and physicians) point to the advantages of having all clinical and laboratory data available during every visit. They also focus on the benefits of bringing clinical decision support tools for preventive care and disease management to physicians at the point of care. Presenting these standard-of-care guidelines during patient visits promises to increase early detection of illness and ensure that patients receive treatments and diagnostic studies that are of proven benefit in most cases. However, for decision support tools to be effective, they must operate in an environment in which physicians have a comprehensive understanding of patients' overall health, including correctly identifying all current diagnoses and risk factors. A good protocol is of little help and may even prove detrimental if it is applied to the care of a patient with an incorrect diagnosis.

Designing the electronic H&P for quality, therefore, goes deeper than simply introducing clinical decision support tools. It requires empowering the medical diagnostic process so that physicians have available a comprehensive history for each patient encounter and the best opportunity to determine accurate diagnoses and select optimal treatments. Fortunately, designing the electronic H&P to effectively meet the requirements for E/M compliance will also fulfill the goal of promoting the diagnostic process.

Ensuring Integrity of Clinical Data

Health policy specialists focus on the storage capabilities of EHRs in ensuring that medical information is not lost and that physicians have access to data obtained at other locations. When considering the data entry aspects of the electronic H&P, the characteristics of two categories of data, objective and subjective, need to be considered. Objective data encompass straightforward factual elements that are captured as short descriptions, numeric values, or check boxes for established criteria. This category includes patient demographic information, procedure and diagnosis codes, graphic sections of clinical records, vital signs, and laboratory results. Subjective data include the less structured, free-text information recorded in the narrative sections of the H&P record.

To ensure data integrity, EHR system design must avoid using any pre-entered clinical information. Although graphic interface designs may have preloaded structure, there must be no automatic entry of clinical information by loading default responses ("negative" or "normal") or by permitting the entry of multiple responses with the click of a single check-box. Narrative interface sections of the H&P record include subjective clinical information. For quality and compliance, designs must ensure that all documented descriptions are individualized to each patient and specific to each particular visit, which requires that systems permit only free-text entry of this clinical information.

The challenge for the sections of the H&P that require free-text entry has been to determine how to collect, process, and analyze these unstructured data. The desire to structure subjective clinical information may have been a driving force in the use of pick lists, sometimes based on standard nomenclature systems such as SNOMED®[7], as an alternative to free-text for physicians to construct pseudonarratives. However, the use of this approach to documentation has proven cumbersome, slow, and imprecise. The conclusion should be that data processing capabilities of EHRs must be treated as secondary to the primary priorities of usability, compliance, providing quality patient care, and even efficiency. Achieving these goals requires the use of free-text language familiar to physicians and patients.

Currently, there are no established standards for extracting specific data from the narrative sections of the H&P record. If health policy eventually determines the need for obtaining quantifiable data from these free-text descriptions, EHR systems will need to include software capabilities, such as natural language processing, to search free-text and extract the desired information in a codified form.

Promoting Appropriate Productivity

In addition to managing the economic pressures of the current payment system, medical practices must have software tools that help them avoid three coding mistakes that can adversely affect productivity. These errors are defined in *Practical E/M* terminology as:

- Overcoding: Submitting an E/M code at a level higher than warranted by the NPP (ie, medical necessity). An example of overcoding is submission of level 4 care for a patient with a sprained ankle or uncomplicated viral upper respiratory infection, which represents overcoding regardless of the amount of care provided or documented because providing high levels of care for minor problems does not meet the definition of medical necessity.

- Underdocumenting: Insufficient documentation for the three key components to support the submitted E/M code. An example of underdocumentation would be submitting a level 4 code for a patient whose severity of illness (medical necessity) warrants a high level of care, but the documentation in the medical record indicates that the physician performed level 3 care (eg, an initial visit whose medical history is documented as detailed rather than comprehensive).

- Undercoding: Submitting an E/M code for care that is lower than the level of care warranted by medical necessity. For example, the physician selects a level 3 code for a patient with a severe illness (eg, uncontrolled lupus).[4(p29)]

In an E/M audit, if an auditor identifies overcoding and/or underdocumenting, there are several degrees of severity for the financial consequences that may be imposed. At the basic level, an audit will reclaim overpayments for all claims it determines to have been submitted improperly. However, the financial penalty can escalate dramatically if Medicare (or a private insurer) elects to "extrapolate" the finite financial penalty from an audit of 50 charts, for example, to the entire population of E/M claims a practice has filed during the previous several years. The third degree of severity results if a Medicare audit imposes added penalties for "fraud," which can occur when the reviewer determines there is a consistent pattern of excessive overcoding or underdocumenting. This determination may be made regardless of whether the improper coding was intentional or unintentional. Current penalties for fraud range from $5,500 to $11,000 per line item. Beyond these three levels of severity, other penalties may also be applied, including exclusion from participation in the Medicare program.

How Devastating Can These Financial Penalties Be?

The December 13, 1995, issue of the *New York Times* included the article "University Agrees to Pay in Settlement on Medicare." The text reported that the "University of Pennsylvania's health system agreed to pay $30 million to settle government complaints that it filed improper bills for doctors' services. . . . The settlement followed a government audit of 100 patients treated in 1993."[8]

The audit of the records of 100 patients had resulted in physicians paying $30 million, a significant portion of which was related to improper E/M coding. This calculates to $300,000 per patient chart (and this is based on a settlement amount, which was significantly lower that the true extrapolated financial penalty). The auditors had extended the results to all the claims submitted during multiple years, a mathematical assumption that was later validated by the courts. The results of this investigation, which subsequently led to the government's program of PATH audits (Physicians at Teaching Hospitals), demonstrates the economic devastation that can result from extrapolation, and it underscores the importance of compliant documentation and coding.

My discussions with physicians and coders in a wide variety of settings indicate that the majority of physicians are probably undercoding. Many do this because of fear that submitting high-level codes could attract insurer attention and lead to audits of E/M services. This strategy does not guarantee protection from audits but does guarantee submitting lower code levels than warranted by the severity of patient illness (NPP). This leads to a downward spiral that must ultimately impair quality and income: undercoding leads to underpayment; the lowered income ultimately causes physicians to spend even less time with their patients, and this can lead to providing lower levels of care than medically indicated by the severity of illness for which the patient is being seen.

The solution to this challenge is correct documentation and coding. *Practical EHR,* like *Practical E/M,* uses compliant methods that eliminate all three of these improper coding practices. Instead, it follows the "Goldilocks Rule" of documentation and coding: based on the severity of the NPP, the code submitted should be not be too high, and not too low, but *just right* (in every case). This is accomplished by constructing the electronic H&P with design and functionality that ensure E/M compliance, including functionality that presents guidance (ie, documentation prompts) to help physicians to identify the appropriate severity of patient illness and then provide and document the level of medical care warranted by the NPP.

This approach brings not only audit protection, but also significant increases in productivity to practices that are not overcoding. These increases result from multiple advantages of having a compliant and efficient record built on the diagnostic process:

■ Optimal EHR designs should help physicians obtain and document medical information with increased efficiency.

■ Security that the record ensures compliant documentation and coding permits physicians to comfortably submit high-level codes for patients with a high NPP, without fearing negative consequences of an audit.

■ Obtaining a comprehensive history during every patient visit allows physicians to become aware of additional potential health problems. In a reasonable percentage of cases, finding additional problems and identifying problems that have a more severe NPP may warrant higher levels of care and coding.

As an important added bonus, this increased productivity for medical practices is accompanied by health benefits for patients and cost savings for the health care system as a whole. Early identification of potentially dangerous health issues allows early intervention, which increases the probability of preventing pending illness and/or successfully managing diseases detected at their earliest stages. These results combine to help physicians achieve health policy goals for EHRs—improved quality of care, increased patient safety, and more cost-effective care.

GOALS FOR FUNCTIONALITY

Current EHRs that include E/M functionality generally use designs and coding software that reflect the traditional approach used to teach physicians E/M documentation and coding: first care for the patient, then document that care, and, last, attempt calculation of an E/M code based on the comprehensiveness and complexity of the three key components (history, examination, and MDM). However, this approach to E/M has proven not only burdensome for physicians during patient care, but also ineffective for achieving E/M compliance. This fundamental compliance challenge is often compounded by the fact that most existing coding software engines fail to consider medical necessity and may also include noncompliant interpretations of coding guidelines, as discussed in detail in Chapter 9.

In contrast, *Practical EHR* functionality introduces an approach proven to facilitate compliant documentation and coding that physicians using EHRs can apply intuitively during patient care. The basic principles underlying this method match physicians' requirements for functionality in an electronic H&P:

1. The design and functionality must promote the diagnostic process and quality care.

2. The approach must work (ie, be usable) for physicians. In other words, the coding process should require no significant additional effort on the physician's part beyond providing good patient care.

3. The functionality invites the physician to identify the NPP as part of the care process. In turn, this determination allows the software to guide the physician, based on compliance standards, to provide the level of care and coding warranted by the medical necessity of the patient's illness.

4. This method integrates documentation and coding into the normal workflow of quality patient care, rather than requiring additional complex mathematical calculations at the end of each patient visit.

5. The software provides physicians with sophisticated tools that facilitate compliance, eliminating the requirement imposed on physicians by the traditional E/M approach for memorizing and applying multiple sets of extensive coding rules.

After 15 years of experience with the E/M system, physicians appreciate that it has been unrealistic and unsuccessful for them to attempt to memorize a vast set of specialized rules that they must then interpret and follow while providing care to patients. This problem is corrected by intelligently incorporating all of the rules into the medical record forms physicians use while seeing patients. The EHR system adds another level of intelligence to this functionality, bringing the capability of error proofing at the point of care to further ensure compliance. This powerful tool is examined in Chapter 11, and its benefits are considered throughout the remainder of Part 3.

The *Practical EHR* protocol for E/M compliance reflects the diagnostic process. It begins with the physician reviewing a comprehensive medical history at the outset of every patient visit. On completion of the history, the physician should have formulated a reasonable differential diagnosis and needs to identify, with the guidance of the software, a preliminary assessment of the NPP and the level of care (according to CPT guidelines) that is medically appropriate for that NPP. With this insight, software tools can indicate the extent of examination and the complexity of MDM appropriate for this level of care (ie, E/M code). Of course, the physician may choose at any time to reassess the NPP and appropriate level of care, based on examination findings and laboratory results identified during this process, with corresponding modifications to the indicated levels of documentation. After completing documentation of MDM, the physician will record a final determination of the NPP. This last step verifies the medically indicated level of care and E/M code that the physician has identified, confirming the compatibility of the level of care and documentation with the degree of medical necessity. At the conclusion of the patient visit, the physician simply needs to record this E/M code for charge entry, along with the appropriate diagnosis code (ie, International Classification of Diseases, Ninth Revision, Clinical Modification codes).

H&P "LOOK AND FEEL"

It is reasonable to consider how the EHR should present the appearance of the completed electronic H&P to physicians. Many existing systems reformulate the graphic interface elements used for capturing information, such as completed medical history questionnaires and check boxes for examination findings, into the pure narrative text form of conventional dictated medical records that physicians traditionally transcribed and stored in paper charts.

However, this appearance is not necessarily an optimal model. Most paper records dictated by practicing physicians exclude significant portions of the comprehensive H&P owing to the time and cost involved in dictating all of the details. Compliance audits of these paper records, or their electronic equivalents, usually reveal that physicians have failed to record negative responses to elements of the PFSH and ROS, including negative responses that must be documented to fulfill compliance requirements. Instead, these transcribed documents usually substitute global statements, such as "otherwise noncontributory," to encompass all the data that were negative and all data that have not been documented and that may or may not have been obtained. This approach to the appearance of the documentation record also usually fails to include pertinent normal findings of the physical examination. For MDM, it frequently lists only the probable diagnoses rather than a differential, and it generally documents only one set of treatment options while failing to present the other options. Finally, in nearly all cases, these records fail to indicate multiple elements of MDM and to document the NPP. In summary, the appearance of conventional dictated records and their electronic equivalents most often demonstrates problem-focused care. In EHRs, this is often the level of care that is shown, regardless of the amount of care the physician may have performed and documented into the data entry interface screens of the electronic H&P and regardless of the level of care that is medically indicated.

Because the quality of care is often a reflection of the character of the medical record physicians use, there is significant benefit in having the "look and feel" of a completed electronic H&P include all of the graphic and narrative design features presented in this chapter and described in detail in the remainder of Part 3.

The electronic comprehensive form that combines graphic and narrative elements for each component of the H&P is efficient, easy to use, and extremely easy and fast to read. Keeping this as the final presentation of the electronic H&P also accurately represents the care process. In addition, for physicians, coders, or attorneys reviewing the medical record, it is far easier and more informative to review the comprehensive document than a pseudotranscription. If a practice were audited, it would have to provide copies of all documents that had been used for data capture anyway because pseudotranscription fails to provide audit-proof documentation. It seems far more reasonable and logical to retain the appearance of the H&P record in the same electronic format the software provides physicians to capture these data. Similarly, it seems unnecessary and counterproductive to create a two-tiered chart that converts this comprehensive recorded documentation into a transcription-type form that duplicates the appearance of the less-than-ideal paper records that EHRs are intended to replace. EHRs might include the additional option of converting the electronic H&P to look and feel like a dictated record for those who prefer the traditional appearance.

SUMMARY

Reaching a desired objective of creating EHRs that work for physicians and patients at the point of care requires setting reasonable and achievable goals for medical record design and functionality. The first three goals for data entry design of the electronic H&P record are that these systems must be usable and flexible for physicians needs, must ensure E/M compliance for documentation of every patient encounter, and must allow sufficient speed of documentation for physicians to meet the constraints imposed by the economics of the current health care system. Designs that achieve these requirements should also naturally help the software fulfill the final three goals for data entry design, which are facilitating quality care, ensuring the integrity of clinical data, and promoting appropriate productivity. Electronic H&P designs must meet all of these goals; they must not compromise compliance and quality to achieve greater speed of documentation or, more important, to achieve greater speed of care. Appendix E provides an in-depth look at the importance of achieving these goals by highlighting the potential quality, compliance, and liability issues that might arise from improper design and/or utilization of an electronic H&P.

The EHR designs should also guide physicians to follow the medical diagnostic process, which physicians need to promote optimal patient care and to ensure compliant documentation and coding. This capability requires EHR functionality to incorporate assessment of the NPP during the care process and electronic H&P design to provide physicians with compliance guidance through documentation prompts. *Practical EHR* also advocates that the final appearance of the completed H&P should include all of the data entry design elements to confirm compliance and reflect the quality care process.

Physicians must at all times respect the principle that our primary mission is to take care of patients, not simply check off boxes on medical record forms as quickly as possible. It must always remain physicians' responsibility to do what is in the best interest of their patients and then to be sure that the medical record reflects that care. One of the most important goals of *Practical EHR* is to have the electronic H&P record design help physicians achieve quality care and compliance as effectively and efficiently as possible.

References

1. Ash J, Bates D. Factors and forces affecting EHR system adoption: report of a 2004 ACMI discussion. *J Am Med Inform Assoc.* 2005;12:89-12.

2. Committee on Quality of Health Care in America, Institute of Medicine. *Crossing the Quality Chasm: A New Health System for the 21st Century.* Washington, DC: National Academies Press; 2001.

3. Clancy C. Keynote address. Presented at: the Second Health Information Technology Summit; September 9, 2005; Washington, DC.

4.   Levinson SR. *Practical E/M: Documentation and Coding Solutions for Quality Patient Care.* Chicago, IL: AMA Press; 2005.

5.   American Medical Association, Health Care Financing Administration. *Documentation Guidelines for Evaluation and Management Services.* Chicago, IL: American Medical Association; 1997:5

6.   American Medical Association. *Current Procedural Terminology.* Chicago, IL: American Medical Association; 2007:9-10.

7.   College of American Pathologists. Systematized Nomenclature of Medicine. Clinical terms, owned and distributed by International Health Terminology Standards Development Organization, 1999. Available at: www.ihtsdo.org/

8.   Johnston, D. University agrees to pay in settlement on Medicare. *New York Times.* December 13, 1995:A18.

chapter 11

Data Entry Parameters and the H&P Design Toolkit

The blueprint for creating an intelligent electronic history and physical examination (H&P) record design should start with a foundation that meets all physicians' data entry goals (discussed in Chapter 10) and at the same time is capable of supporting a broad range of options to meet the preferences of individual physicians. Designing this foundation begins by reexamining two fundamental assumptions of most current software systems: (1) the physician must perform all data entry into the software program (ie, serves as the data entry operator [DEO]), and (2) all data must be entered into the software at the point of care.

OPTIONS FOR DATA ENTRY PERSONNEL

Physician as DEO

A small percentage of physicians are comfortable with entering all clinical data into the electronic H&P record during or immediately following a patient visit. They contend that they type fast enough to maintain maximum efficiency while entering full narrative descriptions into the appropriate sections of the electronic H&P. Physicians comfortable with direct data entry at the point of care also usually believe that placing the computer between themselves and their patients does not interfere with maintaining eye contact or with a patient's sense of having the physician's full attention.

Battleship

Unfortunately, even for the best of typists, entering data into a computer requires frequent eye contact with the computer screen to check for typing errors. Directing attention to the screen and/or keyboard interferes with maintaining attention and eye contact with the patient (and, for most physicians, diverts attention to a far greater extent than writing on paper at the same time they are talking with a patient).

A number of patients have expressed significant unhappiness over this issue, and even questioned whether they would return to their long-time physicians after those physicians had introduced EHRs and placed the laptop between them and their patients to enter data during the visits. Several of these patients observed that the physician spent so much time looking at the computer screen, "I felt like I was playing a game of 'Battleship' with my child." In this game, each player hides behind his or her laptop-shaped playing board and attempts to share as little information as possible with the other player, who is perceived as an opponent. This is not the impression physicians want to convey.

Scribes

After recognizing the limitations imposed by current systems that require typed data entry at the point of care, a significant number of physicians have elected to employ scribes, who remain in the examination room during patient care, recording the medical history questions and answers and details the physician narrates about physical examination findings and medical decision making (MDM). This approach brings the advantage of curing the obstacles to efficiency and patient relations that occur when the physician is the DEO. However, the use of scribes also introduces a number of drawbacks. The practice has to bear the added cost of hiring these trained personnel, all of whom need to have the clinical vocabulary to understand and enter medical terminology into the H&P record. A physician may also be left without data entry assistance whenever the scribe is ill or on vacation. In addition, this practice can lead to patient-relations challenges for a portion of the patient population. Some patients may be uncomfortable with having a nonmedical person in the room during their care and listening to their personal medical issues. Others may also find it distracting and/or confusing when hearing the physician translate clinical information into medical terminology for the scribe to record in the chart.

Using scribes is a "work around" rather than a solution. Instead of correcting the design problems caused by requiring typing for data entry, this choice offers a typing alternative that brings its own costs and compromises.

It is interesting that some academic physicians have assigned their residents the task of being their typing scribes, entering clinical information for them during their care of patients. This attempted solution compounds the data entry imperfections of typing by compromising residents' schedules and their learning experiences.

Alternative Data Entry Mechanisms for Physicians

With the advances in technology, new data entry tools have emerged that translate written or dictated narrative information directly into digital text without requiring the physician to touch a keyboard. This technology permits EHR designers to create data entry solutions that extend beyond the confines of current protocols. These options expand further with the realization that none of physicians' mandates for an optimal H&P record require the physician to be the person entering the data into the computer. Therefore, such technology should be able to offer a broader range of data entry options capable of accommodating physicians who prefer writing or dictating their records, in addition to physicians who prefer to take on the role of DEO. This chapter later examines a full range of the currently available data entry options in greater detail.

Staff and Patients as DEO

Compliance permits, and even encourages, that medical history "may be recorded by ancillary staff or on a form completed by the patient. To document that the physician reviewed the information, there must be a notation supplementing or confirming the information recorded by others."[1(p5)] This option may include direct entry into the computer or use of a data transfer medium for delayed entry, as described subsequently for physicians.

OPTIONS FOR DELAYED DATA ENTRY

For optimal quality, compliance, efficiency, and data integrity, physicians should document their findings during or immediately after providing patient care, before moving on to meet the next patient. Delaying formal documentation, even with the help of brief notes made at the time of a visit, might allow physicians to recall the general idea of a specific encounter 4 to 8 hours later, but it will not allow them to record all the details and nuances of a patient's history and examination and the decision making process.

As an alternative, asynchronous data entry allows physicians to record clinical data on a data transfer medium at the point of care. This recording may involve writing on paper or dictating into a recorder, using a structured template that matches the EHR's data entry screens. At the conclusion of the visit, these transfer media are uploaded to a professional DEO (eg, transcriptionist) who enters the information directly into the software at a later time. With this option, a medical practice may choose whether to hire its own data entry employees or to outsource to a company that provides these services off site.

Messages From Thomas Friedman

In his book *The World Is Flat,* Thomas Friedman emphasized that the introduction of electronic media has allowed near-instantaneous communication among individuals and businesses anywhere in the world, which has created business environments in which people with less highly differentiated skills have "taken the grunt work," leaving more time available for the person in a critical position as "the one who focuses on creative, complex strategies."[2]

Applying this concept to the medical setting, EHRs should be designed to shift the grunt work of data entry away from physicians through the use of creative electronic tools or by transferring such tasks to other people who can perform it for them.

Circumstances Requiring Synchronous Documentation

Some of the interconnectivity and interoperability features of EHRs, when activated, require synchronous entry of several elements of the H&P at the point of care. Therefore, designs that provide for asynchronous data entry must also require that a small amount of clinical information be entered (by the physician or ancillary staff) during or immediately after the patient visit. These special situations involve provision for several types of computerized physician order entry, such as:

- Transmitting orders for laboratory testing directly from the EHR to the patient's testing facility
  - The laboratory needs to receive the list of tests being ordered and the patient's active medical diagnoses.
- Transmitting orders for radiology testing directly from the EHR to the patient's radiology facility
  - The radiology office needs to receive the list of studies being ordered and the patient's active medical diagnoses.

■ Transmitting orders for medications directly from the EHR to the patient's pharmacy

● For initial visits, this requires recording the patient's current medications and medication allergies and entering the prescriptions being ordered in the treatment options section of the MDM component.

● For established patients, this requires review and update of the patient's medications and medication allergies and entering the prescriptions being ordered in the treatment options section of the MDM component.

■ Transmitting orders for diagnostic testing or treatments (eg, an EKG or an immunization) on the day of the visit to other members of the practice's staff

● The appropriate staff member needs to receive the list of tests or treatments ordered

PHYSICIAN TRANSFORMATION

It is almost always uncomfortable for most people to change the way they are accustomed to performing common tasks, particularly tasks that are part of their daily routine. Being required to make adjustments in standard patient care workflow frequently elicits resistance from some physicians and outright defiance from others. Fortunately, asking physicians to use an established and familiar approach to patient care meets far less resistance than offering a new and unfamiliar method. For this reason, most physicians will readily adapt to and accept electronic H&P record designs and data entry protocols that reproduce the diagnostic process they learned and used in medical school, particularly when complemented by sophisticated tools for increased efficiency.

Physicians also become extremely comfortable with their mode of entering data into medical records while evaluating the conditions of patients. To some extent, each physician will be entirely convinced that his or her current data entry technique is the best. In many cases, requiring a physician to use a different and unfamiliar data entry format will meet with significant resistance. Therefore, design efforts that maintain familiarity by closely matching physicians' current tools can also increase acceptance and ease the transition to an "intelligent" electronic record.

ASSEMBLING THE DATA ENTRY TOOLKIT

Chapter 6 introduced three concepts that were used throughout Part 2 to analyze the design and functionality features of existing EHRs: interface, data entry personnel, and data entry format. These concepts can be reapplied as building blocks to reenvision design criteria for each subsection of the electronic H&P to meet physicians' requirements for success. In addition, incorporating error proofing is a new design concept for EHRs. Functionality that enables this innovative fourth concept will help physicians ensure evaluation and management (E/M) compliance and provide medically warranted levels of care.

Interface Options

Interface describes the design features that allow physicians to document clinical information in the medical record. The two general interface categories, graphic and narrative, provide sufficient flexibility to meet documentation requirements for every section of the H&P record. The critical tasks for software designers include designing each interface to meet compliance standards, incorporating documentation prompts to guide care and documentation based on the level of the nature of the presenting problem (NPP), selecting the most appropriate and efficient interface design for each subsection of the record, matching the design and its vocabulary to the needs of the personnel who will be using each interface, and incorporating the variety of tools needed to permit all data entry formats that will improve usability by physicians.

Each of the two medical record interface categories inherently offers different strengths and weaknesses. The *graphic* interface allows rapid documentation of responses from among a predetermined list of possible choices. However, it is inadequate to record detailed individualized responses that cannot be preprogrammed, such as the chronological description of a patient's history of the present illness and details of abnormal physical examination findings.

The *narrative* interface presents a blank section in the electronic H&P screen (or form) to permit the recording of detailed free-text information. This structure offers optimal compliance, quality, and efficiency for patient- and visit-specific documentation of the history of the present illness; details concerning positive responses in the review of systems (ROS) or past, family, and social history (PFSH); examination abnormalities; detailed descriptions of differential diagnoses; and systematic consideration of treatment options. Using free-text would be far too inefficient for documenting long lists of questions and their responses or writing out normal examination findings.

The two interface designs are clearly complementary, and optimal EHR design should offer the type of interface best suited to the information-gathering requirements of each subsection of the EHR.

Examination of the Graphic Interface

Several graphic interface designs are available. As discussed in Chapter 6, compliant graphic interface options include structures with the following:

- Check-box configuration: This interface lists a significant number of pre-entered inquiries (eg, related to medical history) or descriptions (eg, related to examination findings), with check boxes associated with each statement to permit entry of responses such as *yes* or *no* and *normal* or *abnormal*. This type of interface is illustrated in Figure 6.1.
- Blank lines to record concise responses or provide greater detail to enhance check-box responses. This type of interface is also illustrated in Figure 6.1.
- Selection lists for choosing alternatives among multiple possibilities, which come in two basic designs:
  - Restricted list of options, with a single check box next to each selection. Figure 11.1 illustrates the design of this type of selection list.
  - Drop-down menus or pop-up screens provide EHRs with the ability to include far more choices with the addition of a scrolling function. Figure 11.2 illustrates the design of this type of selection list.

FIGURE 11.1

Data Ordered: Single Check-Box Selection List. This sample form is an example of a graphic interface for a cardiologist's selection list of frequently ordered laboratory tests, physiologic tests, and radiologic studies. The interface also provides for free-text entry of other tests that the physician orders less frequently. Note that this "data ordered" design also includes a documentation prompt correlating amount of data (underlined numbers) with medically indicated levels of care based on the NPP. CBC indicates complete blood cell count; CT, computed tomography; EKG, electrocardiogram; and chem 6 and 12, serum chemistry panels.

Data Ordered	1. Minimal or none (level 2) 2. Limited (level 3) 3. Moderate (level 4) 4. Extensive (level 5)		
☒ EKG	☐ Stress test	☒ Echocardiogram	☒ 24-hour Holter monitor
☐ Chest X-ray	☐ Chest CT		
Laboratory	☒ CBC ☐ Chem 6 ☒ Chem 12 ☒ Lipid profile		
Other	Thallium stress test		

FIGURE 11.2

Data Ordered: Drop-Down Menu or Pop-Up Screen. This sample form is an example of a cardiologist's selection list graphic interface that has sufficient room for all commonly or occasionally ordered laboratory tests, physiologic tests, and radiologic studies by adding scrolling capability. The person entering data points and clicks to select desired studies. Note that his data entry design may also include a documentation prompt, similar to that shown in Figure 11.1, on the home screen supporting these menus. CBC indicates complete blood cell count; CT, computed tomography; EKG, electrocardiogram; GI, gastrointestinal; MRI, magnetic resonance imaging; MUGAA, multiple gated acquisition angiocardiography; chem 6 and 12, serum chemistry panels; and VAP, Vertical Auto Profile.

Cardiology studies ▲
Echocardiogram
EKG
MUGAA scan
Stress test
Stress thallium test
24-hour Holter monitor

Radiologic studies
Chest X-ray
Chest CT without contrast
Chest CT with contrast
Chest MRI without gadolinium
Chest MRI with gadolinium
Upper GI series

Laboratory tests
CBC
Chem 6
Chem 12
Lipid profile
VAP test
Myocardial C-reactive protein ▼

Each of the two selection-list designs offers advantages and disadvantages. The check-box approach is quick and easy to use because it presents all common choices on one screen. However, it requires some time and inconvenience to enter tests not included on the list. On the other hand, although the drop-down menu provides a comprehensive list, it can be so extensive that scrolling and searching for multiple tests requires added time and unwelcome effort. Ideally, designers will make approaches available for appropriate sections of the H&P so that physicians can customize the look and operation to their own preferences. An optimal design for most physicians might be to combine the two designs, using check boxes for commonly ordered tests and a drop-down menu listing less common choices. Similarly, a drop-down menu could be divided into two sections, the first listing common tests and the second, accessed by an additional mouse click, listing less frequently ordered tests.

In certain sections of the H&P record, graphic interface designs are essential for maximizing documentation efficiency. The different structures for these templates will match appropriately with different sections. To provide compliance, each graphic design must require individual documentation of the check boxes to confirm each selection, including avoiding the capability for documentation by exception in which responses are preloaded in the check boxes. To promote quality, each template should include all appropriate questions (for history sections) or descriptions (for physical-examination and decision-making sections).

Examination of the Narrative Interface

Free-text entry is, in reality, the only design choice capable of providing a compliant narrative interface that also permits documentation of individualized, patient-specific information. There are two critical considerations for the narrative interface. First, even though physicians need to employ narrative documentation in the specific subsections of the record listed above for compliance and quality purposes, this interface should also be made available as an option in all sections of the H&P as a means of entering unique patient-specific information. Second, for reasons related to E/M compliance, quality care, and integrity of data, the narrative design must avoid use of preloaded pick lists or macros to create pseudonarratives.

Personnel Options

For maximal usability and flexibility, designs should provide for data entry into EHR software by patients and medical staff in portions of the medical history (chief complaint [CC], PFSH, and ROS), when and where it is appropriate. Physicians should also have the option of using professional data entry specialists to enter clinical information into the software, which the physician or others have recorded by writing on paper forms or dictating.

Format Options and Tools

To help physicians become comfortable using EHRs, designs should include both current and innovative data entry tools in a variety of formats to match the full range of physician preferences. Some physicians are content adapting their data entry method to typing on a keyboard and pointing and clicking with a mouse. However, for those physicians who are uncomfortable with this method for data entry, far greater success will be fostered by offering effective tools that use familiar dictation and/or writing formats while allowing data entry by typing and mouse clicking as an option rather than a requirement for using the software.

Most physicians prefer the data entry modality to which they are accustomed. Physicians who dictate at the end of each visit find that this format offers legibility (particularly for physicians who find this compliance requirement unattainable when writing), increased speed compared with typing, and the ability to focus entirely on their patients during visits. These advantages come at the price of high transcription costs, but some physicians eliminate this expense by using voice recognition software. However, errors occur with dictation, regardless of whether software or humans perform the transcription, and proofreading dictated documents is time-consuming.

Physicians who document the H&P by writing their findings during the patient visit believe that writing is even faster than dictation and results in fewer errors. They contend that this approach requires only minimally more time than performing the care alone (because they write while they are asking the medical history questions), and it saves time at the end of the visit that would be used for dictation. It also adds no additional cost to the medical practice. The only drawbacks for data entry by writing are legibility, legibility, and legibility.

Why Do Educators Accept Illegibility?

Illegible handwriting is usually a learned skill. Some physicians have raised it to an art form—being unable to read their own handwriting. However, illegibility is noncompliant (per the first rule of Documentation Guidelines[1]), interferes with quality care, and creates havoc for physicians during audits or in a malpractice investigation. The question arises concerning why medical schools, residency programs, and licensing boards permit this problem to persist. Just as poor, illegible handwriting is noncompliant yet tolerated by the different bodies, the question can be raised about practices that have failed a compliance audit and been placed under a corporate integrity agreement, which requires compliant documentation.

To date, most medical schools have failed to acknowledge their responsibility for teaching compliance and demanding compliant care and documentation by students, residents, and professors. They must recognize the importance of this responsibility in preparing physicians for the practice of medicine. If schools would include legibility as a condition for admission (as long as students are required to write their records), it is certain that all applicants would suddenly learn to write legibly. Continuing to require legible handwriting as a condition for progressing through medical school, residency, and licensing would compel physicians to maintain this skill through the remainder of their careers, resulting in their having the ability to use the full range of EHR data entry tools that will be available to them.

Many physicians may prefer to maintain existing data entry practices rather than abandoning them for direct computer entry techniques that are challenging and cumbersome. Because innovative data entry tools are available that can accommodate all physician preferences for data entry formats, vendors should incorporate these options to facilitate acceptance and success of EHR systems.

Indirect Data Entry Tools

Compliance and quality care considerations mandate that physicians perform all of the actual care and documentation of E/M services (except for the elements of the medical history that they can review after documentation by staff or patients). However, there is no such directive requiring physicians to be the DEO. Therefore, one approach to improve physicians' documentation efficiency involves using high-quality writing or dictation tools as a data transfer medium. To facilitate the indirect data entry process, it is critical that the designs for templates on paper forms precisely match the appearance of the data entry screens of the electronic H&P record. Data entry specialists can then most efficiently transcribe the dictated files or scanned written documents into the software.

Direct Data Entry Tools

For physicians who prefer dictation to record the narrative portions of the H&P component, dictation can be directly transcribed into the EHR at the point of care by using voice recognition software. The new tools available for physicians who prefer writing include directly writing on a tablet personal computer (PC) and using digital pen technology. While these technologies are constantly being improved, their designs must remain compatible with the underlying fundamentals of the comprehensive H&P and the diagnostic process, regardless of the data entry format chosen.

TOOLKIT FOR DATA ENTRY BY WRITING AND DICTATION

Indirect Data Entry Tools

Data Entry Tool 1: Indirect Entry Using Writing and Paper Forms

This approach allows physicians to use a written format for information entry. The physician (and patient, for the CC, PFSH, and ROS of initial visits) completes some or all of the documentation on a compliant paper form that is matched, section for section and word for word, with the comparable screens of an EHR that meets design standards, including E/M compliance, identified in *Practical EHR*. It should use graphic and narrative interfaces appropriately. A professional DEO receives the paper document and enters the data into the patient's file in the EHR. The DEO may be an employee of the medical practice working in the same location or at another office, where he or she receives a scanned electronic version of the document by Internet connectivity. Similarly, electronic transmission allows the data entry function to be outsourced to a professional company at a distant location. In either case, costs are minimized by the structure of the graphic interface designs on these screens and forms. This data should be entered within 24 hours of the patient's visit.

Data Entry Tool 2: Indirect Data Entry Using Paper Forms Plus Dictation Data Entry/Electronic Storage and Retrieval

This hybrid tool combines written and dictation formats for data entry. This tool is similar to tool 1, with the additional feature that narrative portions of the record may be dictated. Thus, the physician would use a pen to fill in the check-box graphic templates on appropriate paper forms and indicate that any narrative sections have been dictated (as illustrated in Figure 11.3). Paper documents would be uploaded to a DEO, and dictation might be uploaded to a separate transcription specialist. Both employees would enter their respective components into the same patient record, preferably within 24 hours of a patient visit and/or before the claim is billed.

Advantages of Indirect Data Entry Tools

Multiple benefits are provided by these two indirect data entry tools. In addition to the fact that entering the documentation by writing or dictation is generally faster that typing on a keyboard or using mouse clicks, professional DEOs have lower cost and higher motivation for the task than most physicians. These tools shift a less complex task away from physicians and free their time for more productive, medical tasks, as shown in Table 11.1.

It is highly recommended that images of the original paper documents and audio files of the dictation should be stored electronically in each patient's chart. This practice is essential for providing immediate availability of the patient's clinical information before it has been transcribed into the

Physical Examination Section of a Specialty-Specific Examination for Ear, Nose, and Throat, compliant with 1997 Documentation Guidelines. This example demonstrates how the physician would fill in the check boxes of the graphic section and then check another box to confirm narrative dictation of the abnormal examination findings. This form also illustrates the use of a documentation prompt to guide compliant care and documentation warranted by the patient's NPP. Note also that vital signs are handwritten (by the physician or clinical assistant).

Physical Examination:	**Ear, Nose, Throat**							

General (at least 3 measures of vital signs) measure of
BP sitting or standing ___/___mm Hg

HT _5_ ft _9_ in   WT _163_ lbs
BP supine ___/___mm Hg

Pulse _76_/min; regular or irregular

Respirations___/min   Temperature___°F (or___°C)

			nl / abnl				nl / abnl
	General appearance	*Stature, nutrition*	☒ ☐	Neck	Masses and trachea	*Symmetry, masses*	☒ ☐
	Communication, voice	*Pitch, clarity*	☒ ☐		Thyroid	*Size, nodules*	☒ ☐
Head, face	Inspection	*Lesions, masses*	☒ ☐	Eyes	Motility and gaze	*EOMs, nystagmus*	☒ ☐
	Palpation/percussion	*Skeleton, sinuses*	☒ ☐	Respiratory	Respiratory effort	*Inspiratory-expiratory*	☒ ☐
	Salivary glands	*Masses, tenderness*	☒ ☐		Auscultation	*Clear*	☐ ☐
	Facial strength	*Symmetry*	☒ ☐	CVS	Heart auscultation	*Heart rate, sounds*	☐ ☐
ENT	Pneumo-otoscopy	*EACs; TMs mobile*	☒ ☐		Peripheral vascular system	*Carotid palpation, auscultation*	☒ ☐
	Hearing assessment	*Gross/Weber/Rinne*	☒ ☐	Lymphatics	Neck, axillae, groin, etc.	*Adenopathy absence*	☒ ☐
	External ear and nose	*Appearance*	☒ ☐	Neuropsych	Cranial nerves	*II-XII*	☒ ☐
	Internal nose	*Mucosa, turbs*	☐ ☒		Orientation	*Person, place, time*	☐ ☐
	After decongestion†	*Septum, OMCs*	☐ ☒		Mood and affect	*Comments*	☒ ☐
	Lips, teeth, gums	*Mucosa, dentition*	☒ ☐		Romberg†		☐ ☐
	Oral cavity, oropharynx	*Tonsils, palate*	☒ ☐		Tandem Romberg†		☐ ☐
	Hypopharynx	*Piriform sinuses*	☒ ☐		Past pointing†		☐ ☐
	Larynx (mirror)	*Structure, mobility*	☒ ☐		☒ See attached dictation		
	Nasopharynx (mirror)	*Choanae*	☒ ☐				

1. Problem-focused = 1-5 elements (level 1) 2. Expanded = 6-11 elements (level 2) 3. Detailed = 12 or more elements (level 3)
4. Comprehensive = document every element in basic *areas and* at least 1 element in each optional (shaded) area (level 4 & 5)
†Optional

Abbreviations: abnl, abnormal; CVS, cardiovascular system; EAC, external auditory canal; EOMs, extra-ocular movements; nl, normal; OMCs, osteo-meatal complex; TM, tympanic membrane; and turbs, turbinates.

Note that, in accordance with the documentation prompt for level 4 initial visit care, the physician has (examined and) documented each required element (those not indicated as optional by a dagger) in the nonshaded areas and at least one element in each of the shaded areas.[3(p135)]

T A B L E 11.1

Effectiveness of Professional DEO Compared With Physician for Data Entry Into Computer[3(p195)]

	Physician as DEO	**Professional DEO**
Ability to enter data rapidly	Poor	Excellent
Accuracy in entering data	Poor	Excellent
Effective use of physician time and productivity	Low	High
Impact on efficiency of care	Negative	None
Impact on physician-patient relationship	Negative	None
Cost of the DEO	Very high	Low

Abbreviation: DEO, data entry operator.

EHR: it is important in the event of an emergency or answering a call related to the patient on the day of the visit. Saving this information also provides a means of checking original documentation in the event of data entry error by DEOs or transcriptionists. These electronic versions of the original documents add a layer of protection in the event of a compliance audit or a professional liability investigation. If a question is raised about the validity and originality of the electronic clinical descriptions, the original documents and dictation file provide proof of what the physician actually wrote and dictated.

These indirect documentation tools also provide a significant advantage by broadening the population of physicians and administrators who, from a usability perspective, will feel comfortable bringing an EHR system into their practice. These tools make adoption of EHRs feasible for all physicians, including physicians who do not want to become proficient typists, who do not want to place a laptop between themselves and their patients, and/or who are reluctant to relinquish working with familiar and comfortable established formats. This expansion of the candidates for EHRs affects not only small medical practices, but also large groups that may have one or more reluctant physicians who are opposed to adoption of EHRs. In regional health information organizations (RHIOs), using these hybrid tools can also allow physicians who prefer not to purchase software systems to upload their nonelectronic documentation so that it can be entered into the system's central server, and their patients' clinical information can be shared with all other participants in the RHIO.

Disadvantages of Indirect Data Entry Tools
Physicians and administrators should have few if any objections to using data transfer media when using effectively designed templates that ensure compliance and promote efficiency. The primary objection should be the cost of the DEOs and transcriptionists, and this concern can be reasonably addressed. First, practices can minimize this cost by using well-designed paper forms with graphic interface designs in all appropriate portions of the record. Further, as emphasized in Table 11.1, the costs of DEOs and transcriptionists are significantly less than the cost of physician time to accomplish the same task. Finally, the savings realized by using an EHR system instead of paper charts significantly exceeds the cost of DEOs; that is, although using the indirect data entry tools comes with a labor cost, that cost is less than the practice was spending previously for storing and retrieving patient charts.

Although these indirect data entry tools offer an important transitional alternative, some of the direct data entry tools (particularly tools 3 and 6) provide all of the same advantages while addressing the drawbacks. In addition, they offer the important benefit of immediate transcription of the clinical information into the appropriate section of the electronic H&P.

Direct Data Entry Tools

Data Entry Tool 3: Dictation With Voice Recognition Software
This solution for documenting narrative components of the H&P seems attractive to many current EHR developers, because it enables them to provide physicians with a dictation format as an alternative to data entry

of free-text using a keyboard or mouse. This tool is available for direct data entry at the point of care. The software automatically converts physicians' dictation into digital text in the appropriate location of the electronic form, eliminating the need for the physician to use the keyboard for the narrative sections of the H&P.

Advantages of Voice Recognition Software
In many ways, voice recognition software duplicates the characteristics of dictation with human transcription described for data entry tool 2. It also offers the advantage of retaining an audio wave file of the dictation to provide security if the software makes transcription errors. Compared with transcription, the data entry is instantaneous, eliminating a step for uploading data stored on a microprocessor and waiting hours for the dictation to be entered into the patient's chart. Following initial purchase of the software, this tool also eliminates the ongoing cost of transcription.

Disadvantages of Voice Recognition Software
With any dictation system, there is concern about accuracy of the conversion of the spoken word into a digital (typed) document. There is a learning curve for use of this software because physicians must "train" the software to recognize their voices and speech patterns. The software also trains the physician to speak at a certain rate and, to some degree, with a specific voice pattern to maximize accuracy. When using this software, corrections need to be made immediately when an error appears on screen during dictation. Stopping to correct errors costs time and can become distracting, particularly if the tool is used in the presence of a patient. Therefore, as with any dictation approach, most physicians will likely prefer to dictate after a visit has concluded. It is hoped that accuracy rates will continue to improve as this technology evolves in the medical environment.

Data Entry Tool 4: Active Mouse Entry on Check-Box Forms
In current systems that require or permit physicians to act as DEO, there has been significant attention given to physician complaints about the effort required to fill in check boxes on graphic templates, such as the one illustrated in Figure 11.3. These concerns center on the physical exam screens, which are completed after providing the care (screens for questions on medical history for the PFSH and ROS are easily recorded one at a time, as the patient answers them). Using the mouse to click one box at a time to record a completed physical examination is inefficient and awkward. However, as noted in Part 2, current design attempts to address this problem, using tools for documentation by exception, generate potential issues with compliance, reliability of data, and quality of care.

Existing technology for using the mouse offers an effective solution, allowing physicians to check a series of boxes individually and rapidly. For example, for a series of normal findings, such as the first nine rows on the left side of Figure 11.3, the user should be able to click on the highest normal box in the series, hold down the mouse clicker, and roll or drag the pointer down through the next eight normal boxes by moving the mouse downward on the mouse pad. Any time the documentation calls for a different entry, such as designating the two "abnormal" findings in the 10th and 11th rows on the left, the mouse is released, moved to the correct position, and clicked (or clicked and rolled) in the correct boxes. Similiarly, boxes must be left unmarked for examination elements that were not performed. This function is familiar to anyone who works with word processors. It permits individualized documentation that fulfills compliance requirements while conveying an accurate picture of each patient's health. For physicians who want to enter data directly into the computer, this function will prove invaluable for the graphic interface elements of the examination.*

Advantages of Active Mouse Entry
This tool uses existing software capabilities in an effective way that greatly increases efficiency and eliminates a menial task, while still permitting individualized documentation that meets criteria for compliance and data integrity. There should be no significant learning curve for using this familiar tool correctly.

Disadvantages of Active Mouse Entry
Physicians using this technology obviously must pay attention to the computer screen to ensure that they are moving the mouse appropriately for accurate documentation. This activity may cause some distraction if a physician is asking a patient medical history questions and looking at the computer screen at the same time.

Data Entry Tool 5: Tablet PCs With Handwriting Recognition
Introducing the tablet PC to EHR design adds another existing technology that expands flexibility to promote physician acceptance and increases data entry efficiency for narrative sections of the H&P record. Using tablet PC software reintroduces direct physician entry with handwriting as the format. For the narrative sections of the H&P record, physicians can write directly on the screen, and, assuming reasonable legibility, the software converts handwritten free-text into digital text. This tool should also have the capability of duplicating the benefits of active mouse entry by running a stylus down the screen over a series of check boxes, allowing physicians to enter an "X" in every box touched by the stylus. The tablet PC offers a full range of data entry format capabilities to meet physician preferences, including writing on the screen, dictating into the microphone for transcription (voice recognition or human transcriptionist), typing on the keyboard, and using the mouse.

Advantages of the Tablet PC
The tablet PC works like an "electronic clipboard," which should be familiar to almost every physician. It is flat, like a clipboard, so it removes the visual barrier of the vertical screen of a laptop computer interposing between physicians and patients. By providing a full range of data entry format capabilities, the tablet PC fulfills usability and flexibility requirements.

Disadvantages of the Tablet PC
Illegibility remains a significant potential barrier for using the written format for narrative entry. Even when the handwriting is legible, if the software misreads a word or phrase and enters inaccurate information,

---

* As with any documentation feature, physicians must document carefully to accurately record the history obtained or examination performed. Each box that is checked attests that the care was provided and indicates the findings. These tools should never be used to document inaccurately, to avoid the potential negative consequences of documentation-by-exception approaches.

the physician will need to interrupt the patient interaction to correct the error(s), a process that could prove disruptive if it occurs too frequently. This hardware is also more costly than a desktop PC, which should be considered a relatively minor concern compared with the scope of the total EHR investment and the range of benefits for multiple approaches to direct data entry by physicians. However, the cost for additional hardware and the need to protect against theft might become factors if practices want additional tablet PCs in their waiting rooms so that new patients can use them to complete the survey questions for direct entry of the PFSH and ROS into their medical charts.

Data Entry Tool 6: Digital Pen

The digital pen is a sophisticated integration of hardware and software technology that converts handwritten analog information created using "pen and paper" into digital data, enabling the data to be utilized in various applications. The digital pen is used in conjunction with digital paper (also known as *interactive paper*), which is patterned with barely-visible microdots, for creating digital files capable of storing images of handwritten documents. The printed dot patterns on the digital paper identify the position coordinates on the paper, and the microcamera in the pen captures a digital snapshot of these unique patterns to store the position of written or printed information, including handwriting, relative to the micro dots. The digital pen converts the analog information (handwritten order forms and memos, clinical charts, etc.) into digital data and stores it in its built-in memory. Once stored in the pen's built-in memory, the information can be easily uploaded to a PC, EHR, or other IT devices.

The use of digital pen technology for data capture with EHRs requires the integration of additional form-generating software to pre-print identical images of the EHR's data entry screens onto the digital paper. The pen is capable of capturing the form itself as well as any data entered, including marks in check box areas and handwriting in the free-text narrative sections. The microdots can also be programmed to include information identifying the screen being duplicated, patient identifying information, and the date.

When a physician (or a staff member or a patient) uses a digital pen for data entry and then places the digital pen in its docking station, all the information that was captured by the pen is immediately uploaded to the appropriate portion of the corresponding screens in the patient's chart in digital form. Any marks made in the check boxes of the digital paper appear as Xs in the corresponding boxes on screen. Any text written in the narrative sections of the digital paper are converted to typed text that appears in the corresponding section of the appropriate EHR screen. This conversion of written text to typed digital text parallels the process used in the tablet PC.

This tool has an additional feature that should eliminate one of the concerns with the use of tablet PCs for handwriting recognition. Although the software still has the potential to misread a word or phrase and perform incorrect digital entry, the digital pen safeguards the integrity and accuracy of the data by also uploading a digital image of the written document into the patient's electronic folder in the EHR. If there is ever a question about the information that the physician or patient intended to document, the original handwritten form can be recreated from the visual file. Because the captured handwritten information is also the original and true information entered by the user, this feature should lessen concerns about transcription errors because the documentation can always be verified by printing and reviewing the digitized image of the original handwritten form. This extra protection for data integrity, compliance review, and potential liability review is similar to that available when using data entry tool 1, which saves electronic files of scanned handwritten documents.

Advantages of the Digital Pen
The digital pen allows physicians to use a real clipboard and "pen and paper" as a data transfer medium. The digital pen also allows a physician with legible handwriting who prefers writing for data entry to introduce an EHR into patient care while maintaining familiar habits for data entry and patient interaction. This tool can also be used for checking boxes in the graphic sections of the record in combination with voice recognition software or a digital recorder for dictation of the narrative sections of the record. Finally, the digital pen provides an effective way for patients to complete their forms for demographic information and the medical history portions of initial patient visit. It is easy for the patients to use because it is no different from writing on conventional paper forms, and all their documentation is automatically entered directly into the EHR. This technology offers an efficient and economical solution for direct entry of written information.

Disadvantages of the Digital Pen
Illegibility remains a significant potential barrier for physicians using the digital pen for narrative documentation. Even when the writing is legible, the software might make some transcription errors. In addition to having data-integrity protection from the backup file that preserves a digitized image of the actual handwritten form, practices can consider having the converted or print document reviewed and corrected by professionals (eg, transcriptionists), who can compare the print version with the digitized image of the paper form. Because most of the converted or handwritten-turned-print information will be accurate, the corrections should require minimal time and, therefore, incur relatively minimal cost.

According to a software developer for digital pen technology, there are also some challenges in programming the underlying forms because of the differences in EHR designs owing to lack of standardized H&P record interfaces. However, this issue should diminish with transition to the "recognized interoperability standards,"[4] mandated in President Bush's second executive order on health information technology to facilitate interoperability for sharing data among EHRs from different practices and with patient health records.

Data Entry Tool 7: Direct Entry With Keyboard and Mouse
This tool is the conventional approach for EHR systems, using a desktop or laptop and assigning the physician to be the DEO. This form of entry may also be extended to patients. The medical practice could make a kiosk available in the office, allowing patients to directly enter demographic and insurance information and elements of their medical history into an electronic screen or laptop.

Disadvantages of Direct Entry With Keyboard and Mouse
As discussed in Part 2, problems for physicians using this mode of data entry include increased time to document meaningful and individualized narrative information and potential interference with patient interactions. Problems for patients entering personal information include the cost

of the additional equipment and the difficulty encountered by patients who are uncomfortable, or uncomfortably slow, using a computer. Therefore, at present, practices that invest in such technology might find that a significant majority of their patients cannot successfully use direct computer entry. They must provide office personnel to give individual assistance in completing the forms on the computer, or they must provide an alternative approach for patients who are not as familiar with computers (eg, providing a digital pen or paper forms from which data can be entered by staff later).

Data Entry Tool 8: Internet Portal for Patients to Enter Their Data

This tool extends direct data entry by patients beyond the office waiting room, allowing them to enter their personal information over the Internet through a secure portal. Patients comfortable with using computers and the Internet will be able to enter the same scope of data described for tool 7 while at home or in another location before their office visit.

Advantages of an Internet Portal

In addition to allowing patients the option of entering all the necessary information before they go to the office for an appointment, the Web portal provides additional opportunities for communication between the practice and its patients. It can provide information about the physicians and staff, practice policies, payment responsibilities, and preparation for diagnostic tests and procedures. Additional options include making available information about particular diseases treated by the practice and their management. Some practices are now using portals for secure e-mail communications from patients with inquiries about their medical conditions and replies from physicians.

Disadvantages of an Internet Portal

This approach introduces added cost for the maintenance of the Web portal. It also confronts the reality that a majority of patients will be uncomfortable using this approach or will prefer not to invest their personal time to perform tasks related to a medical visit.

FUNCTIONALITY AND PROTOCOL

The *Practical EHR* methodology includes the application of two principles for EHR functionality that are needed to help physicians integrate E/M documentation and coding into patient care and the medical diagnostic process:

- Assessment of the NPP must be included as part of E/M services. This consideration allows the physician's judgment to determine the appropriate levels of patient care and, subsequently, to ensure that the levels of documentation and coding reflect this care.

- Error-proof functionality provides feedback in each section of the H&P to ensure that all documentation meets the compliance standards of Current Procedural Terminology (CPT®) coding and the Documentation Guidelines.

Practical EHR Method

The *Practical EHR* method follows the *Practical E/M* method, which builds compliance principles into the traditional diagnostic and therapeutic approach physicians learn for providing quality patient care. Experience has proven it is impractical and unsuccessful to rely on physicians to memorize and apply the large sets of CPT rules and Documentation Guidelines while providing E/M care. An EHR that does not successfully address E/M compliance will not effectively serve physicians or patients. It also fails to meet current Certification Commission for Healthcare Information Technology (CCHIT) functionality guidelines that require an EHR "to have the ability to select an *appropriate* [italics added] CPT Evaluation and Management code based on data found in a clinical encounter,"[8] because appropriate codes must include consideration of medical necessity. Therefore, to assist and guide physicians in this process, the electronic H&P must incorporate on-screen documentation prompts that guide the provision and documentation of care at the level warranted by the NPP.

This protocol calls for obtaining a comprehensive medical history during every patient visit to obtain a complete picture of the patient's current health and provide the insight needed to reasonably assess the NPP. At this point, an NPP documentation prompt, illustrated in Table 11.2, helps physicians make an initial determination of the severity of the patient's problems and the level of E/M care warranted by that severity of illness. On completion of this step, physicians know (with the help of additional documentation prompts) the *medically indicated* level of physical examination and complexity of MDM that must be performed and documented to meet or exceed quality and compliance standards. Physicians may, of course, reconsider the severity of the NPP on the basis of examination findings and medical test results, and that reconsideration is included in this protocol.

Focusing on the NPP in this approach puts concern for the patient at the center of E/M care, where it belongs. In addition, documentation and coding become an integral part of the process of providing care, not a set of

TABLE 11.2

Sample Documentation Prompt for the Nature of the Presenting Problem (NPP) for the Initial Outpatient Visit or Outpatient Consultation Service*

Level	Description
1. Self-limited or minor (level 1)	A problem that runs a definite and prescribed course, is transient in nature, and is not likely to permanently alter health status OR has a good prognosis with management/ compliance.
2. Low severity (level 2)	A problem in which the risk of morbidity without treatment is low; there is little to no risk of mortality without treatment; full recovery without functional impairment is expected.
3. Low to moderate (level 2)	A problem in which the risk of morbidity without treatment is low to moderate; there is low to moderate risk of mortality without treatment; full recovery without functional impairment expected in most cases, with low probability of prolonged functional impairment.
4. Moderate severity (level 3)	A problem in which the risk of morbidity without treatment is moderate; there is moderate risk of mortality without treatment; uncertain prognosis OR increased probability of prolonged functional impairment.
5. Moderate to high (levels 4 and 5)	A problem in which the risk of morbidity without treatment is moderate to high; there is moderate risk of mortality without treatment; uncertain prognosis *or* increased probability of prolonged functional impairment.
6. High severity (levels 4 and 5)	A problem in which the risk of morbidity without treatment is high to extreme; there is a moderate to high risk of mortality without treatment *or* high probability of severe, prolonged functional impairment.

*This prompt combines Current Procedural Terminology (CPT) definitions of the NPP and descriptors for each level of care. The midlevel CPT descriptors for "low to moderate" and "moderate to high" are not specifically defined in CPT coding. They were presented in *Practical E/M* by developing language that places the severity between low and moderate for the first intermediate definition and between moderate and high for the second.[3(p46)] administrative tasks performed after care is completed. Guiding physicians to use this approach and providing them with the proper tools to do so achieve one of physicians' most important goals for EHR adoption: it makes the "E/M problem" go away.

The Role of the NPP in "Crossing the Quality Chasm"

Among its conclusions in *Crossing the Quality Chasm,* the Institute of Medicine reports that "Employers—particularly the Leapfrog Group—are demanding adoption of technology to support quality, and will likely further expand their standards to encompass additional standards of quality and patient safety."[6]

It is reasonable to propose that a minimum threshold of quality requires that each patient receive at least the level of care warranted for the severity of his or her illness at the time of the visit, as indicated by the published compliance standards of the American Medical Association and its specialty societies. For EHRs to fulfill their quality mandate and ensure that physicians meet this standard of care, they must provide physicians with effective tools to consider (and document) the NPP at the point of care and to apply this insight as guidance for appropriate intensity of care.

There are two categories of prompts that designers can build into the electronic H&P record to provide this guidance for compliance and quality: passive and active.

Passive Guidance

Passive guidance places compliance criteria on the screen in the form of documentation prompts, and it relies on physicians to correctly interpret and follow that guidance. The prompts give physicians an analysis of the various levels of care that correlate with different severities of illness. In the physical examination template illustrated in Figure 11.3, the physician would have made an initial assessment of the NPP and level of medically indicated care before performing the physical examination. The documentation prompt, which is specific for the type of service being provided, is located at the bottom of the template. It advises physicians of the extent of examination that is medically indicated for each level of care. If, for example, the physician determined that the NPP was moderate, thereby warranting level 3 care, the documentation prompt informs the physician that it is medically indicated to examine and document 12 or more elements of the examination. Additional examples of prompts with passive guidance appear in Figure 7.2 (for the history of present illness) and Figure 11.1 (illustrating the data-ordered section of MDM).

Active Guidance

For physicians who enter data directly into a desktop or tablet PC, active guidance can supplement passive prompts for tracking the amount of care documented for those sections of the H&P that use graphic interface designs with check boxes. This functionality begins after the medical history is obtained, with the physician actively selecting the appropriate level of NPP from the type of prompt shown in Table 11.2. The software shares this choice with the active documentation prompts, allowing them to keep track of the level of care as the physician enters the documentation, check box by check box, providing visual reinforcement when the medically indicated level of care has been provided (or exceeded). As an example of the appearance of an active prompt, Figure 11.4 illustrates a design that uses a horizontal bar showing CPT criteria with a sliding element above the bar that moves to the right as check boxes are completed.

FIGURE 11.4

Example of an Active-Guidance Design for the Physical Examination Template Shown in Figure 11.3. A horizontal bar graph with a moving indicator at the top helps physicians visualize the level of care as it is performed and documented. The box with the asterisk corresponds to the severity of the nature of the presenting problem (NPP) the physician determined after obtaining the medical history, which can be adjusted at any time thereafter, depending on subsequent findings. The numbers in parentheses correspond to the elements of the examination for each level of care as identified in Figure 11.3.

NPP Minor (1-5)	NPP Low or low to moderate (6-11)	NPP Moderate* (12 or more)	NPP Moderate* to high or high (all major elements,1 of each minor)

There are multiple design options available for active prompts, and designers should exercise their creativity to make the designs logical and easy for physicians to interpret. In selecting the wording for these prompts, it is critical to indicate that the goal is to provide a *medically indicated* level of care; it is not documentation for the purpose of achieving a code level.

Error Proofing ("Poka-yoke")

The electronic H&P brings the potential for error-proofing functionality when physicians use one of the direct data entry tools. The software can incorporate the rules of the Documentation Guidelines to protect physicians from omitting details required for absolute compliance. For example, when the patient enters the PFSH and ROS components of the medical history, "to document that the physician reviewed the information, there must be a notation supplementing or confirming the information recorded by others."[1(p6)] In the PFSH sections, the patient is asked to provide details of all positive responses. The software can alert physicians to any positive responses that lack such details and call for the documentation of further information. Before allowing completion of this section, the software should require that every positive PFSH response with details be recorded. It should also require physicians to initial or electronically sign the screen to attest that they reviewed the information entered by the patient.

The ROS portion of the H&P calls for similar error proofing. In this section, patients check boxes if they have any listed symptoms or signs, but they are not equipped to offer appropriate medical details about their positive responses. The physician must use appropriate questions to elicit these details and then document the findings. Software functionality can ensure that physicians enter explanations into the narrative section for each symptom that the patient checked as positive. As in the PFSH section, before allowing the completion of the ROS, the software should require that the physician record details for every positive response. It should also require a physician signature to confirm that all patient-entered information has been reviewed.

Incorporating E/M compliance into H&P record design puts physicians onto the road to quality care by empowering the diagnostic process. Designs for usability, flexibility, and efficiency give physicians the freedom to drive on that highway at high speed and in any lane they choose. Error proofing can be considered the concrete "Jersey Barriers" that keep physicians from accidentally driving off the road. Incorporating this functionality brings an additional level of intelligence to documentation, ensuring compliance and encouraging adherence to the diagnostic process.

Introducing "Poka-yoke"

At the Fourth National Health Information Technology Summit in March 2007, Michael Barr, MD, vice president for Practice Advocacy and Improvement, American College of Physicians (ACP), discussed concerns and problems encountered by practices using current EHRs based on information gathered through ACP's Center for Practice Innovation. He also presented a partial "EHR wish list" of quality standards physicians require for the next generation of EHRs, including a number of principles central to *Practical EHR*: (1) multiple options for data entry, (2) appropriate data entry by personnel other than physicians, (3) standardized presentation for the data, and (4) guidance to address incomplete information (ie, error proofing).

Barr projected a slide titled "EHR—Poka-yoke" with a quote from Wikipedia. It explained perfectly the idea of EHR software having the functionality to keep physicians on course for care and documentation:

> "**Poka-yoke** (pronounced 'POH-kah YOH-keh') is a Japanese term that means 'fail-safing' or 'mistake-proofing'—avoiding (*yokeru*) inadvertent errors (*poka*) is a behavior-shaping constraint, or a method of preventing errors by putting limits on how an operation can be performed in order to force the correct completion of the operation. The concept was formalised, and the term adopted, by Shigeo Shingo as part of the Toyota Production System. Originally described as *Baka-yoke*, but as this means 'fool-proofing' (or 'idiot proofing') the name was changed to the milder *Poka-yoke*. An example of this in general experience is the inability to remove a car key from the ignition switch of an automobile if the automatic transmission is not first put in the "Park" position, so that the driver cannot leave the car in an unsafe parking condition where the wheels are not locked against movement."[7]

As the electronic H&P record is analyzed section by section in the remaining chapters of Part 3, the potential for incorporating poka-yoke error proofing is one of the central design themes.

Overview of the H&P Record Design Toolkit

Table 11.3 summarizes the various design and functionality tools presented in this chapter and how they apply to the electronic H&P record.

T A B L E   11.3

Toolkit Synopsis

Design tools	Tool	Usefulness
Interface	Graphic	CC, PFSH, ROS, Physical examination
		Data reviewed, data ordered
		Risk of presenting problem
		Risk of diagnostic tests
		Risk of management options
		NPP
	Narrative	Details of ROS positive responses
		HPI
		Details of abnormal examination findings
		Impressions, management options
Data entry personnel	Patient	Initial visit CC, PFSH, ROS
	Staff	Established visit update of PFSH, ROS
		Small portion of HPI
	Physician	Review and provide details of PFSH and ROS
		All other medical documentation
Data entry format	Tool 1, indirect writing only	Writing on paper, paper delivered or scanned; data entry operator inputs into computer
	Tool 2, indirect writing and dictation	Writing on paper, dictating into digital recorder; DEO for writing; transcriptionist for dictation
	Tool 3, dictation with voice recognition software	Direct entry of free text (short answers and narrative sections)
	Tool 4, active mouse entry	Rapid direct entry of check boxes in graphic sections, used with tool 7
	Tool 5, tablet PC	Mouse or stylus entry for check boxes and drop-down menus; keyboard or writing for free text
	Tool 6, digital pen	Writing on paper with direct transfer to computer
	Tool 7, keyboard and mouse	Mouse for check boxes and drop-down menus; keyboard for written text
	Tool 8, Internet portal	Patient access for entering history (and demographic) data from home or other site; also offers interactive communication with patients
Functionality *Practical EHR*	E/M compliance	Integrates NPP
Error proofing	"Poka-yoke"	Ensure all indicated care has been documented

Abbreviations: CC, chief complaint; DEO, data entry operator; EHR, electronic health record; E/M, evaluation and management; HPI, history of the present illness; NPP, nature of the presenting problem; PC, personal computer; PFSH, past, family, and social history; and ROS, review of systems.

SUMMARY

Practical EHR advocates that EHR designs should provide a complete spectrum of data entry options so that medical practices can satisfy the personal data entry preferences of all physicians while reaping the common benefits of electronic data storage and retrieval.

The data entry toolkit should allow only designs that, when used as intended, guarantee fully compliant documentation and promote quality care. The toolkit includes graphic and narrative interface designs, options for all allowed data entry personnel, and multiple possible data entry modalities. These tools can accommodate physicians who prefer to write their H&P reports (who can do so legibly), prefer dictation, and prefer direct data entry into the computer. The overall impact of this variety of choices is that, given these options, many physicians will select hybrid approaches that include some writing, some dictation, and/or some direct computer entry. The data input design should provide so much flexibility that physicians currently performing and recording a quality H&P will feel that the software is able to fit their personal documentation and practice style, not require changing them.

Data entry tools that meet compliance, quality, and usability standards include those listed in Table 11.4.

TABLE 11.4

Data Entry Tools

Data Entry Tool	Description
Indirect data entry	
Tool 1	Writing on paper, scanning for software entry by DEO
Tool 2	Writing on paper and dictating on recorder for entry by transcriptionist
Direct data entry	
Tool 3	Dictation and voice recognition software
Tool 4	Active mouse entry (used with tool 7)
Tool 5	Tablet PC
Tool 6	Digital pen
Tool 7	Keyboard and mouse for direct entry, including option of a kiosk for patients
Tool 8	Internet portal for patient entry of data from home or other site

Abbreviations: DEO, data entry operator; and PC, personal computer.

The key to effective and usable H&P record designs is building on functionality that includes the NPP as the CPT coding measure of medical necessity for E/M services, which allows physicians to focus on patient care as their central mission, while documentation and coding compliance become easily integrated into the process through the use of documentation prompts for guidance. This approach fulfills a primary physician goal of solving the E/M documentation and coding challenge.

References

1. American Medical Association, Health Care Financing Administration. *Documentation Guidelines for Evaluation and Management Services.* Chicago, IL: American Medical Association; 1997.

2. Friedman TL. *The World Is Flat: A Brief History of the Twenty-first Century.* New York, NY: Farrar, Straus and Giroux.

3. Levinson SR. *Practical E/M: Documentation and Coding Solutions for Quality Patient Care.* Chicago, IL: AMA Press; 2005.

4. Second executive order on health information technology. www.whitehouse. gov/news/releases/2006/08/20060822-2.html. Accessed June 26, 2007.

5. Levinson SR. Practical E/M Methodology. In: *Practical E/M: Documentation and Coding Solutions for Quality Patient Care.* Chicago, IL: AMA Press; 2005:49-56.

6. Committee on Quality of Health Care in America, Institute of Medicine. *Crossing the Quality Chasm: A New Health System for the 21st Century.* Washington, DC: National Academies Press; 2001:31.

7. Poka-yoke. http://en.wikipedia.org/wiki/Poka-yoke. Accessed February 2, 2008.

chapter 12

Design Solutions for the Medical History Component

The *Practical EHR* method recognizes the clinical value of obtaining a comprehensive medical history at the outset of every visit. This essential step gives physicians insight into a patient's overall health status and their current medical concerns, and both of these perspectives are needed to appreciate the nature of the presenting problem(s) (NPP) and to develop a rational differential diagnosis. Finally, any issues in the patient's health history (past, family, and social history [PFSH] and review of systems [ROS]) that the physician identifies as relevant for the current visit and/or future care should subsequently be identified in the diagnosis (ie, impression) portion of the medical decision making (MDM) section of the EHR. Physicians should also be able to carry these issues forward to a "patient profile" section of the EHR for permanent reference. By identifying all significant (acute and chronic) health concerns in the impressions section, the MDM documentation supports the NPP. From a quality care perspective, this information will be available for immediate reference during subsequent care. In addition, moving all *significant* issues to active consideration facilitates medical history updates of the patient's health status during future visits. This enables the MDM portion of each visit to be synchronized with the patient profile section in the EHR. Just as new medical problems are added to the profile for a complete record, resolved problems noted in the MDM should also be updated in the patient profile to reflect the change in status for that visit.

The compliance and quality requirements for the PFSH and ROS differ significantly between an initial outpatient visit and an established outpatient visit. There are also minor differences for inpatient and nursing home established visits. Therefore, the design features for these components of the medical history will be considered separately for different types of service.

CHIEF COMPLAINT, PFSH, AND ROS: INITIAL VISIT

The PFSH and ROS are the elements of the history that create the portal for physicians into the world of comprehensive patient care. These elements provide the setting of each patient's personal story. When physicians review these elements first, they are guided into a more holistic approach, appreciating the entire background picture as a foundation of the patient's health before delving into the problems leading to the current visit. Often, this background setting offers clues that provide insight into present health issues. At other times, the information directs attention to possible medical problems that, although unrelated, may be of equal or greater significance than the issues surrounding a patient's chief complaint (CC).

In terms of quality and compliance, obtaining and documenting a complete PFSH and ROS are critical steps in distinguishing comprehensive from problem-focused care. This medical history information also provides the insights that allow physicians to determine the nature of the full spectrum of the patient's problems, to derive accurate differential diagnoses, and to identify health issues warranting counseling and preventive services.

For these sections of the electronic history and physical examination (H&P) record, the Documentation Guidelines[1] has suggested the starting point for a design that is efficient and compliant. The Guidelines advise that physicians can obtain this information through the use of a questionnaire, which is completed by a member of the staff or by the patients themselves. It also adds the caveat (for error-proofing design) that physicians must supplement patients' positive responses with appropriate medical information and must confirm review of the negative responses.[1(p6)]

Physician efficiency is maximized for these subsections of the H&P record by designating patients, whenever appropriate, to record their own responses to selected questions. Using graphic interface designs that guide patients to provide *yes* or *no* responses and short answers to direct questions facilitates ease of documentation for patients and ease of review by physicians. Of course, the questions should be written in nonmedical terms for patients' ease of comprehension. Review of patient responses is extremely easy for physicians because they can immediately identify and focus exclusively on the positive responses. This design is so efficient that in the occasional case when all of the patient's responses are negative, the total physician time for reviewing a well-designed check-box interface (plus placing initials for confirmation of review) usually requires fewer than 30 seconds for the CC, the complete PFSH, and the complete ROS.

For compliance, quality care, and data integrity, it is critical for these designs to require patient documentation of a response to each question. For graphic interface tools that provide check-boxes for entry, this means the patient must enter information in one of the boxes adjacent to each question. *Practical EHR* rejects alternative design options that offer a list of choices, each with just a single check-box, accompanied by instructions to check only boxes with positive responses. Such designs will fail a compliance audit, and they fail to provide reliable clinical information because absence of documentation is not the same as active documentation. When fields are left blank, there is no way to ascertain if the response was really *No* or whether the patient did not read or understand the questions. In addition, when all responses are negative, the whole page is blank, and physicians do not know whether the patient even looked at the form.

Finally, all positive responses in these sections require additional detailed explanation. The PFSH design encourages patients to provide further information in adjacent free-text areas, and often these additional descriptions are sufficient. However, the staff or the physician should obtain and document any further information deemed appropriate. For the ROS section, each positive sign or symptom should be treated like a mini-history of the present illness (HPI), with questions about the onset, progression, and details of the problem. Therefore, rather than having the design direct patients to provide further details, it is important for physicians to make the appropriate inquiries and document further information in this section.

Goals for Design: CC, PFSH, and ROS

The goals for design of the CC, PFSH, and ROS sections of the EHR are shown in Table 12.1.

Chief Complaint (CC)

The *Current Procedural Terminology* (*CPT*®) coding system[2] and the *Documentation Guidelines for Evaluation and Management Services*[1] define *chief complaint* (CC) as "a concise statement describing the symptom, problem, condition, diagnosis or other factor that is the reason for the encounter, usually stated in the patient's own words."[2(p1)] This inquiry calls for a short answer from the patient, which a design template can elicit with a brief question on a computer screen or on a paper form. The CC is commonly located as the initial medical question, where it allows patients to start telling their history by recording the principal reason for the present visit.

TABLE 12.1

Design Goals for the CC, PFSH, and ROS Sections of an EHR

Goal	Design Features to Meet the Goal
Efficiency	1) Patient* enters data directly into computer or to data transfer medium (paper) 2) Use appropriate graphic interface options for patient data entry 3) Patient should elaborate on positive responses for PFSH section 4) Physician must review and may further elaborate on PFSH responses; must investigate all positive ROS responses; requires efficient documentation tools a) Brief descriptions of details for positive PFSH responses b) Narrative descriptions of details for positive ROS responses 5) Physician reviews and signs to attest review
Compliance	1) CC must be a short narrative by the patient 2) PFSH: Ask about at least one element of each of the three subcomponents a) Patient and/or physician must enter brief descriptions of details for positive responses 3) ROS: Ask about at least one element of at least 10 organ systems a) Physician must enter narrative descriptions of details for positive responses
Quality	1) PFSH: Include all pertinent questions to obtain a true comprehensive review appropriate for medical care in general and for physicians' specialty in particular (no added physician time to obtain) 2) ROS a) Include all organ systems and all pertinent questions (particularly detailed in physician's specialty) for a comprehensive picture of patient's health b) Each positive response calls for a mini HPI to assess signs and symptoms
Usability	1) Patient entry by writing on paper or using keyboard and mouse 2) Physician entry by writing, dictating, and/or using keyboard and mouse
Data integrity	Require individual documentation to indicate positive responses (no preloaded responses or multiple response capabilities) in all graphic templates
Error proofing	1) Requires documentation of details for each positive PFSH and ROS response 2) Requires physician signature attesting to review of CC, PFSH, and ROS

*When appropriate, ancillary staff may assist patients in entering responses.

Abbreviations: CC, chief complaint; HPI, history of present illness; PFSH, past, family, and social history; and ROS, review of systems.

Design for Compliance, Quality, and Efficiency

This section needs to ask a straightforward, open-ended question about why the patient is seeking medical attention. Because it asks the patient to provide a concise free-text response, the design must consist of a small section of two or three blank lines that follow the inquiry. This question must use everyday language patients can easily understand; it would be inappropriate to ask "What is your chief complaint?" Flexibility permits physicians to enter their own choice for an inquiry. Personal experience over many years has found consistent success by having the paper or electronic form ask "What problem(s) are you here for today?" Patients readily understand this question, and they generally respond to it with brief, direct answers. In addition, this phrasing also invites patients to list more than one problem, which ensures that the physician is aware of all of their active concerns. Figure 12.1 illustrates the fundamental design requirement for the CC as it might appear on an electronic screen and a comparable paper transfer medium.

FIGURE 12.1

Template for Recording the Chief Complaint (CC). Short-answer type of graphic interface design for the chief complaint for an electronic format (A) and a paper format (B).

A

> **Chief Compliant: What problem(s) are you here for today?**
>
> Cough, check up on diabetes

B

> **What problem(s) are you here for today?**
> *Cough, check-up on diabetes*

Past Medical History

The *CPT* codebook describes *past medical history* as "a review of the patient's past experiences with illnesses, injuries, and treatments that includes significant information about:

- Prior major illnesses and injuries
- Prior operations
- Prior hospitalizations
- Current medications
- Allergies (eg, drug, food)
- Age-appropriate immunization status
- Age-appropriate feeding/dietary status"[2(p3)]

Design for Compliance, Quality, and Efficiency

The Documentation Guidelines advise that physicians can fulfill the requirement for a "complete" PFSH by documenting "at least one specific item from each of the three history areas"[1(p9)] (ie, past medical history, family history, and social history). Of course, most physicians do not believe that asking just one question in each of these subsections (eg, "Do you have any allergies?") meets the definition of being *complete*, contributes adequately to obtaining a *comprehensive* medical history, or, most important, meets the requirements for providing optimal medical care. Although this minimum requirement might meet the E/M compliance criterion for a "complete" PFSH, *Practical EHR* recommends obtaining a thorough PFSH that satisfies physicians' own quality standards.

Compliance Is a Beginning, Not an End

Providing designs that incorporate all of the past medical history information physicians want into a template that elicits and records this information is a prime example of the fact that fulfilling compliance requirements is only the starting point for an intelligent EHR design. Compliance requirements provide a foundation on which physicians are able to build additional inquiries based on their professional and personal standards for quality care.

Data entry capabilities must allow patients and staff to enter information comfortably into each of the several subsections of the past medical history form, paper or electronic. These need to combine appropriate check-box templates and brief free-text sections, as illustrated in Figure 12.2. The critical

F I G U R E   12.2

Sample Design for Past Medical History Portion of the Record. Sample graphic design combining short-answer, free-text sections (allergies, operations, and medications) with a check-box template (past experience with medical illnesses). Patients are asked to complete details for the medical illnesses checked as *Yes* in the lines next to and/or below the check-boxes; physicians must review these responses and document further details as appropriate. Paper and electronic forms should have comparable appearance.

What problems are you here for today?	List any allergies to medications:
(chief complaint section)	

Past Medical History

1) Please check "Yes" or "No" to indicate if you have any of the following illnesses; for "Yes" answers, please elaborate.

	Yes	No			Yes	No	
Diabetes	☐	☐	_____	Stomach problems	☐	☐	_____
High blood pressure	☐	☐	_____	Allergies	☐	☐	_____
Thyroid problems	☐	☐	_____	Kidney problems	☐	☐	_____
Heart disease/cholesterol problems	☐	☐	_____	Neurologic problems	☐	☐	_____
Respiratory problems	☐	☐	_____	Other diagnoses	☐	☐	_____
Bleeding disorder	☐	☐	_____				

2) Please list any operations (and dates of surgery) you have ever had

3) Please list any current medications (including amounts and times taken per day)
(include aspirin, antacids, vitamins, hormone replacement, birth control, herbal supplements, and over-the-counter medications of any kind.)

factor for usability and flexibility requirements is that the graphic interface design of the past medical illnesses portion of the design must be completely customizable, inviting physicians to list the diseases they want included in medical records.

Social History

The CPT coding system describes the *social history* as "an age-appropriate review of past and current activities that include significant information about:

- Marital status and/or living arrangements
- Current employment
- Use of drugs, alcohol, and tobacco
- Level of education
- Sexual history
- Other relevant social factors"[2(p3)]

Designs for this section must accommodate full flexibility to permit questions that are appropriate for the medical specialty, the patient's age, and the physician's personal preferences.

Design for Compliance, Quality, and Efficiency

As described for the past medical history, the Documentation Guidelines require notation of only one item from the social history to contribute to the requirements for a complete PFSH. The graphic interface illustrated in Figure 12.3 shows that the design needs to allow for check-box *Yes* and *No* responses and short-answer explanations from patients, which can be supplemented by the physician. This section must also be completely customizable so that physicians can choose the type of social history information they want to obtain from patients. Pediatricians, for example, will commonly select significantly different questions from those selected by an internist, and an infectious disease specialist will likely want to inquire about a variety of environmental factors different from those of interest to an occupational disease specialist.

FIGURE 12.3

Sample Design for the Social History Portion of the Record. This sample template combines check-box and short-answer data entry options. Patients are asked to complete details for the situations marked *Yes* in the lines next to and/or below the check-boxes; physicians must review these responses and document further details as appropriate.

Social History:	Yes No	Please list details below:
Do you use tobacco?	☐ ☐	List type and how much: _____
If no, did you use it previously? When did you quit?	☐ ☐	List type and how much: _____
Do you drink alcohol?	☐ ☐	List type and how much: _____
Do you use recreational drugs?	☐ ☐	List type and how much: _____
What is your occupation and working conditions? _____		

Family History

The CPT codebook describes the *family history* as "a review of medical events in the patient's family that includes significant information about:

■ The health status or causes of death of parents, siblings, and children

■ Specific diseases related to problems identified in the CC or HPI, and/or ROS

■ Diseases of family members that may be hereditary or place the patient at risk[2(p2)]

The design of the family history portion of the EHR must also accommodate full flexibility to permit questions that are appropriate for the medical specialty, the patient's age, and the physician's personal preferences.

Design for Compliance, Quality, and Efficiency

The Documentation Guidelines require notation of only one item from the family history to meet the requirements for a complete PFSH. The graphic interface for the sample family history template illustrated in Figure 12.4 shows questions related to health status or cause of death of

F I G U R E 1 2 . 4

Sample Design for the Family History Portion of the Record. This sample template incorporates CPT coding system recommendations and parallels the elements of the family history taught to medical students. It can be expanded and/or modified to suit each physician's personal preferences. When used in paper format, it should also include a signature box for physicians to attest their review of all sections of the CC and PFSH.

Family History

1) Please indicate the health status for each of the following close relatives, If deceased, list age and cause of death.

Father: _____

Mother: _____

Siblings: _____

Children: _____

2) Please check "Yes" or "No" to indicate whether any close relatives have any of the following illnesses. If yes, please indicate which relationship of individual(s) who have the problem.

	Yes	No	
Diabetes	☐	☐	_____
Allergy	☐	☐	_____
Cancer	☐	☐	_____
Heart disease	☐	☐	_____
Bleeding disorder	☐	☐	_____
Anesthesia problems	☐	☐	_____

	Completed by:	Reviewed by:

immediate relatives and a list of familial diseases that could have implications for the health of a patient. Designs should have the ability for expansion or constriction to meet individual preferences.

For all sections of the PFSH that permit data entry by patients, the Documentation Guidelines direct that physicians must add a notation "supplementing or confirming the information recorded by others."[1(p6)] In practical terms, this instructs physicians to review all patient documentation, address any positive responses that call for further detail, and provide a signature attesting to the review. Figure 12.4 provides a "Reviewed by" box that should be included for physician signature (or initials) when the practice provides patients (or staff) with paper forms for documentation and then scan the forms for indirect data entry by a data entry operator or provides patients with a digital pen for direct data entry. Paper forms usually have all three subcomponents of the PFSH on one page, which requires only one signature to confirm a complete review. Alternatively, the signature portion may reside on the electronic screen for practices using direct data entry tools such as a web page on a website or tablet PC.

Review of Systems (ROS)

The *CPT* codebook describes the *ROS* as "an inventory of body systems obtained through a series of questions seeking to identify signs and/or symptoms that the patient may be experiencing or has experienced."[2(p4)] It also identifies 14 organ systems that may be investigated and indicates that the value of this review is that is helps physicians "define the problem, clarify the differential diagnosis, identify needed testing, or serves as baseline data on other systems that might be affected by any possible management options."[2(p4)]

Design for Compliance, Quality, and Efficiency

The Documentation Guidelines advise that to perform a complete ROS, there must be a review of at least 10 of the 14 organ systems. Because the Guidelines do not list a minimum requirement for the number of inquiries per organ system, it seems that achieving a complete ROS requires documentation of responses to at least one question asked concerning signs and symptoms in each of the 10 or more organ systems. However, the Documentation Guidelines implies the appropriateness of more extensive inquiries for "those systems with positive or pertinent negative responses."[1(p8)]

A common error in ROS record design is inclusion of questions related to specific diagnoses rather than signs or symptoms (eg, "Do you have heart failure?") Such questions are appropriate for the past medical history, but they do not qualify as elements of the ROS. A common error committed by physicians is in assuming that an inquiry about associated signs and symptoms documented in the HPI may be considered as satisfying the documentation requirements for the ROS. Although the Documentation Guidelines state that "the CC, ROS, and PFSH…may be included in the description of the history of the present illness,"[1(p6)] the same inquiries are not counted twice; the *associated signs and symptoms* that are related to the presenting problem are elements of the HPI, while only the symptoms that are unrelated to the HPI are considered part of the "inventory of body systems"[1(p8)] that comprises the ROS.

For purposes of compliance, to achieve a complete ROS the Documentation Guidelines require that all of the questions relating to the 10 or more organ systems must be asked. While the Guidelines allow some of the information to be documented as "all other systems negative," this documentation shortcut is permitted only when the physician has documented responses for all systems that have positive and "pertinent negative responses."[1(p8)] Unfortunately, compliance reviews repeatedly demonstrate that physicians who use this documentation shortcut almost invariably document only responses related to the system directly involved with the present illness, overlooking several related systems that require complete documentation of responses to pertinent questions. For example, if the CC is cough, most physicians using this shortcut generally document only questions related to the respiratory system and report all others as negative. However, for compliance and quality, at least 10 systems must be investigated, and individual responses should be documented for all *pertinent* "systems," which in this example include not only the respiratory system, but also eyes, ears, nose, mouth, and throat; cardiovascular; gastrointestinal; allergic/immunologic; constitutional; and psychiatric. These systems are pertinent because medical problems in any of them could cause or contribute to the patient having a cough.

To avoid such challenges and compliance pitfalls, *Practical EHR* recommends that the medical record design incorporate multiple questions in all systems specified by the *CPT* codebook and allow the patient to fill in the *yes* or *no* check-box answers for each one. This approach avoids concerns about considering elements documented in the HPI section, bypasses the need for the all-others-negative option, and guarantees compliant documentation for this section. It is also clinically helpful for physicians to be able to refer to a previous record and confirm which questions elicited negative responses.

Using a graphic interface design, as shown in the example in Figure 12.5, provides an efficient documentation mechanism for patients and allows physicians to make a rapid review of the responses. The template design must also permit physicians to customize the questions listed.

Quality care and compliance mandate that a physician address all positive patient responses. In addition to check-boxes for *yes* and *no* responses, the sample template in Figure 12.5 includes a third check-box, labeled *Current*, which allows patients to identify positive responses that relate to the CC. This extra box assists the reviewing physician by indicating that he or she can defer detailed questioning on current symptoms until the HPI is obtained. However, all positive signs and symptoms that are unrelated to the HPI require individual investigation. Each of these becomes a mini-HPI, with screening questions performed and documented by the physician (in a narrative section located next to each symptom or, as shown, in a free-text box beneath the check-box section). Each positive response offers an opportunity for providing meaningful care. If a patient with a CC of an ankle injury gives a positive response to the ROS inquiry about chest pain, the physician must ascertain whether this is a stable and established problem under appropriate medical supervision or if it is a new problem that warrants routine, urgent, or emergency evaluation.

FIGURE 12.5

Sample Design for the ROS Portion of the Record. This sample form shows a two column approach that is most appropriate for fitting all review of systems (ROS) questions on a one-page paper transfer medium. In this paper situation, it is suggested that for any boxes checked *yes* by the patient (and not also checked as current), the physician should write the descriptive term as a descriptive header in the narrative section and then add the details; eg, if the patient checks the *yes* box for cough, the physician should write or dictate the word "Cough" followed by the relevant history obtained. The corresponding EHR screen for the electronic form should have a similar appearance for consistency, ease of transferring information, and efficient review characteristics.

1) Please check "Yes" or "No" to indicate whether you presently have any of the following symptoms.

2) For any "Yes" responses, please check the "Current" box if this symptom relates to the reason for your visit today.

Category	Symptom	Yes	No	Current	Symptom	Yes	No	Current
General	Chills	☐	☐	☐	Weight loss or gain	☐	☐	☐
	Fatigue	☐	☐	☐	Daytime sleepiness	☐	☐	☐
Allergy	Sneezing fits	☐	☐	☐	Environmental reaction	☐	☐	☐
Neurology	Headache	☐	☐	☐	Weakness	☐	☐	☐
	Passing out	☐	☐	☐	Numbness, tingling	☐	☐	☐
Eye	Eye pain/pressure	☐	☐	☐	Vision changes	☐	☐	☐
	Watery/itchy eyes	☐	☐	☐				
Ear, nose,	Hearing loss	☐	☐	☐	Dizziness	☐	☐	☐
	Nasal congestion	☐	☐	☐	Sinus pressure/pain	☐	☐	☐
	Hoarseness	☐	☐	☐	Neck lump	☐	☐	☐
	Throat clearing	☐	☐	☐	Throat pain	☐	☐	☐
Respiratory	Cough	☐	☐	☐	Coughing blood	☐	☐	☐
	Wheezing	☐	☐	☐	Shortness of breath	☐	☐	☐
Heart	Chest pain	☐	☐	☐	Palpitations	☐	☐	☐
	Ankle swelling	☐	☐	☐	Waking up short of breath	☐	☐	☐
Gastrointestinal	Difficult swallowing	☐	☐	☐	Heartburn	☐	☐	☐
	Abdominal pain	☐	☐	☐	Nausea/vomiting	☐	☐	☐
	Bowel irregularity	☐	☐	☐	Rectal bleeding	☐	☐	☐
Genitourinary	Frequent urination	☐	☐	☐	Painful urination	☐	☐	☐
	Blood in urine	☐	☐	☐	Prostate problems	☐	☐	☐
Blood; lymph	Swollen glands	☐	☐	☐	Sweating at night	☐	☐	☐
	Bleeding problems	☐	☐	☐	Easy bruising	☐	☐	☐
Endocrine	Feel warmer than others	☐	☐	☐	Feel cooler than others	☐	☐	☐
Musculoskeletal	Joint aches	☐	☐	☐	Muscle aches	☐	☐	☐
Skin	Rash	☐	☐	☐	Hives	☐	☐	☐
	Itching	☐	☐	☐	Skin or hair changes	☐	☐	☐
Mental health	Depression	☐	☐	☐	Anxiety or panic	☐	☐	☐

List any other symptoms or medical concerns:

☐ Details dictated | Reviewed by:

> **Triage**
>
> When a patient responds *yes* to the ROS inquiry about chest pain, the physician's primary responsibility is to determine the potential for this patient to have a serious health problem, before evaluating the patient's CC, eg, ankle injury or ear pain. Asking the patient several directed questions will allow any physician to determine whether the chest pain is a long-standing symptom that is currently managed by the patient's physician or a new or exacerbated problem warranting current intervention.
>
> If the chest pain is of sufficient concern, the visit should be interrupted in favor of arranging for immediate transportation to the office of the patient's physician or to the emergency department. Care for the CC can be deferred.

The narrative section also provides physicians the added benefit of combining multiple positively-indicated (checked *yes*-boxes) symptoms from several organ systems into a meaningful mini-HPI, thus allowing them to explore the multiple and related manifestations of a single illness. For example, if the graphic section illustrated in Figure 12.5 were to demonstrate positive responses for 1) *fatigue* and *weight gain* in the General-section; 2) *feeling cooler* than others in the Endocrine-section; and 3) *dry skin* and *brittle hair* changes in the Skin-section, an astute physician could combine these findings in the narrative section and then consider additional relevant questions that could lead to a possible diagnosis of hypothyroidism.

The ROS template is a section of the electronic H&P record in which creative design can clarify the documentation and introduce error proofing. In designs that locate the narrative section beneath the graphic interface, any positive check-box response that is unrelated to the HPI (ie, the *Current* box is not also checked) should automatically generate a matching header in the free-text area. For example, when the *yes* box is checked for cough, the computer screen should automatically show COUGH in the free-text area. For error proofing, the software should guide the physician to this narrative section and remind or require (as the practice elects) that some amount of descriptive information be entered before the physician can proceed to the next positive response. Each positive check-box response should have some descriptive entry before the software permits the physician to sign the section and proceed to the final portion of the medical history (the HPI), unless the physician choose to override this compliance and quality protection.

Medical practices may also provide patients an option for direct entry of the ROS through the use of a kiosk in the office, a tablet PC, or a Web portal. In these cases, the screen design for the form may provide a single column of questions with scrolling functionality. As the patient checks the *yes* boxes, the software can create a matched header for the physician in the free-text area, unless the patient also checked the *Current* box.

PFSH AND ROS: FOLLOW-UP VISITS

For promoting quality care through a realistic assessment of the NPP during each encounter, *Practical EHR* recommends a *complete* PFSH and a *complete* ROS for established patient visits, just as for initial visits. The Documentation Guidelines facilitate optimal efficiency for this effort by permitting the patient or a physician's clinical staff member to document this information.

A variety of software design options are available for obtaining and documenting this updated information compliantly and efficiently albeit several have certain intrinsic weaknesses. One conventional option is to have patients complete another comprehensive PFSH and ROS questionnaire (paper or electronic) at every return visit. However, this option becomes tedious and time-consuming for patients and physicians. It is repetitious for patients, while physicians must again review all the same positive responses to ascertain if there has been any change in the status of each positive symptom; eg, it is necessary to find out if the patient's headache may have become much worse. A second option is to show patients the responses from their initial visit and ask them to indicate any changes since that visit. This approach also creates significant paperwork and additional time when practices provide patients with copies of old documents and new paper forms. It may work better when the patient is directly reviewing and entering data into the software at a kiosk or using a tablet PC, particularly if the electronic screen can allow the patient to indicate for each persisting symptom whether it has also changed in character.

The Documentation Guidelines offer an alternative approach to repeating the extensive questions used during initial patient visits, which is highly effective and efficient for physicians and patients. It suggests that, "A ROS and/or a PFSH obtained during an earlier encounter does not need to be re-recorded if there is evidence that the physician reviewed and updated the previous information."[1(p6)] This alternative for obtaining the complete PFSH and ROS during established patient visits recognizes that the importance of updating this background information is to determine whether significant new health concerns have developed since the patient last visited this physician's office. It relies on physicians obtaining a complete PFSH and a complete ROS at the time of the patient's initial visit, ie, if the physician documented a low-level "pertinent" PFSH and ROS during the initial visit, an update of "no change" in that history results in a low-level "pertinent" update. This approach also requires that the physician has listed all *significant* concerns as active issues in the MDM section of the record during previous visits.

With this foundation, *Practical EHR* suggests that a most effective approach to the PFSH and ROS during follow-up visits is to have the physician or a member of the clinical staff ask the patient at the beginning of a visit whether there has been any significant change in the patient's general health since the previous visit. Because all active problems from previous visits are already identified in the record and will be addressed during the HPI, this inquiry enables the physician to learn whether any aspect of the patient's health that was previously normal has become a problem.

The Importance of Asking the Right Questions

Most physicians recognize that if patients are simply asked "Has there been any change in your health since you were here 2 months ago?" most of the time, the answer will be *No*, because the patient does not know the type of information being sought. Using more directed questions, which include examples of the type of information considered medically relevant, will more frequently result in appropriate responses. Physicians can then pursue the details of such changes to update the patient's health picture. For example, a patient could be asked: "Mr X, since you were here on May 2, have you had any changes in your general health, such as a visit to a doctor's office or the hospital, a new diagnosis, or a change in your medications?" After the patient's response, the follow-up question is: "Have you had any new health symptoms, such as chest pain, shortness of breath, or severe headache?" It is often helpful to review the patient's complete medication list as it is easy to forget changes in type or dosage.

With this guidance, patients can provide critically important health information that affects their care. The information can be helpful to specialists and consultants in the care they provide and also in directing patients back to their primary physicians for problems unrelated to the specialty practice. One of the common

continued

benefits of this inquiry is discovering that the introduction of a new medication correlates with the onset of the new symptoms that is the reason for a patient's visit. This knowledge can lead to an immediate probable answer for the patient's concerns and may also save the time and cost of more extensive evaluations.

Designs of EHR systems can incorporate questions that allow the clinical staff to easily obtain and document this information. Although designs could also guide patients to provide this information in structured templates (electronic or paper), my own experience strongly suggests that having a physician or clinical staff member ask these questions proves more efficient and effective for obtaining meaningful information.

Design for Compliance, Quality, and Efficiency

The first two design options considered for updating the PFSH and ROS rely on reusing or reviewing and modifying the appropriate forms illustrated in Figures 12.2 through 12.5. The Documentation Guidelines instructs about the compliance requirements for the "update" approach, indicating "the review and update may be documented by: describing any new ROS and/or PFSH information or noting there has been no change in the information; and noting the date and location of the earlier ROS and/or PFSH."[1(p6)] Because a follow-up visit always references information from the patient's previous visit to the physician's office, the location of the previous visit is intrinsically obvious. The design for this update needs to include a fill-in-the-blank for the date of the previous visit. For added quality, specific documentation of the patient's current list of medications and allergies can prove beneficial because patients find it challenging to recall all medication changes. Furthermore, identifying medication and allergy changes allows the update of a patient profile section, which is helpful at the end of the visit for safely prescribing additional medications without risk of allergic response or drug-drug interactions. Figure 12.6 illustrates a data entry design that can be used for the type of update described in the Documentation Guidelines.

FIGURE 12.6

Sample Design for Updating the PFSH and ROS in the Electronic Record. This sample form presets the condition that there has been "no change" since the date of the previous visit, and it requires the physician or staff member to enter that date. It then provides a narrative interface, introduced by the word "except," for entry of free-text descriptions of any changes. FH indicates family history; PFSH, past, family, and social history; and ROS, review of systems.

PFSH: No change since last visit, date: ____/____/____ ☐ Details dictated
(including visits to physician office or hospital, new diagnosis, and/or change in medication)

Except _____

New allergies* _____   Existing allergies* _____

Current medications* _____

Reviewed by _____

ROS: No change since last visit, date: ____/____/____ ☐ Details dictated
(including symptoms such as chest pain, shortness of breath, headache)

Except _____

Reviewed by _____

*The sections of the PFSH update for documentation of new allergies, existing allergies, and current medications may be included for quality; they are not required for evaluation and management compliance.

Compliance Requirements for Different Types of Service
Although outpatient visits and home visits likely occur with significant time between visits, other types of established visits occur on a daily or relatively frequent basis. Logic dictates that although new signs and symptoms may occur at any time, changes in the PFSH are unlikely to occur on a day-to-day basis. Following this logic, the Documentation Guidelines provide that "for certain categories of E/M services that include only an interval history, it is not necessary to record information about the PFSH. Those categories are subsequent hospital care...and subsequent nursing facility care."[1(p9)] Therefore, a comprehensive history for these two types of established visit services (involving CPT codes 99231-99233 and 99307-99310) requires an update of only the ROS, not the PFSH.

Goals for Design: Update of PFSH and ROS at Follow-up Visits

The goals for design of the update of records for the PFSH and ROS sections of the EHR are shown in Table 12.2.

TABLE 12.2

Design Goals for PFSH and ROS Updates in an EHR

Goal	Design Features to Meet the Goal
Efficiency	1) Staff or physician enters update information directly into computer or on data transfer medium (paper or recorder) 　a) Alternatively, may use a form for data entry by the patient 2) Appropriate use of narrative interface for entry of free text 3) Nurse or other clinical staff member obtaining a review places signature; physician also signs to attest review
Compliance	1) Update must include date of previous visit, documentation of changes or of "no change," and signature that physician has reviewed If use repeat of extensive initial visit forms, physician must review all questions, supplement positive responses, and sign to attest review
Quality	1) Indicating changes in general health provides a thorough picture of factors influencing the HPI and an opportunity to identify other issues as well 2) Physician obtains and documents details of any changes
Usability	Physician entry by writing, dictating, or using keyboard and mouse
Data integrity	All information relates to changes since previous visit (no copying or bringing forward of documentation from previous visits as if it were original information and the result of repeated inquiry)
Error proofing	Requires physician signature attesting to having reviewed the updated records

Abbreviation: HPI, history of present illness; PFSH, past, family, and social history; and ROS, review of systems.

HISTORY OF PRESENT ILLNESS (HPI)

Obtaining and documenting the HPI is the springboard for quality care, bringing to bear the physician's knowledge, experience, and insights. Particularly in more complex cases, knowledge of the multiple permutations of the natural course of various illnesses allows the use of creative questions that lead to differentiating one possible diagnosis from many others. The *Bates' Guide* defines the clinical focus of the *HPI* as a "complete, clear, and chronologic account of the problems prompting the patient to seek care."[3] This core clinical theme is echoed in the compliance criteria of the *CPT* codebook and the Documentation Guidelines, which both describe the HPI as "a chronological description of the development of the patient's present illness from the first sign and/or symptom (or from the previous encounter) to the present."[1(p7)]

The *Bates' Guide, CPT* codebook, and Documentation Guidelines also recommend inclusion, in the chronological history, of descriptions of eight characteristics of the principal symptoms: location, quality, severity, duration, timing, context, modifying factors, and associated signs and symptoms. (Note: The *Bates' Guide* describes seven characteristics but adds the eighth, "duration," as a subcomponent of timing.) It is an unfortunate consequence of the focus on "counting" to determine the intensity of a service that E/M compliance calculations, particularly those performed by EHR software coding engines, have almost exclusively concentrated on whether physicians have documented four or more of the eight elements (required to achieve an "extended" HPI rather than a "limited" one), often to the exclusion of considering whether they have, in fact, obtained and documented a chronological description of the patient's present illness (ie, an actual medical history).

Confining questions to the status of some of the eight elements present at the time of a visit creates a two-dimensional *snapshot* of the patient's status on that date, rather than a three-dimensional holograph of the course of the illness and the factors that have influenced it. *Practical EHR* returns the focus of the HPI to obtaining and documenting a chronological description of the course of each patient's illness, with secondary consideration of the eight elements. In other words, physicians must obtain and document a true *history* of the course of an illness. The electronic H&P record design should prompt physicians to trace the chronological course of the illness to satisfy criteria for quality and compliance.

Eliciting an HPI vs Taking a Snapshot

Physicians are taught that a quality HPI begins with a question about how and when the current problem began. As the patient describes the onset, a good physician will select guiding questions to determine the severity, location, timing, or other appropriate aspects of the beginning of the illness and will then inquire, "What happened next?" Proceeding step-wise from one significant event to the next, physicians are able to elicit a timeline of an illness and its effects on the patient and responses to any previous attempts at treatment.

In contrast to a true medical history, a report of a present illness that describes only some of the eight elements without describing the chronological course of the illness provides only a verbal *snapshot* of the patient's condition on the date of the visit. It lacks understanding of all the significant events that occurred between the onset and the visit.

Design for Compliance, Quality, and Efficiency

Documenting a true HPI requires a narrative interface design that provides physicians with a *clean slate* whereby free-text is used to record the individualized story of each patient's medical concerns. Depending on each physician's preferences, tool(s) for documenting a free-text history may consist of blank lines on a paper transfer medium, a blank dictation or voice recognition file, or typing into a free-text box on a computer screen. Regardless of the format, compliant designs should permit input of only patient-specific information; they should not include preloaded clinical information.

To help physicians obtain the "extended" HPI required to complete the recommended comprehensive medical history, the design for the HPI document should also include a *documentation prompt*, passive or active, that conveys the Documentation Guidelines requirements for the HPI. Each prompt needs to be specific to the type of service being performed. The elements of a meaningful prompt should include the following:

- A list of the eight elements of the HPI (because physicians should not be required to memorize the list)
- Guidance that reports the levels of care, based on the NPP, that are appropriate for a "limited" HPI, which records a "chronological description" and includes one to three HPI elements
- Guidance that reports the levels of care, based on the NPP, that are appropriate for an extended HPI, which records a chronological description and includes four to eight HPI elements
- Guidance that an alternative option for recording an extended HPI may consist of "the status of at least three chronic or inactive conditions"[1(p7)]

Going beyond compliance, *Practical EHR* recommends that to promote quality care, an extended HPI is appropriate for every visit. For seemingly straightforward and low-severity problems, this level of history confirms there are no underlying severe conditions and can be performed relatively quickly. For more complex conditions, a thorough HPI is essential for initiating the diagnostic process.

Protocol for a Fundamental Extended HPI

A reasonable and efficient basic extended HPI can be an effective starting point for illnesses that initially seem to be of low severity, providing sufficient detail to determine whether more extensive inquiry is indicated. This approach develops logically when initiating an HPI by inquiring when the problem began (establishing *duration*). The course of essentially every significant presenting symptom can be further clarified by learning the *severity* of the problem ("Is the symptom mild, moderate, or severe?") and its *timing* ("Is the symptom constant or intermittent? How long do individual episodes last? How much time passes between episodes?"). In addition, physicians almost invariably find it appropriate to inquire about *associated signs and symptoms* in every case. Investigating the time course of a patient's illness, while including at least these four characteristics of the HPI, creates a solid foundation for an effective HPI during the majority of patient visits. Beyond this, physicians' expertise will guide the depth and breadth of further questioning, including additional elements of the HPI (the remaining four elements are location, quality, context, and modifying factors) as indicated.

In creating the most efficient designs for this section of the record, it is important to appreciate that most of a physician's time in obtaining and documenting a high-quality HPI should be devoted to interacting with the patient. Many physicians who prefer writing are able to document the entire history as they obtain it, ie, their "additional" time for documentation is zero. For physicians who prefer to dictate their records at the conclusion of the visit, most contend that it takes relatively little time to record the HPI. Finally, although many physicians report that typing free-text information directly into the computer requires significantly more time and effort compared with writing and dictating, this option should be available for physicians who want to use the keyboard during or immediately after a patient visit.

As an option, EHR systems may facilitate a small amount of increased efficiency by permitting a member of the clinical staff to obtain and document selected preliminary information related to the HPI. Specifically, having a nurse or medical assistant ask for an overview of the duration, timing, and severity of the problem can start the patient thinking from a historical perspective and give physicians preliminary insight as they begin to obtain a detailed HPI.

Is it compliant for a nurse to obtain a portion of the HPI?

In the spring 2007, articles in the publication "Part B News" reported that the Centers for Medicare & Medicaid Services (CMS) raised the question of whether a nurse may obtain and document a portion of the HPI. While the Documentation Guidelines do not specifically state that ancillary staff may record the HPI (as they do for the PFSH and ROS), there is no clause that specifically prohibits the staff from performing this function.

From a compliance and quality perspective, physicians need to obtain the HPI because this information is essential for performing the diagnostic process. Nevertheless, reviewing preliminary information obtained by another health care provider as a starting point for a thorough HPI does not preclude the diagnostic process and/or violate CPT guidelines or Documentation Guidelines. Furthermore, the Documentation Guidelines state that assistants may obtain and record the ROS, and part of the ROS can include obtaining a mini HPI for any positive response (which physicians must later review and develop further as indicated). The matter that needs to be considered is if compliance permits a nurse to obtain and record the details of a patient's chest pain during the ROS, why would it not be equally appropriate and compliant for the same nurse to record preliminary information about a patient's CC of 2 days of a stuffy nose?

The question of staff recording portions of the HPI should clearly be stated and resolved by the CMS. In the future, if CMS officially incorporates this restriction as another noncompliant E/M policy, participating physicians will be advised to conform to this ruling. (At the time of this writing, I have no knowledge of commercial insurers adopting a similar position.)

Regardless of whether physicians obtain the entire HPI or build on preliminary information recorded by the clinical staff, electronic H&P record designs should guide physicians to obtain a true chronological timeline of the patient's illness, and they should provide data entry tools that make it quick and easy to document patient-specific information in the EHR. Figure 12.7 shows a sample of a simple narrative interface for data entry of the HPI. This sample design combines the ability for documentation of free-text with the additional feature of helpful documentation prompts.

FIGURE **12.7**

Sample Design for the HPI Portion of the Record. This sample form includes lines for documenting on a paper form (for example, using a digital pen) for physicians who prefer to write. On the computer screen, the design would simply provide a blank data field for entering free-text. Added features include a section (optional) for preliminary information obtained by a member of the clinical staff and documentation prompts to remind physicians about the chronological description, guidelines for the number of HPI elements associated with each level of care, and a list of the eight elements of the HPI. The chief complaint section is included only on established patient visits (because it appears separately on the form completed by patients during initial visits).

Present Illness	Chronology with: 1. One to three elements (level 2) 2. Four to eight or the status of elements or three chronic conditions (level 3, 4, or 5) or, the status of three or more chronic or inactive conditions (1) duration, (2) timing, (3) severity, (4) location, (5) quality, (6) context, (7) modifying factors, (8) associated signs and symptoms
Chief complaint	
(History from nurse)	
History from physician	

Goals for Design: HPI

The goals for design of the HPI section of the EHR are shown in Table 12.3.

TABLE **12.3**

Design Goals for the HPI Section of an EHR

Goal	Design Features to Meet the Goal
Efficiency	1) Narrative interface that promotes optimal speed for documenting a meaningful, individualized medical history through entry of free text 2) Clinical staff may obtain and document preliminary overview information*
Compliance	1) Documentation prompt guides obtaining a "chronological description" 2) Documentation prompt guides obtaining appropriate number of elements 3) Documentation prompt lists the eight elements of the HPI
Quality	Free-text entry encourages and facilitates documenting the individualized course of each patient's medical problems
Usability	Physician entry by writing, dictating, or using keyboard/mouse
Data integrity	Free-text narrative enhances documentation of each patient's individualized information
Error proofing	None

Abbreviation: HPI, history of the present illness.

*This option is currently under reconsideration by CMS, as noted in sidebar, "Is it compliant for a nurse to obtain a portion of the HPI?"

DATA ENTRY TOOLS AVAILABLE FOR THE MEDICAL HISTORY

Significant time savings are realized by having patients record the appropriate sections of their own medical histories, as permitted by the Documentation Guidelines. To optimize usability for patients entering their own information, EHR systems should provide effective options for patients to write directly on a paper template or to enter information directly into the software. The potential writing options offered may include scanning of the paper for entry by a data entry operator (tool 1, Chapter 11) or writing with a digital pen for direct transfer of an image and transcription into the EHR (tool 6, Chapter 11). The advantages of the digital pen include ease of use without training, lower cost than using data entry personnel, and immediate information transfer for availability to the physician in a digital format at the time of the visit. Although allowing patients to write directly onto a tablet PC (tool 5, Chapter 11) is a possible option, it may be a suboptimal choice. It is more costly, has a risk of equipment damage or theft, and requires patients to correct transcription errors made by the software, which would be slow and cumbersome with current technology and requires training for many patients.

Additional direct data entry options for patients include typing and mouse clicking at a computer terminal in the office (tool 7, Chapter 11) or via an Internet portal directly from home or another location (tool 8, Chapter 11). These options should prove effective for physicians and patients. However, they have higher initial and maintenance costs, many patients will find their use relatively slow and challenging, and, at present, a significant percentage of patients will require assistance using this option. It seems likely that for the foreseeable future, a majority of patients will prefer using a pen and paper to working with a keyboard and mouse, so physicians providing electronic entry tools will likely benefit by maintaining a direct or indirect writing option as well.

All physician entries in the medical history section of the EHR involve narrative descriptions. These descriptions range from brief explanations of details in the PFSH sections to mini-HPIs for positive responses in the ROS, to telling a detailed story of the presenting problems in the HPI. A basic premise of *Practical EHR* is that designs should provide writing tools for physicians who prefer to write, transcription tools for physicians who prefer to dictate, and (exclusively) compliant direct data entry options for physicians who want to enter data directly into the computer. Furthermore, each tool should be sufficiently easy to use that physicians may use a hybrid approach, combining two or three of the tools for different sections of the record. To provide this full range of tools, EHR companies need to include at least one of the data entry tools for each of the three data entry formats:

- Writing format
  - Writing on paper with scanning to a professional data entry person for synchronous or asynchronous entry into the computer
  - Digital pen
  - Tablet PC
- Dictation format
  - Dictating into a digital recorder with subsequent uploading to a professional transcriptionist for asynchronous entry into the computer
  - Dictating into a computer microphone for synchronous transcription by voice recognition software

- Computer format
  - Typing free-text into the appropriate sections of the medical history screens

FUNCTIONALITY OF THE MEDICAL HISTORY COMPONENT OF EHRs

Practical EHR Method

The *Practical EHR* method begins with the foundation of a *comprehensive* medical history for every visit. According to the CPT definition, a comprehensive medical history includes a CC, a *complete* PFSH, a *complete* ROS, and an *extended* HPI. The designs described in this chapter *automate* the first three of these components at the appropriate levels of care. For initial visits, the design requires patients to document their CC and a complete PFSH and ROS. During follow-up visits, the forms guide physicians or their clinical staff to obtain and document the CC and update the PFSH and ROS as the first steps of the visit. Because these designs intrinsically provide for the highest level of medical history for the first three components, they require no documentation prompts.

The CPT descriptors for the HPI differ for different types of service. Therefore, the office staff needs to identify the correct type of service at the start of each visit. They must enter this information into the software so that it can provide physicians with correct forms and documentation prompts. The type of service also guides the selection of the correct paper forms for patients and physicians using them as data transfer media.

For the HPI, EHR designs should add *documentation prompts* to the HPI section of the record to inform physicians of requirements for obtaining and documenting an extended HPI. *Passive* functionality provides these prompts on screen and on any paper documentation tools as illustrated in Figure 12.7. The option of *active* functionality would include additional documentation steps for the HPI section, requiring physicians to check up to three boxes to indicate when compliance criteria are met. The first box attests that the HPI includes a chronological description, the second attests that it includes four or more of the eight elements of the HPI, and the third indicates situations when physicians review the status of at least three chronic or inactive conditions instead of obtaining a conventional HPI. The design for a prompt executing this active functionality could have the following appearance:

> - HPI includes a chronological description and 1 to 3 elements of the HPI
> - HPI includes a chronological description and 4 to 8 elements of the HPI
> - HPI includes status of 3 or more chronic or inactive conditions

The software's coding engine would implement the following interpretations based on the boxes checked:

- All boxes unchecked: no HPI obtained
- First box checked: *brief* HPI obtained
- Second box checked: *extended* HPI obtained
- Third box checked: *extended* HPI obtained

Error Proofing

Medical practices using direct data entry, by keyboard and mouse and/or one or more of the direct data entry tools described in Chapter 11, can benefit from software designs that are able to detect areas of the medical history that have not been fully documented. The software should be able to assist with ensuring compliance by confirming that all appropriate sections of the medical history have been completed before permitting physicians to proceed to the next section of the record.

For initial visits, the software should identify any portions of the CC, PFSH, or ROS that the patient may have not completed, including answers to the *Yes* or *No* check-boxes and details for all positive responses in the PFSH. It should also confirm that the physician has provided some supplemental information for each positive patient response in the ROS. Error proofing should also ensure that the physician signs the *Reviewed by* box at the end of the PFSH section and the ROS section to attest to reviewing all patient-recorded information. Similarly, for documentation during follow-up visits, the software should require completion and signing of updates to the PFSH and ROS.

For medical practices that use indirect data entry through writing on paper forms and/or dictation (tools 1 and 2, Chapter 11), most data will be entered in the software after the time of the visit. In these circumstances, software error proofing can provide only delayed notification of incomplete sections of the record. If a physician subsequently completes the record, the software must identify all changes and additions by date and time. This delayed documentation might create potential compliance issues in case of an audit. Therefore, although it will be valuable for the software to alert physicians when such omissions occur when using these data entry tools, optimal error protection requires vigilance by physicians and staff to ensure that patients, staff, and physicians complete all appropriate portions of the record during each visit.

SUMMARY

A comprehensive medical history is the cornerstone of quality medical care. Without an effective PFSH and ROS, physicians are simply evaluating a CC, which is problem-focused care. Instead, understanding the entire scope of a patient's health background allows physicians to assess and treat the whole patient. This information marks the difference between just treating a lung and understanding the context of the overall health of a person who happens to have a respiratory complaint on the date of a visit. The additional medical history expands scientific analysis and adds the art of medicine to medical care. The comprehensive history is also essential for accurately determining the NPP, which is the key that allows physicians to solve the challenge of E/M compliance.

Software designs for the medical history component of the electronic H&P that can facilitate efficiency for obtaining and documenting a comprehensive medical history without a significant additional investment of physicians' time must also follow *CPT* principles for compliance and promote excellence for patient care. Achieving these combined goals calls for tools that allow patients and staff members to document the CC, PFSH, and ROS elements of the medical history. The choices for optimal documentation tools available to help patients perform this task include using paper forms matched to the corresponding software screens (ultimately entered by a professional data entry operator), digital pen technology, and direct keyboard and mouse options using an electronic kiosk, tablet PC, and/or Internet access.

Physicians require full flexibility for modifying electronic medical history screens to meet their practice preferences. Software designs should also provide multiple options for data entry, with at least one choice available for writing on paper, dictating, and entering data directly via keyboard or mouse for each section of the medical history.

Practical EHR functionality requires proper design of a combination of graphic and narrative interface elements to ensure obtaining and documenting the CC, a complete PFSH, and a complete ROS. Documentation prompts need to be included for the HPI section to provide guidance for obtaining and documenting an extended HPI. Software systems should also include error-proofing functionality that directs physicians to obtain supplementary clinical information for all positive ROS responses, provide details for positive PFSH findings that patients have not adequately explained, and complete the signature-boxes attesting to their review of information entered by patients and staff.

Combining these design and functionality principles allows physicians to have access to a comprehensive medical history for every visit in the most efficient manner possible while maintaining compliance and promoting effective differential diagnoses and accurate preliminary assessment of the NPP.

References

1.   American Medical Association, Health Care Financing Administration. *Documentation Guidelines for Evaluation and Management Services.* Chicago, IL: American Medical Association; 1997.

2.   American Medical Association. *Current Procedural Terminology (CPT®).* Chicago, IL: American Medical Association; 2007.

3.   Bickley LS, Szilagyi PG. *Bates' Guide to Physical Examination and History Taking.* 8th ed. Philadelphia, PA: Lippincott Williams & Wilkins; 2004:4.

Design Solutions for the Nature of the Presenting Problem

After obtaining an effective medical history, physicians have usually derived a probable differential diagnosis. At the same time, they have also developed a reasonable appreciation of the severity of the patient's medical problem. The amount and scope of clinical information available to physicians at this point in a patient visit is significantly more extensive than those conveyed by the vignettes that the *Current Procedural Terminology* (*CPT®*) manual[1] provides in Appendix C to illustrate the correlation between the nature of the presenting problem (NPP) and different levels of evaluation and management (E/M) services. The *CPT* manual emphasizes the importance of this assessment by advising that "Clinical examples of the codes for E/M services are provided to assist physicians in understanding the meaning of the descriptors *and selecting the correct code* [italics added]."[1(p1)] The need for including (and documenting) a judgment about the NPP during most E/M services is underscored by the fact that the *CPT* manual includes a description of the severity of the NPP for every type of E/M service that relies on performing and documenting the three key components (history, examination, and medical decision making).

INTEGRATING THE NPP INTO SOFTWARE DESIGN

Despite the recommendation in the *CPT* manual for physicians to use the NPP as guidance in determining the medically indicated level of care (as illustrated by the clinical examples), the traditional approach to teaching physicians about E/M documentation and coding has given little attention to this critically important "contributory factor,"[1(p2)] instead focusing almost exclusively on the three "key" components. It is probably as a result of this omission that nearly all current electronic health record (EHR) systems have failed to consider medical necessity (as determined by the NPP) into the design and functionality.

In contrast, the *Practical EHR* method calls for EHR software to incorporate tools (documentation prompts) that help physicians determine and report the severity of the NPP. It also recommends additional prompts that guide physicians to provide and document the levels of care warranted by the NPP. From a quality-care perspective, integrating medical necessity guidance into EHR design also helps physicians actuate the medical diagnostic process during patient care.

The *Practical EHR* Method Parallels CPT Instructions

Guidance in the *CPT* manual describes this two-step approach in its introduction to Appendix C. (1) For identifying the NPP and relating it to the appropriate level of care, the *CPT* manual states: "The Clinical Examples when used with the E/M descriptors [ie, descriptions of the severity of the NPP] . . . provide a comprehensive and powerful tool for physicians to report the services provided to their patients [ie, submit correct E/M codes]."[1(p437)] (2) After determining the level of care warranted by the NPP, physicians are next instructed that "the three key components . . . must be met and documented in the medical record to report a particular level of service."[1(p437)] In other words, once physicians determine the appropriate level of care, this information should guide the level of care provided and documented.

Because the *Practical EHR* method recommends a comprehensive medical history during every encounter to help physicians determine the severity of the NPP, this guidance for providing and documenting the medically indicated level of care applies to ensuring the appropriate extent of physical examination and the appropriate complexity of medical decision making.

Of course, the design of the history and physical examination (H&P) record must also permit physicians to reassess the severity of the NPP and appropriate level of care during the physical examination and medical decision making because examination or laboratory findings may alter clinical impressions. The physician may determine an increase in the severity of the NPP and the warranted level of care if more serious problems are revealed (eg, finding severe abdominal tenderness and guarding in a patient whose medical history suggested only viral gastroenteritis). Similarly, a physician may determine it is appropriate to lower the NPP and indicated level of care if findings rule out more serious problems (eg, finding absence of abdominal tenderness and guarding in a patient whose medical history suggested appendicitis).

The physician's final assessment of the NPP, which is documented by checking the appropriate box on the design template (Figure 13.1), occurs at the conclusion of an encounter, after the physician has completed documenting medical decision making. Because the *CPT* manual's definitions of the severity of NPP are subjective, active documentation of the NPP reflects the physician's professional determination of the severity of the patient's illness at the time of the visit. When this assessment is compatible with the history, examination findings, clinical impressions, and management plans, it provides powerful support for medical necessity to justify the level of care in case of an audit.

DESIGN FOR COMPLIANCE, QUALITY, AND EFFICIENCY

Integration of the NPP into electronic H&P record design is an innovative development that is essential for satisfying two of physicians' primary EHR needs: generating high-quality clinical charts and achieving compliant E/M documentation. The first requirement in attaining this goal is for software designers to create a screen that provides physicians with all the information they require to identify the severity of the NPP and the associated levels of care. The software designers must also include definitions of the two intermediate levels of NPP, low to moderate and moderate to high. The *CPT* manual uses these two descriptors frequently in describing the severity of

NPP associated with many levels of care, even though they are not specifically defined in the *CPT* manual. Implementing the definitions suggested in
Practical E/M is recommended:

■ Low to moderate severity: "A problem where the risk of morbidity
without treatment is low to moderate; there is low to moderate risk
of mortality without treatment; full recovery without functional
impairment is expected in most cases, with low probability of
prolonged functional impairment"[2]

■ Moderate to high severity: "A problem where the risk of morbidity
without treatment is moderate to high; there is moderate risk of
mortality without treatment; uncertain prognosis *or* increased
probability of prolonged functional impairment"[2]

NPP Sample Screens With Integrated Documentation Prompts

An effective design for the NPP part of the record must also include
documentation prompts, which will incorporate CPT coding guidelines
linking the level of the NPP to the level of care (E/M code) warranted by
the severity of the patient's illness for each type of service. As with the
three key components, *CPT*'s descriptors for the NPP vary for each type of
service. Therefore, EHR designers must customize the prompts on the NPP
screen to reflect the type of service (E/M) Figures 13.1, 13.2, and 13.3 illustrate

F I G U R E   13.1

Sample Design for Documentation Prompt for NPP, Outpatient Initial Visit. This form includes *Current
Procedural Terminology* (*CPT®*) definitions for the basic levels of the nature of the presenting problem (NPP)[1(p3)]
plus proposed intermediate-level NPPs. It also includes documentation prompts that link the severity of the NPP to
indicated levels of evaluation and management services (E/M), based on CPT descriptors.

	NPP Level	Indicated Level of Care	Problem Descriptor
☐	Minor	level 1	A problem that runs a definite and prescribed course, is transient in nature, and is not likely to permanently alter health status; *or* has a good prognosis with management and compliance
☐	Low	level 1	A problem in which the risk of morbidity without treatment is low; there is little to no risk of mortality without treatment; full recovery without functional impairment expected
☐	Low-moderate	level 2	A problem in which the risk of morbidity without treatment is low to moderate; there is low to moderate risk of mortality without treatment; full recovery without functional impairment expected in most cases, with low probability of prolonged functional impairment
☐	Moderate	level 3	A problem in which the risk of morbidity without treatment is moderate; there is moderate risk of mortality without treatment; full recovery without functional impairment expected in most cases, with low probability of prolonged functional impairment
☐	Moderate-high	levels 4, 5	A problem in which the risk of morbidity without treatment is moderate to high; there is moderate risk of mortality without treatment; uncertain prognosis or increased probability of prolonged functional impairment
☐	High	levels 4, 5	A problem in which the risk of morbidity without treatment is high to extreme; there is moderate to high risk of mortality without treatment, *or* high probability of severe prolonged functional impairment

FIGURE 13.2

Sample Design for Documentation Prompt for NPP, Consultation. This screen is similar to the outpatient initial visit; however, there is one difference in the documentation prompt (shaded) portion of the screen. For consultation visits, CPT descriptors indicate that when the nature of the presenting problem (NPP) is low severity, level 2 care is warranted as opposed to level 1 for initial outpatient visits.

	NPP Level	Indicated Level of Care	Problem Descriptor
☐	Minor	level 1	A problem that runs a definite and prescribed course, is transient in nature, and is not likely to permanently alter health status; *or* has a good prognosis with management and compliance
☐	Low	level 2	A problem in which the risk of morbidity without treatment is low; there is little to no risk of mortality without treatment; full recovery without functional impairment expected
☐	Low-moderate	level 2	A problem in which the risk of morbidity without treatment is low to moderate; there is low to moderate risk of mortality without treatment; full recover without functional impairment expected in most cases, with low probability of prolonged functional impairment
☐	Moderate	level 3	A problem in which the risk of morbidity without treatment is moderate; there is moderate risk of mortality without treatment; full recovery without functional impairment expected in most cases, with low probability of prolonged functional impairment
☐	Moderate-high	levels 4, 5	A problem in which the risk of morbidity without treatment is moderate to high; there is moderate risk of mortality without treatment; uncertain prognosis or increased probability of prolonged functional impairment
☐	High	levels 4, 5	A problem in which the risk of morbidity without treatment is high to extreme; there is moderate to high risk of mortality without treatment, *or* high probability of severe prolonged functional impairment

the information that should be included on NPP screens for the three types of office outpatient services, providing physicians with definitions for levels of NPP plus documentation prompts based on *CPT*'s E/M descriptors to help physicians identify the associated level of care. As recommended for all sections of the H&P record, the design of paper documents used as data transfer media should include the same information and should have the same appearance as the software screens to ensure effective data entry by digital pen or data entry professionals.

Other types of service call for appropriately customized NPP screens and documentation prompts. For some, such as initial hospital care (ie, inpatient admissions) and inpatient subsequent care visits, there may be fewer than five levels of care. Some types of service, such as inpatient subsequent care visits, substitute entirely different NPP definitions. Figures 13.4 and 13.5 illustrate sample designs for inpatient admission service and subsequent care visits, demonstrating the differences from outpatient office care. The screen design and documentation prompts for inpatient consultation services are identical to those for outpatient consultation services, shown in Figure 13.2. As designers create these special screens, it will be critical for them to carefully follow all CPT descriptors for each type of service and each level of care to provide physicians with accurate information they need to ensure compliant documentation. Appendix D provides a table that summarizes the CPT descriptors, correlating severity of NPP with levels of care

FIGURE 13.3

Sample Design for Documentation Prompt for NPP, Outpatient Established Visit. This form indicates the same definitions for severity of the nature of the presenting problem (NPP) as in Figure 13.1, with the addition of a definition for "minimal," which applies only to this type of service. CPT descriptors for E/M services require association of different levels of care for this type of service for minor, low, and low to moderate severity NPPs, as shown in the shaded documentation prompts.

NPP Level	Indicated Level of Care	Problem Descriptor
☐ Minimal	level 1	A problem that may not require the presence of the physician, but service is provided under the physician's supervision
☐ Minor	level 2	A problem that runs a definite and prescribed course, is transient in nature, and is not likely to permanently alter health status; *or* has a good prognosis with management and compliance
☐ Low	level 2	A problem in which the risk of morbidity without treatment is low; there is little to no risk of mortality without treatment; full recovery without functional impairment expected
☐ Low-moderate	level 3	A problem in which the risk of morbidity without treatment is low to moderate; there is low to moderate risk of mortality without treatment; full recovery without functional impairment expected in most cases, with low probability of prolonged functional impairment
☐ Moderate	level 3	A problem in which the risk of morbidity without treatment is moderate; there is moderate risk of mortality without treatment; full recovery without functional impairment expected in most cases, with low probability of prolonged functional impairment
☐ Moderate-high	levels 4, 5	A problem in which the risk of morbidity without treatment is moderate to high; there is moderate risk of mortality without treatment; uncertain prognosis or increased probability of prolonged functional impairment
☐ High	levels 4, 5	A problem in which the risk of morbidity without treatment is high to extreme; there is moderate to high risk of mortality without treatment, *or* high probability of severe prolonged functional impairment

FIGURE 13.4

Sample Design for Documentation Prompt for NPP, Initial Hospital Care. There are only three levels of care described for this type of service.

NPP Level	Indicated Level of Care	Problem Descriptor
☐ Low	level 1	A problem in which the risk of morbidity without treatment is low; there is little to no risk of mortality without treatment; full recovery without functional impairment expected
☐ Low-moderate	level 1	A problem in which the risk of morbidity without treatment is low to moderate; there is low to moderate risk of mortality without treatment; full recovery without functional impairment expected in most cases, with low probability of prolonged functional impairment
☐ Moderate	level 2	A problem in which the risk of morbidity without treatment is moderate; there is moderate risk of mortality without treatment; full recovery without functional impairment expected in most cases, with low probability of prolonged functional impairment
☐ Moderate-high	level 2	A problem in which the risk of morbidity without treatment is moderate to high; there is moderate risk of mortality without treatment; uncertain prognosis or increased probability of prolonged functional impairment
☐ High	level 3	A problem in which the risk of morbidity without treatment is high to extreme; there is moderate to high risk of mortality without treatment, *or* high probability of severe prolonged functional impairment

F I G U R E   13.5

Sample Design for Documentation Prompt for NPP, Subsequent Hospital Care. The subsequent care inpatient descriptors for the nature of the presenting problem (NPP) differ dramatically from those for outpatient office visits and initial evaluations. This template emphasizes the importance of screens providing accurate documentation prompts, based on CPT descriptors for each type of service. There are only three levels of care described for this type of service.

Nature of Presenting Problem(s)		
	Indicated Level of Care	Description of Usual Condition of the Patient
☐	level 1	Usually the patient is stable, recovering, or improving
☐	level 2	Usually the patient is responding inadequately to therapy or a minor complication has developed
☐	level 3	Usually the patient is unstable or has developed a significant complication or a significant new problem has developed

for each type of service that includes consideration of the three key components. This simplified table could serve as another effective model for EHRs (ie, EHRs that include a pop-up of *CPT* definitions for each level of NPP, if and when the physician clicks on the level-indicator).

Of note, the only types of service that currently use the special NPP descriptors shown in Figure 13.5 are subsequent hospital care visits (CPT codes 99231-99233) and subsequent nursing facility care visits (CPT codes 99307-99310).

Establishing the NPP as a Basis for Solving the Compliance Challenge

As discussed in Chapter 7, the two fundamental principles that can create major problems for medical practices in the event of an E/M audit by the Centers for Medicare & Medicaid Services or related agencies are:

- If a service (or a portion of a service) was not documented, it was not performed[3]
- "Medicare will not pay for services that are not medically necessary."[4]

The *Practical EHR* method recognizes that the converse of these statements is also true. Medicare will pay for services that are medically necessary, and when the level of medical necessity is documented, physicians attest that this assessment was done. Therefore, when the medical record establishes a reasonable assessment of the NPP that is consistent with the remainder of the documentation, it becomes the physician's judgment that establishes the degree of medical necessity, not an auditor's. When a physician has also properly documented the three key components (without the use of noncompliant EHR cloning tools, such as copy and paste and generic macros), an auditor's only option is to give the physician credit for compliant care and documentation.

> ### Auditors' Response to Compliant Documentation, Including the NPP
>
> A number of years ago, I had the opportunity to provide E/M audit training and tools to auditors for several Medicare carriers. Several months after completing their training, I returned to each carrier separately to verify their success and answer any questions. After completing the review, I asked the auditors to analyze charts with designs similar to those presented in this section of the book. They contained complete documentation, including all elements of medical decision making and documentation of the NPP. All auditors uniformly confirmed that these charts were absolutely compliant and could not be legitimately downcoded. Equally convincing was the fact that at each location, the auditors invariably asked the same follow-up question: "Why doesn't every physician use these medical record tools? It makes my job so much easier!"
>
> This is the type of compliance review physicians want to hear from a reviewer. This assurance of compliance achieves one of physicians' primary EHR goals, while also facilitating quality care. It is a primary reason for including the NPP as an essential component of EHR design.

DESIGN AND FUNCTIONALITY FOR PHYSICIANS WORKING WITH A PAPER DATA TRANSFER MEDIUM

Physicians who prefer not to perform direct keyboard data entry will be using a paper data transfer medium or a digital pen to write portions of their H&P documentation, with or without supplemental dictation. They will document their final impression of the NPP at the conclusion of each encounter, by checking the box appropriate for their assessment of the severity of the NPP. Therefore, this documentation section should be placed at the end of the H&P record, following the medical decision making section. However, physicians should first consider the NPP for reference after obtaining the medical history. Guidance to perform the preliminary appraisal of the severity of the NPP at this appropriate time may come simply with instruction and training or it may be guided by a reminder on the paper form located just above the physical examination section. This could convey a message similar to the following: "Reminder: Refer to the NPP Section for preliminary assessment level of care warranted by severity of NPP before performing the physical examination."

DESIGN AND FUNCTIONALITY FOR PHYSICIANS PERFORMING DIRECT DATA ENTRY

Software designers have a much greater opportunity for creativity in developing screens for the NPP. Even though the critical NPP documentation section with check-boxes will be placed as the final documentation section of each encounter, the software should be able to provide pop-up windows that open the NPP screen at appropriate times. For the most effective use of this information, a window should open with the NPP at the conclusion of the medical history, before the physician moves to the screen for documenting the physical examination. There should also be a function key or toolbar icon available to open this window at any time from the examination and medical decision making sections in case physicians want to review the NPP and reassess the indicated level of care.

Passive Guidance

For designs providing passive guidance, the pop-up windows should have an appearance similar to the screens shown in Figures 13.1 to 13.5, but with the check boxes inactivated at this stage. Physicians will refer to the screen after documenting the medical history and apply the guidance from the shaded documentation prompts when using the examination and medical decision making sections of the EHR. They should also have the ability to recall the pop-up window at any time for guidance and/or to modify the initial impression of the severity of NPP. In systems providing passive guidance, physicians need to be instructed that subsequent changes in their assessment of the NPP may call for reconsideration of the levels of physical examination and or the complexity of medical decision making that correspond to the medically indicated level of care.

Active Guidance

For designs providing active guidance, the pop-up windows should also have active check boxes. These NPP templates will require physicians to indicate their preliminary assessment of the NPP following documentation of the medical history. The software will have the functionality to transfer this information to documentation prompts that provide active guidance, such as the active prompt illustrated in Figure 11.6 for the physical examination. The software must have the ability for physicians to reopen these active screens so that they can modify initial assessments when indicated.

Active guidance introduces the potential for interactivity between the software and physician, not only with the design of the documentation prompts for physical examination and medical decision making, but also for feedback if an assessment changes. For example, if during an initial visit, the physician's preliminary assessment of the NPP is "moderate," the physician should appropriately provide a detailed examination. However, if review of the laboratory findings reveals unexpectedly abnormal results that lead the physician to conclude there is an increased severity of the NPP to "moderate to high," the software should alert the physician that the level of physical examination and medical decision making warranted by the NPP might have been affected by this change.

SUMMARY

Integrating the NPP into the patient care process serves two crucial roles for promoting quality care for every patient visit and ensuring E/M compliance. First, after obtaining a comprehensive medical history, preliminary assessment of the severity of the NPP enables physicians to follow CPT guidelines for providing and documenting medically indicated levels of care. Second, including documentation of the physician's final clinical judgment of the severity of the NPP at the end of the visit establishes the medical necessity for the level of care performed.

To meet physicians' EHR requirements, successful EHR software designs must incorporate NPP guidance and documentation tools into the H&P

record to ensure compliance and promote the diagnostic process. The content and appearance of these NPP tools on EHR screens and on paper transfer media need to be compatible to promote usability and flexibility for all physicians, regardless of the potential data entry formats used. After completing the medical history and making preliminary assessment of the severity of the NPP and indicated level of care accomplished, physicians can resume the normal sequence of completing the physical examination and medical decision making, while relying on the documentation prompts in those sections of the EHR to confirm that the amount of care provided and documented meets or exceeds the CPT guidelines for the severity of the patient's NPP. Documentation of the physician's final assessment of the NPP occurs at the conclusion of the visit.

References

1. American Medical Association. *Current Procedural Terminology (CPT®).* Chicago, IL: American Medical Association; 2007.

2. Levinson SR. *Practical E/M: Documentation and Coding Solutions for Quality Patient Care.* Chicago, IL: AMA Press; 2005:46.

3. Department of Health & Human Services; Centers for Medicare & Medicaid Services. "Examples of Situations in Which Physician is Liable." In: *Medicare Claims Processing Manual.* Part 3, Section 7103.1(I). Available at: www.socialsecurity.gov/OP_Home/ssact/title18/1862.htm#act-1862 Accessed July 1, 2007.

4. Social Security Online. Compilation of the Social Security Laws. Section 1862(a)(1)(a). www.socialsecurity.gov/OP_Home/ssact/title18/1862.htm#act-1862. Accessed July 1, 2007.

chapter 14

Design Solutions for the Physical Examination Record

At this stage of the diagnostic process, after analyzing the severity of the nature of the presenting problem (NPP) and the appropriate level of care for the current medical visit, physicians return to performing the physical examination. Physicians should be skilled at examining the body area(s) directly related to patients' medical concerns at the time of the visit. However, compliance and quality measures call for physicians to perform more than a problem-focused examination when the NPP is of low to moderate severity or greater. The medical record should guide them to provide and document the level of examination warranted by the NPP. To accomplish this, the design of the examination component of the history and physical examination (H&P) record must meet five important goals:

1. A data entry template customized for each physician's specialty and personal preferences
2. A design interface that permits maximally efficient documentation of normal findings in the unaffected or asymptomatic body areas and organ systems
3. A design that also facilitates efficient documentation of "specific relevant negative findings of the examination of the affected or symptomatic body area(s) or organ system(s)."[1(p11)] This feature addresses the Documentation Guidelines' instruction that "notation of 'abnormal' without elaboration is insufficient"[1(p11)] documentation for the symptomatic organ systems.
4. A documentation interface that facilitates descriptive narrative recording of the specific abnormal findings of the affected or symptomatic body area(s) or organ system(s) and "abnormal or unexpected findings of the examination of any asymptomatic body area(s) or organ system(s)"[1(p11)]
5. Guidance to describe the extent of examination warranted by the NPP

The first of these five goals satisfies H&P record requirements for usability and flexibility. Achieving the remaining four goals fulfills the requirements for compliance and efficiency. The final goal also reflects the need to include the NPP in guiding appropriate levels of care, while the other requirements derive directly from the 1995 and 1997 editions of the Documentation Guidelines.

DESIGN FOR COMPLIANCE, QUALITY, AND EFFICIENCY

The Documentation Guidelines[1] published in May 1997 extended and superseded the 1995 version. Most of the significant changes in the 1997 version apply to the physical examination component, including the introduction of "greater clinical specificity"[1(p1)] and changed documentation requirements for the general multisystem examination. The Guidelines also noted that "for the first time, content and documentation requirements have been defined for examinations pertaining to 10 organ systems."[1(p1)] (There are 11 single organ system examinations listed when the different examination templates for male and female genitourinary specialty examinations are separately considered.) It is important to note that "the content of these examinations was developed with the assistance of representatives from the specialties that frequently perform these examinations."[1(p1)]

Types of Examination Defined in the 1997 Documentation Guidelines[1]

1) General multisystem examination

Single organ system examinations

2) Cardiovascular
3) Ear, nose, mouth, and throat
4) Eyes
5) Genitourinary (female)
6) Genitourinary (male)
7) Hematologic, lymphatic, and immunologic
8) Musculoskeletal
9) Neurologic
10) Psychiatric
11) Respiratory
12) Skin

Under the 1995 Documentation Guidelines, the descriptions for levels of care duplicated the *qualitative* definitions in the *Current Procedural Terminology* (*CPT*®) manual. These descriptions included the terms *limited examination, extended examination,* and *complete examination of a single organ system* and they remain *subjective.* As a consequence, the 1995 Documentation Guidelines left physicians, consultants, and auditors without a uniform *quantitative* set of criteria for evaluating the levels of care for the physical examination. To avoid these problems, *Practical EHR* strongly recommends that physicians and software developers use the recognized *objective* standards in the 1997 Documentation Guidelines,[1] which provide a blueprint for designs that impart audit protection by meeting strictly defined compliance standards. They can then be further customized to meet physicians' individual preferences yet remain compliant. Furthermore, documenting on the basis of the 1995 guidelines, which lack specified examination elements, usually requires free-text to describe all normal and abnormal findings. In contrast, using the specified elements of the 1997 examination guidelines encourages the use of an effectively designed check-box interface that allows for a much faster documentation of all normal findings.

Components of the Examination Template

In medical school, physicians learn to perform and document a *comprehensive* physical examination, including positive and negative physical examination findings for every organ system. With increasing experience and expertise, they learn to perform the extensive levels of examination rapidly and effectively. Although almost all physicians acknowledge the importance of accurately documenting the details of all abnormal examination findings on the date of the visit, the challenge for EHRs and medical software engineers has been to provide data entry designs that allow rapid documentation of all normal findings without disrupting the flow of a visit. It is particularly time-consuming for physicians to use a narrative approach for documenting the details of normal examination findings, regardless of whether they type, write, or dictate the report. The specificity of the examinations described in the 1997 Documentation Guidelines enables EHR developers to create screens with the user-friendly *graphic interface*, which allows rapid documentation of normal examination findings and the abnormal findings that require further description. This graphic interface must also be combined with a narrative interface for physicians to record detailed descriptions of all abnormal findings.

Time Trials for the Physical Examination Section of the EHR

The documentation prompts included in the examination section guide physicians to provide the medically indicated level of care based on the selected NPP. The time needed to provide this care depends on the skills and habits of each physician. Similarly, the efficiency for free-text entry of visit-specific abnormal findings depends on the number of significant abnormalities and the extensiveness of the physicians' narration, regardless of whether the physician uses a written, dictated, or keyboard entry format.

On the other hand, the speed of documentation of normal examination findings directly relates to the design of the data entry screens (and paper transfer media). The goal is to provide tools constructed based on the 1997 Documentation Guidelines to ensure compliance that also allow completion of individualized documentation of normal findings in the symptomatic and asymptomatic organ systems in 15 seconds or less.

Achieving the five goals for the examination screens calls for a template design that combines three components: (1) a check-box graphic interface for indicating the areas examined and whether the findings were normal or abnormal, (2) a free-text narrative space for recording details of all abnormal findings and documenting the examination of additional areas not listed in the check-box portion, and (3) a documentation prompt matched to the type of service. This design provides guidance for the extent of examination medically indicated (according to CPT descriptors) for each potential level of care a physician may have identified on the basis of the NPP. These components are illustrated in the sample form shown in Figure 14.1, a sample "Ear, Nose, Mouth, and Throat" single organ system examination template.

Documentation Prompt Section for the Examination Template
Because the CPT descriptors differ for each type of service and among several of the specialty examinations, EHR designers must include documentation prompts with the correct guidelines for levels of care for each type of

examination and for each type of service. To illustrate the significance of these differences, Figure 14.2 shows a compliant documentation prompt for the established outpatient visit service, which contrasts with the prompt for the initial visit pertaining to the same single organ system examination shown in Figure 14.1.

FIGURE 14.1

Sample Ear, Nose, Mouth, and Throat Single Organ System Examination Template. This is an example of the physical examination section of the electronic record for an initial outpatient visit, based on the 1997 Documentation Guidelines, for the ear, nose, mouth, and throat single organ system examination. The column shown in italics is a recommended additional section, which allows the graphic interface to also provide documentation of the significant normal findings related to the symptomatic body area(s). The exam elements marked with asterisks are added as options for the physician. This feature is discussed in the "Customization 2" section later in the chapter.

Physical Examination   Ear, Nose, Throat (initial visit)

General   (at least 3 measures of vital signs)   HT ___ ft ___ in   WT ___ lbs

BP sitting-standing ___/___ mm Hg   BP supine ___/___ mm Hg

Pulse ___/min   regular - irregular   Respirations ___/min   Temperature ___ °F (or °C)

			nl	abnl				nl	abnl
	General appearance	*Stature, nutrition*	☐	☐	**Neck**	Masses and trachea	*Symmetry, masses*	☐	☐
	Communication and voice	*Pitch, clarity*	☐	☐		Thyroid	*Size, nodules*	☐	☐
Head/face	Inspection	*Lesions, masses*	☐	☐	**Eyes**	Motility and gaze	*EOMs, nystagmus*	☐	☐
	Palpation/percussion	*Skeleton, sinuses*	☐	☐	**Respiratory**	Respiratory effort	*Inspiratory-expiratory*	☐	☐
	Salivary glands	*Masses, palpation*	☐	☐		Auscultation	*Clear*	☐	☐
	Facial strength	*Symmetry*	☐	☐	**CVS**	Heart auscultation	*Rhythm, heart sounds*	☐	☐
Ears, nose, throat	Pneumo-otoscopy	*EACs; TMs mobile*	☐	☐		Periph vasc system	*Edema, color*	☐	☐
	Hearing assessment	*Gross/Weber/Rinne*	☐	☐	**Lymphatic**	Neck/axillae/groin/etc.	*Adenopathy absence*	☐	☐
	External ear and nose	*Appearance*	☐	☐	**Neurological/ psychological**	Cranial nerves	*II-XII*	☐	☐
	Internal nose	*Mucosa, turbs*	☐	☐		Orientation	*Person, place, time*	☐	☐
	After decongestion†	*Septum, OMCs*	☐	☐		Mood and affect	*Comments*	☐	☐
	Lips, teeth, gums	*Mucosa, dentition*	☐	☐		Romberg*		☐	☐
	Oral cavity, oropharynx	*Tonsils, palate*	☐	☐		Tandem Romberg*		☐	☐
	Hypopharynx	*Piriform sinuses*	☐	☐		Past pointing*		☐	☐
	Larynx (mirror)	*Structure, mobility*	☐	☐					
	Nasopharynx (mirror)	*Choanae*	☐	☐		☐ See attached			

1. Problem focused = 1-5 elements (level 1)   2. Expanded = 6-11 elements (level 2)   3. Detailed = 12 or more elements (level 3)
4. Comprehensive = document every element in basic areas *and* at least one element in each optional (shaded) area (levels 4 and 5)   *Optional

Abbreviations: abnl, abnormal; CVS, cardiovascular system; EAC, external auditory canal; EOMs, extra-ocular movements; nl, normal; OMCs, osteo-meatal complexes; TM, tympanic membranes; and turbs, turbinates.

F IGURE   14.2

Sample Compliant Documentation Prompt for an Established Outpatient Visit. Example of the physical examination documentation prompt, based on the 1997 Documentation Guidelines, for the ear, nose, mouth, and throat for an *established patient* outpatient visit.

> 1. Problem focused = 1-5 elements (level 2)   2. Expanded = 6-11 elements (level 3)   3. Detailed = 12 or more elements (level 4)
> 4. Comprehensive = document every element in basic areas *and* at least one element in each optional (shaded) area (level 5) *Optional

Narrative Section of the Examination Template

The middle component of the examination form presents a straightforward narrative interface, which permits physicians to record efficiently the exact details of all abnormal examination findings. The provision for free text allows physicians to "paint a verbal picture" of the significant abnormalities they observe or to precisely describe the sounds, feel, or smell of a particular finding. These detailed and precise descriptions provide the degree of clarity that allows physicians or other members of the health care team to assess and monitor the progress of the patient's illness and response to treatment from one visit to the next.

Useful and Usable Descriptions

Physicians learn the importance of precise descriptions in supporting diagnoses and monitoring the course of an illness and its care. The most useful imagery conveys meaningful patient-specific information from one visit to the next and from one physician to another. The use of specific adjectives may not only define the extent of a clinical problem, but also suggest the correct diagnosis. Some examples relying on the different senses include the following:

Visual: "There is diffuse inflammation of the upper portion of the right tympanic membrane (TM), severe at the superior annulus. The posterior TM is bulging with a 5-mm area of dark yellow exudate"

Auditory: "Prominent fine crackling rales throughout the base of the left lung; fail to clear following cough"

Tactile: Multiple smooth, oblong, rubbery, nontender, 1- to 3-cm mobile lymph nodes in the left anterior cervical and left axillary regions

It is important for designers to recognize that it is not possible to create this type of patient-specific and visit-specific descriptive narrative of abnormal findings by using check-boxes, pick-lists, or preloaded macros. Providing such tools leads instead to recording generic descriptions such as "inflamed" (for visual), "rales" (for auditory), and "adenopathy" (for tactile). Limiting documentation to such imprecise terminology is likely to influence physicians to evaluate their patients less precisely (because they would be unable to document any detailed descriptions), which tends to disrupt the diagnostic process and lead to increasing reliance on diagnostic studies in lieu of thorough physical examination. Even when physicians appreciate all the subtleties of examination findings for their patients at the time of a visit, the inability to record a detailed and precise description of what they see, hear, and feel means that all these critical clinical observations and interpretations will be lost to the physicians' care of these patients for all subsequent encounters.

It is, therefore, important for physicians to emphasize the value of these narrative descriptions; realize that only a small amount of time is required to write, dictate, or type these free-text details; and insist that software vendors provide only a narrative interface for documenting the abnormal findings of the physical examination.

Graphic Section of the Examination Template

The upper portion of the examination template presents a graphic interface. For each single organ system or multisystem examination, the elements listed must incorporate all of the examination components described in the 1997 Documentation Guidelines. These are listed by organ system and combined with check-boxes to indicate *normal* or *abnormal* for each area examined. Simply checking the *Normal* boxes is sufficient for documentation of all normal findings related to *asymptomatic* organ systems. However, the Documentation Guidelines impose an additional compliance requirement that "*relevant negative findings . . . of the **affected or symptomatic** [bold added] body areas should be documented.*"[1(p11)] Although physicians may complete this task by entering free-text descriptions into the narrative section of the template, *Practical EHR* design incorporates an additional feature into the graphic interface for increased efficiency in recording these pertinent normal findings. As illustrated in the third column of the graphic section of Figure 14.1, this design adds a brief description (shown in italics) of what a physician would consider the *normal* findings for each examination element. On this sample form, a check mark in the normal box for "General appearance" conveys the physician's indication that the patient's "stature and nutrition" appear normal. Similarly, checking the normal box for lips, teeth, and gums allows the physician to report that the "mucosa and dentition" have no abnormality. This added description saves the time of separately typing, dictating, or writing these normal findings in the narrative section. Physicians should customize these additional descriptions to reflect their preferences.

Goals for Design: Physical Examination

The goals for design of the physical examination section of the EHR are shown in Table 14.1.

TABLE 14.1

Design Goals for the Physical Examination Section of an Electronic Health Record (EHR)

Goal	Elements to Meet the Goal
Efficiency	1) Graphic interface corresponds to examinations described in the 1997 Documentation Guidelines. It permits rapid documentation of elements examined and whether findings are normal or abnormal, and it includes a brief explanation of the physician's meaning of normal.
	2) Narrative interface promotes optimal speed for documenting a meaningful individualized description of all abnormalities through entry of free text. (This section also permits documentation of additional findings not programmed into the graphic section.)
Compliance	1) Graphic section includes all elements required for every single organ system examination. For a general multisystem examination, it must include all elements of at least 9 of 14 organ systems.
	2) Documentation prompt provides guidance on extent of examination warranted, based on physician's preliminary assessment of the severity of the nature of the presenting problem (NPP) and corresponding medically indicated level of care.

T A B L E 14.1, cont'd.

Goal	Elements to Meet the Goal
Quality	1) On review of a prior encounter, a physician can easily and quickly identify normal and abnormal physical examination findings by visually scanning the check-box portion of the template. 2) Free-text entry encourages and facilitates documenting a detailed description of abnormal findings specific to the visit. 3) This documentation permits a physician to closely monitor changes in findings from visit to visit.
Usability	Availability of all entry options: writing, dictating, and using keyboard and mouse
Data integrity	Free-text narrative facilitates documentation of patient-specific and visit-specific information.
Error proofing	Software functionality should require physicians to provide narrative description of all abnormal findings.

DESIGN ENHANCEMENTS FOR THE GRAPHIC INTERFACE SECTION

The narrative interface portion of the examination template can have the same appearance for all 12 examination templates described in the 1997 Documentation Guidelines. This is simply a blank section for entry of free-text descriptions of all the abnormal findings of the physical examination and any additional findings for examination elements not included in the graphic section.

Nevertheless, the 1997 Documentation Guidelines strictly define the content required for the graphic section of the templates. They provide a rigid baseline standard for single organ system examinations. These templates must include all listed elements to allow documentation of a *comprehensive* level of examination. This requirement is the basis for appreciating that, even though the Documentation Guidelines permit any physician to use any one of the defined examinations, it is almost certain that specialists will be the only physicians to use the single organ system examinations designated for their specialties. For example, logic dictates that only specialists in neurology and neurosurgery will find it appropriate to use the neurological examination template. It is unlikely that a physician specializing in another field would find the requirements for this examination to be appropriate for patient care.

However, the Documentation Guidelines allow a degree of flexibility for reducing the number of organ systems included in the general multisystem examination. This is fortunate because the majority of physicians practice in specialties that do not have an appropriate single organ system examination available. They must, therefore, rely on the multisystem examination as the foundation for their own customized examination forms. Although this template includes examination descriptions for elements of all 14 organ systems, E/M compliance requires performance and documentation of a minimum of only 9 of these systems to achieve a comprehensive multisystem examination. This flexibility is important because there are elements of the multisystem examination that many physicians might find inappropriate or unnecessary to include in their patient care. Gastroenterologists, for example, would usually prefer not to perform a musculoskeletal examination, and rheumatologists would usually prefer not to perform an abdominal examination. Therefore, because of the more liberal Documentation Guidelines' requirements for multisystem examination, physicians may eliminate as many as five of the organ systems from their own care and template and still be able to provide and document comprehensive care that is suitable to their specialty. Alternatively, these rarely performed examination elements can be removed from the primary-examination–screen and be relegated to a separate pop-up window, which physicians can access as needed.

Customization of the Graphic Section

Designing screens (and matched paper transfer media when desired) that can meet each physician's specialty and practice preferences for documentation of the physical examination involves customization on a practice-by-practice or physician-by-physician basis.

Customization 1: Selecting an Appropriate Examination Template

Each physician should consider two issues when selecting which of the available templates is optimal for his or her practice. First, an appropriate template should include all or most of the common body areas the physician examines in the majority of patients. Even more important, the critical factor in making a correct decision is to exclude from consideration any single organ system examination templates that require examination of areas of the body that would be inappropriate for the specialty or outside the scope of the physician's expertise. Because the Documentation Guidelines require that *all* listed areas in single organ system templates must be examined and documented when performing a comprehensive-level examination, the presence of any inappropriate examination areas should disqualify that template as a choice.

The majority of physicians will find that most single organ systems contain a requirement to examine one or more organ systems that would be inappropriate for their practices. These physicians should, therefore, select the general multisystem examination and modify and optimize it to meet their needs. This option provides the flexibility for eliminating inappropriate examination elements, completely or on a case-by-case basis.

Customization 2: Adding Elements to the Basic Template (Multisystem or Single Organ System Examinations)

For increased documentation efficiency, each physician can supplement the basic template selected in Customization 1 by incorporating additional examination elements they commonly evaluate when caring for patients. For example, most otolaryngologists should find the template labeled "Ear, Nose, Mouth, and Throat Examination" to be appropriate for their practices. However, some of these specialists frequently perform additional examination elements that are not included on the standard template, such as clinical tests of balance function. Adding these elements to the graphic portion of the examination template greatly increases the physician's speed of documenting findings in patients with balance problems.

Although these additional documentation elements increase efficiency, care must be taken that they do not inadvertently disrupt the compliance features of these forms. To avoid this potential complication, any additional elements should include an identifying label to indicate that they are not elements of the defined examination template. For example, the ear, nose, and throat examination record shown in Figure 14.1 includes several elements not included in the examination defined in the 1997 Documentation Guidelines. Each of these is marked with an asterisk to remind physicians (and reviewers in an audit) that documenting these elements does not "count" toward the E/M compliance requirements for documentation. In other words, checking one of the boxes marked with an asterisk does not count for the purpose of supporting a selected level of care (E/M code). Conversely, leaving one or more of the optional elements unmarked does not have a negative effect on satisfying the comprehensive examination requirement for documenting all elements in a given anatomic area. The elements shown with this customization in Figure 14.1 are as follows:

- After decongestion (a subheading under the internal nose examination, which allows the physician to indicate the appearance after spraying a decongestant in the nose to shrink the membranes)
- Romberg,* Tandem Romberg,* and Past pointing* (balance tests in the neurological/psychological section of the examination)

In summary, using the asterisk or some other identifier to label elements added to the defined template allows physicians to increase documentation efficiency yet be able to ignore such elements for purposes of E/M compliance.

Customization 3: Separate Screen for Rarely Used Systems From the Multisystem Examination Template

Most physicians whose specialty is not listed among the 11 single organ system examinations will choose the general multisystem examination template and customize it to fit their needs and preferences. Although this template provides physicians with the ability to document examination findings for as many as 14 organ systems, even the highest-level examination (ie, comprehensive examination for level 5 service) requires only that a physician's care and documentation "should include at least nine organ systems or body areas."[1(p12)] The Documentation Guidelines also advise, "For each system/area selected, all elements of the examination identified by a bullet (■) should be performed, unless specific directions limit the content of the examination. For each area/system, documentation of at least two elements identified by a bullet is expected."[1(p12)]

Placing the defined examination elements for all 14 organ systems on one screen requires too much text and becomes too cluttered for rapid documentation. However, the flexibility of the multisystem examination guidelines permits exclusion of as many as five of the listed body areas or organ systems from physicians' customized electronic forms, and sufficient documentation still remains in the graphic section to document level 4 and level 5 care. Therefore, physicians can request that the vendor remove from the primary template as many as five body areas that they would rarely, if ever, examine in their usual patient population. For example, some family practitioners, many internal medicine specialists, and most regional specialists will elect to exclude a female genitourinary examination that requires pelvic examination from the screens of their customized electronic forms. In addition, many physicians who do not frequently see patients with trauma may elect to remove the lengthy musculoskeletal examination components from the primary screen of the electronic form as well.

All of the removed examination elements should be relegated to a secondary and optional element of the electronic form, which is retained in the background of the software system. The organ systems stored on this screen can be accessed if any of these areas are examined. For physicians entering data directly into the computer, these rarely used organ systems can appear in an optional feature in the electronic form on a separate pop-up screen. When a physician accesses the pop-up window and documents the examination elements in one or more of these organ systems, these should be transferred to the primary screen of the electronic form with the check-boxes for these examined elements checked. For physicians documenting their check-boxes using a digital pen or paper as a data transfer medium, the less frequently examined areas may be placed on a separate paper form that is used only when needed.

Figures 14.3 and 14.4 show examples of how a primary care physician or internist might customize a general multisystem examination template. Figure 14.3 contains the most commonly used of the 14 organ systems. Figure 14.4 illustrates the screen of the secondary or optional portion of the electronic form, which in this case contains the examination elements for the following organ systems: GU male, GU female, and musculoskeletal. An internist might access this hidden screen, for example, when evaluating patients who experience trauma to an extremity, seek care for pain in the lower part of the back, or complain of neurological symptoms.

Customization 4: Adding Brief Descriptions of Normal Findings

Software designers should create an area in the graphic interface section for physicians to provide the terms they usually use to describe normal findings for each of the defined examination elements included in this check-box section, which can be added to the EHR. Although this additional information is not part of the standardized examination templates indicated by the Documentation Guidelines, *Practical EHR* advises including these descriptions to fulfill the requirement for documenting "relevant negative findings of the affected or symptomatic body area(s) or organ system(s)."[1(p11)] For examination of symptomatic body areas, simply reporting normal fails to satisfy this Documentation Guidelines requirement. The addition of these brief descriptions is compliant, improves quality by conveying a more complete picture of the features the physician actually examined, and increases efficiency compared with entering free-text descriptions of the relevant negative findings in the narrative section of the template.

DATA ENTRY TOOLS AVAILABLE FOR THE PHYSICAL EXAMINATION RECORD

Because the physical examination template combines two data entry interface designs, physicians may use different tools for entering information in each section.

Graphic Interface Section With Check-Boxes

For physicians who document the findings directly into the computer in the graphic-interface section, the active mouse entry tool (tool 4, Chapter 11) should prove a most valuable asset. Because compliance requires that each box be documented individually, physicians seek a software tool that provides a more efficient mode of checking the boxes than moving the mouse to individually click a normal or abnormal box for each separate examination element. The active mouse tool saves time by permitting a continual series of entries of normal findings (or a series of abnormal findings), one box after another. When using this software design, the physician positions

FIGURE 14.3

General Multisystem Examination Template. This is an example of the physical examination section of the electronic record for an initial outpatient visit, based on the 1997 Documentation Guidelines, for the general multisystem examination. Due to the large number of elements that can be examined and documented, this template is illustrated in two separate figures (this one and Figure 14.4); this figure shows the most commonly examined organ systems that are listed on the primary screen of the electronic form.

Physical Examination:

General Multisystem Exam

General (at least 3 measures of vital signs)
BP sitting-standing ___ / ___ mm Hg
Pulse ___ /min regular - irregular
HT ___ ft ___ in   WT ___ lbs
BP supine ___ / ___ mm Hg
Resp ___ /min   TEMP ___ °F (or °C)

System	Element	Normal/AB	System	Element	Normal/AB
General	General appearance – Stature, nutrition	☐ ☐	**Chest/**	Breast Inspection – Symmetry, color	☐ ☐
Eyes	Conjunctivae & Lids – Appearance, color	☐ ☐	**Breasts**	Breast/Axillae palp – Nodules, masses	☐ ☐
	Pupils & Irises – Size, reactivity	☐ ☐	**GI/ABD**	Masses/Tenderness – Palpation	☐ ☐
	Optic Discs – Fundi, vessels	☐ ☐		Liver/Spleen – Size, tenderness	☐ ☐
ENT	Ears & Nose, External – Appearance	☐ ☐		Hernia eval – Inspection, palpation	☐ ☐
	Otoscopy – Canals, tymp membranes	☐ ☐		Anus/Rectum/Perin – Appearance, palpation	☐ ☐
	Hearing – Response to sound	☐ ☐		Stool Blood Test – Eval when indicated	☐ ☐
	Internal nose – Septum, mucosa, turbs	☐ ☐	**Lymph**	Neck/Axillae/Groin/Other – Adenopathy	☐ ☐
	Lips, Teeth & Gums – Mucosa, dentition	☐ ☐		(circle areas examined; requires exam in 2 or more regions)	
	Oropharynx – Mucosa, tonsils, palate	☐ ☐	**Skin/**	Inspection – Head, trunk, RUE	☐ ☐
Neck	Masses & Trachea – Symmetry, masses	☐ ☐	**Subcu**	LUE, RLE, LLE	☐ ☐
	Thyroid – Size, nodules	☐ ☐		Palpation – Head, trunk, RUE	☐ ☐
Resp	Respiratory effort – Inspiratory-expiratory	☐ ☐		LUE, RLE, LLE	☐ ☐
	Chest palpation – Movement	☐ ☐		(circle areas examined)	
	Chest percussion – Sound	☐ ☐	**Neuro**	Cranial nerves – II - XII	☐ ☐
	Auscultation – Lung sounds	☐ ☐		Deep tendon reflexes – Knee, ankle, Babinski	☐ ☐
CVS	Heart palpation – Rhythm	☐ ☐		Sensation – Light touch	☐ ☐
	Heart auscultation – Sounds	☐ ☐	**Psych**	Judgment & Insight – Subjectively	☐ ☐
	Carotid arteries – Pulsation	☐ ☐		Orientation – Person, place, time	☐ ☐
	Abdominal aorta – Pulsation	☐ ☐		Memory – Recent & remote	☐ ☐
	Femoral arteries – Pulsation	☐ ☐		Mood & Affect – Comments	☐ ☐
	Pedial pulses – Pulsation	☐ ☐			
	Edema,Varices, LE – Appearance	☐ ☐			

☐ Continued on supplemental page   ☐ Abnormal findings dictated

1. Problem focused = 1-5 elements (level 1)   2. Expanded = 6-11 elements (level 2)   3. Detailed = 12 or more elements (level 3)
4. Comprehensive = document two (or more) elements in each of nine (or more) systems (level 4 or 5)   *Optional

Abbreviations: abnl, abnormal; CVS, cardiovascular system; EAC, external auditory canal; ENT, Ear, Nose & Throat; EOMs, extra-ocular movements; GI/ABD, Gastrointestinal/Abdomen; LE, Lower Extremity; LLE, Left Lower Extremity; LUE, Left Upper Extremity; nl, normal; Neuro, neurological; Psych, psychiatric; RESP, respirations; RLE, Right Lower Extremity; RUE, Right Upper Extremity; and Subcu, Subcutaneous.

Separate Screen for Less Commonly Examined Systems or Body Areas. This illustrates the less commonly examined elements that a physician would have assigned to the secondary and optional element of the electronic form, which could appear as a pop-up when needed. In this example, the exam elements for GU male, GU female, and musculoskeletal are included in the optional section. For physicians using a digital pen or paper as a data transfer medium, these elements would be provided on a separate sheet of paper that would be accessed only when needed.

Physical Examination:		General Multisystem Exam (continued)	Normal/AB					Normal/AB
GU/	Scrotal contents	Appearance, palpation	☐ ☐	**MSKEL**	RT Upper extremity	Inspec., palp., percussion	☐ ☐
Male	Penis	Appearance, palpation	☐ ☐			Range of motion	☐ ☐
	Prostate	Palpation	☐ ☐			Stability or laxity	☐ ☐
GU	Ext genitalia	Appearance, palpation	☐ ☐			Muscle strength & tone	☐ ☐
Female	Urethra	Inspection	☐ ☐		LT Upper extremity	Inspec., palp., percussion	☐ ☐
(PELVIC)	Bladder	Palpation	☐ ☐			Range of motion	☐ ☐
	Cervis	Palpation	☐ ☐			Stability or laxity	☐ ☐
	Uterus	Palpation	☐ ☐			Muscle strength & tone	☐ ☐
	Adnexa/Paramet	Palpation	☐ ☐		RT Lower extremity	Inspec., palp., percussion	☐ ☐
MSKEL	Head & Neck	Inspec., palp., percussion	☐ ☐			Range of motion	☐ ☐
		Range of motion	☐ ☐			Stability or laxity	☐ ☐
		Stability or laxity	☐ ☐			Muscle strength & tone	☐ ☐
		Muscle strength & tone	☐ ☐		LT Lower extremity	Inspec., palp., percussion	☐ ☐
	Spine, ribs, pelvis	Inspec., palp., percussion	☐ ☐			Range of motion	☐ ☐
		Range of motion	☐ ☐			Stability or laxity	☐ ☐
		Stability or laxity	☐ ☐			Muscle strength & tone	☐ ☐
		Muscle strength & tone	☐ ☐			☐ **Abnormal findings dictated**	

**1. Problem focused = 1-5 elements (level 1)   2. Expanded = 6-11 elements (level 2)   3. Detailed = 12 or more elements (level 3)
4. Comprehensive = document two (or more) elements in each of nine (or more) systems (level 4 or 5)   *Optional**

Abbreviations: abnl, abnormal; GU, Genitourinary; MSKEL, musculoskeletal; nl, normal; Palp, Palpation; Inspec, Inspection; RT, Right; and LT, Left.

the mouse to place the cursor on the first *Normal* box, clicks and holds the mouse button, and moves the cursor down the page, entering check marks through each consecutive *Normal* box. The physician releases the button when reaching an element that was not examined, and therefore must remain unchecked, or when reaching an element that requires a check in the box indicating that the finding was *abnormal.* Through a series of active mouse movements that check multiple boxes, combined with individual clicks and elements left blank (when not examined), the physician can rapidly and accurately document the findings for all areas examined.

Physicians working with a tablet PC (tool 5, Chapter 11) have another option for rapid individualized documentation of multiple check-boxes. With an image of the check-box interface on the screen (such as the sample shown in Figure 14.3), a stylus can be used to touch the screen to individually check appropriate *normal* and *abnormal* responses. This design should also offer the alternative functionality of an active stylus entry, allowing physicians to place the stylus on the first check-box and move it down the screen when there is a series of *Normal* or *Abnormal* boxes, thereby checking each box in the same manner as the active mouse entry actively checks a series of boxes. As with the active mouse entry, it is physicians' responsibility to perform the care and correctly document all normal and abnormal findings, while leaving check-boxes unchecked for unexamined areas.

Physicians who write on paper to document the check-box section can effectively use indirect data entry with a professional data entry operator (DEO; tool 1, Chapter 11) or direct data entry by using a digital pen (tool 6, Chapter 11). The design increases the speed of documentation by giving physicians the ability to check a series of boxes by moving the pen to create a line down the page through a series of *Normal* boxes. The DEO can easily interpret this line as a series of checked boxes. The programmer should permit the software to interpret the line through a series of boxes created by a digital pen as a series of individually checked boxes.

Narrative Interface Section for Free-Text Entry

The final task for physicians in the physical examination section of the EHR is to document all abnormal findings, with appropriate detail, in the narrative section of the template. Although it is extremely easy for someone reading the check-box section to identify the areas of the physical examination that were abnormal, it is the narrative section that paints a thorough and precise verbal picture of the abnormal findings. The narrative description's details and accuracy also provide a reliable baseline for comparing the patient's status during subsequent examinations, regardless of whether the patient receives care from the same or another physician.

In some circumstances, physicians will want to provide a more detailed description of pertinent normal findings in the narrative section to enhance the quality of care. For example, if a patient seeks care because of pulmonary symptoms and auscultation reveals normal lung sounds, it may be advantageous to document this finding in a more detailed narrative than just checking the box for normal breath sounds. It would be relevant, for example, to add "no rales or rhonchi; inspiratory and expiratory breath sounds symmetrical." This information would be meaningful for monitoring the patient's clinical course through subsequent visits.

Because the criteria for compliance and quality mandate that this section of the examination record must provide for entry of free-text descriptions specific to each patient and each visit, software systems should offer physicians a choice among the full range of data entry options for maximum flexibility and efficiency. Physicians who use the keyboard for data entry should have the option of typing the details of all abnormal findings directly into the H&P record (tool 7, Chapter 11). Physicians who dictate their narratives should be able to use a digital recorder with a transcriptionist for asynchronous data entry (tool 2, Chapter 11) or dictation with voice recognition software for direct entry into the software (tool 3, Chapter 11). Physicians who write their narratives may use indirect entry by writing on paper and having asynchronous data entry by a DEO (tool 1, Chapter 11), synchronous entry by writing on a tablet PC (tool 5, Chapter 11), or synchronous entry by writing on specialized paper with a digital pen (tool 6, Chapter 11).

FUNCTIONALITY OF THE
PHYSICAL EXAMINATION RECORD

Practical EHR Method

Physicians perform the physical examination after obtaining a comprehensive medical history and making a preliminary assessment of the NPP and the medically indicated level of care. Because the Documentation Guidelines for the examination vary for each type of service and each of the 12 defined examinations, the rules are too extensive for physicians to memorize. It would be unreasonable and excessively time-consuming for physicians to interrupt patient care to seek guidance on these rules by reviewing a coding manual during every patient visit. As an effective alternative, *Practical EHR* screens provide documentation prompts specific to the type of examination and type of service on every physical examination form. These prompts report the examination requirements associated with each level of care that physicians might identify on the basis of severity of the NPP.

Passive functionality provides physicians with these prompts on the examination screen of the EHR and on any paper forms used as transfer media. Awareness of the medically indicated extent of examination guides physicians to perform and document an amount of care appropriate to the NPP. Examples of passive documentation prompts for the physical examination record are shown in Figures 14.1, 14.2, and 14.3.

The option of adding *active* functionality, in addition to the passive prompts, can be considered for physicians recording the graphic portion of the examination form directly on the computer, onto a tablet PC, or on paper using a digital pen with data immediately transferred to the computer. Figure 11.4 illustrates one possible design of a sample active prompt that would appear on the computer screen of the physical examination record.

Error Proofing

When applying the principles described for the design of physical examination templates, there is one aspect of the documentation that clearly benefits from the addition of error-proofing capability. For physicians performing one of the types of synchronous data entry, the software should have sufficient sophistication to ensure that for every element of the examination identified as *abnormal* in the graphic section, the physician has entered a corresponding description of the abnormal findings in the narrative section. This requires the software to recognize each examination component identified as *abnormal*, create a corresponding category in the narrative section, and confirm that the physician has entered corresponding information for each of these categories. The software programming should be straightforward for physicians using direct keyboard entry or writing on a tablet PC; the design will require some added creativity for physicians using voice recognition software and this capability may not be available for physicians using the digital pen. This error-proofing functionality should confirm that the physician has entered narrative descriptions for each abnormal response before permitting the physician to proceed to the next section of the record.

SUMMARY

The physical examination section of the intelligent EHR should include templates based on the standards of the 1997 Documentation Guidelines.[1] This structure ensures compliant documentation when combined with compliant *passive* or *active* documentation prompts that are correlated with the patient's NPP and medically indicated levels of care.

An effective design for a compliant physical examination template combines a graphic check-box interface with a narrative interface section and a documentation prompt to guide compliance. The check-box section allows rapid documentation of all areas examined and identification of whether each finding is normal or abnormal. The narrative section requires a free-text description to document the details of the abnormal findings. It is important for physicians to select the examination template design most appropriate for their own specialty and the nature of their practice. Additional EHR design features should include customization of the graphic section for documentation of additional examination elements that are not included in the descriptions provided in the 1997 Documentation Guidelines, customization of the multisystem examination, and adding descriptions that characterize normal examination elements to increase the speed of documenting normal findings for symptomatic body areas.

Designs should provide physicians a choice among data entry tools, including using keyboard entry, dictating, writing, or a combination of these tools for different sections of the form. The check-box design features should require no more than 15 seconds for physicians to indicate the areas examined and whether they were normal or abnormal. The speed of narrative documentation is subject to multiple variables, including the number and extent of abnormal findings and the efficiency of the data entry format the physician uses. When combined with documentation prompts, electronic examination record forms designed in this manner that also add error-proofing functionality help ensure compliance and appropriate levels of care, while promoting high-quality, individualized descriptions of all significant findings.

Reference

1.   American Medical Association & Health Care Financing Administration. *Documentation Guidelines for Evaluation and Management Services.* Washington, DC: Health Care Financing Administration; 1997.

chapter 15

Design Solutions for Medical Decision Making and Final Nature of the Presenting Problem

Since the introduction of the evaluation and management (E/M) documentation and coding system in 1992, the greatest conceptual and practical challenges for physicians to achieve compliance have come from the medical decision making (MDM) component and from the lack of consideration of the nature of the presenting problem (NPP). Tools and methods that can enable electronic health records (EHRs) to address the NPP issues have been presented in preceding chapters. This chapter introduces designs that integrate MDM compliance into the electronic history and physical examination (H&P) record. At the end of this chapter, the final reassessment of the NPP component of the EHR will be examined as the final step in the compliant E/M documentation and coding process.

One of the unfortunate consequences of the generally unsatisfactory conventional approaches to MDM documentation has been the failure of software designers to provide screens that require, or even to allow, physicians to document all subcomponents of MDM. To ensure that documentation of MDM meets compliance and quality requirements, it is the responsibility of physicians to define and set design requirements for each of the nine elements that must be considered and documented to consistently record compliant MDM. EHRs must be designed to recognize and incorporate these parameters while avoiding the intrinsically noncompliant features discussed in Chapter 9. The EHR screens for this section of the record must enable physicians to accomplish documentation of decision making that accurately reflects their diagnostic process during each patient visit and provides valid authentication that they have exercised the level of decision making appropriate for the nature of each patient's disease process at the time of the visit.

IDENTIFYING CURRENT MDM CHALLENGES

As introduced in Chapter 9, four challenges have inhibited the ability of physicians to master compliant documentation for this key component of the H&P record, regardless of whether they are using written, dictated, or electronic records:

1. Nontraditional documentation categories defined in the *Current Procedural Terminology* (*CPT®*) manual[1]

2. CPT categories calling for quantitative assessment but having only qualitative descriptors

3. Failure to provide separate documentation for treatment plans and data ordered

4. Complex coding calculations

The designs for EHRs must successfully address all four of these issues to help physicians achieve compliant documentation of MDM. The failure to create designs that resolve these issues has been a consistent barrier to meeting one of physicians' primary EHR goals, which is to make the E/M compliance problem disappear.

Challenge 1: Nontraditional Documentation Categories

The *CPT* manual defines MDM as "the complexity of establishing a diagnosis and/or selecting a management option."[1(p7)] This complexity is determined by evaluating a combination of three subcomponents: (1) the number of possible diagnoses and/or management options considered; (2) the amount and/or complexity of medical data obtained, reviewed, and analyzed; and (3) the risks of complications, morbidity, comorbidities, and/or mortality.

All coders and most physicians are aware of the primary documentation rule, derived from the Centers for Medicare & Medicaid Services(CMS) claims processing manual, that if medical information was not documented, it is considered not done.[2] Yet, reviews of most physicians' current medical records reveal that insufficient information is recorded to meet the CPT requirements for compliant MDM documentation.[1] First, rather than documenting the range of possible diagnoses and treatment options, a significant number of physicians have fallen into the habit of documenting only one primary diagnosis and one selected treatment option. This tendency is probably the result of increasing economic pressure, which reduces the amount of time available for extensive documentation. The second problem is that traditional E/M coding courses fail to instruct physicians to document four of the elements required for reporting the complexity of MDM[2]:

■ Risk of complications, morbidity and/or mortality, and comorbidities associated with the patient's presenting problem(s)

■ Risk of complications, morbidity and/or mortality, and comorbidities associated with the diagnostic procedure(s)

■ Risk of complications, morbidity and/or mortality, and comorbidities associated with the possible management options

■ Complexity of medical records, diagnostic tests, and/or other information that must be obtained, reviewed, and analyzed[1(p7)]

It is interesting that although conventional E/M training courses usually inform physicians that these are MDM elements, nearly all fail to advise physicians that they need to be *documented* in the medical record. Failure to document these subjective assessments leaves the evaluation of risks and complexities to the discretion of a reviewer, rather than placing it where it belongs, in the judgment of the physician caring for a patient.

Challenge 2: Evaluating Subjective Elements of MDM

The CPT descriptions of the subcomponents of MDM include four elements that are supposed to measure the "amount" or "number" of items documented in the medical record. However, neither the *CPT* manual nor the two versions (1995 and 1997) of the Documentation Guidelines has offered *quantitative* values to supplement the currently available qualitative descriptions in the *CPT* manual. Therefore, physicians have only the subjective terms "minimal or none," "limited," "moderate," and "extensive"[1(p8)] to describe the *amount* of data ordered and/or reviewed and, similarly, only "minimal," "limited," "multiple," and "extensive"[1(p8)] to describe the *number* of diagnoses or management options.

Documenting the complexity of data (ordered and reviewed) and evaluation of the three types of risk (presenting problems, diagnostic procedures, and treatment options) also allows for only a subjective analysis. The Documentation Guidelines[3] provide the Table of Risk to show examples of different levels of risk, but no examples are provided to illustrate different levels of data complexity. The lack of *objective* measures for these four MDM elements makes the need to document these elements even more important because once a physician records this judgment in the record it must be accepted by a reviewer, provided that it is reasonable.

Challenge 3: Combined Documentation of Treatment Options and Data Ordered

Conventional medical record designs, whether based on the concepts of the "comprehensive H&P" or the alternative SOAP (subjective data, objective data, assessment, plan) note, traditionally conclude their decision making design with sections for "impressions" (or "assessment") and "plans." Physicians list the differential diagnoses in the impressions section, and they use the plans category to record their recommendations for diagnostic tests (such as laboratory tests, radiologic studies, and diagnostic procedures) and for treatments (such as medications, physical therapy, or surgical intervention). However, for purposes of E/M compliance, listing data to be obtained together with recommended therapies creates an additional level of confusion for physicians in determining the number of treatment options. It is inconvenient and difficult to count only some of the items listed under the heading of plans as *treatments* while counting others as *amount of data*.

An additional and more subtle challenge results from the fact that data ordered are most often listed in a straightforward manner, without consideration of possible alternative testing options. When data ordered are listed together with treatments, it is common to find that physicians, in a similar manner, list only the primary treatment ordered, without documentation of other treatment options considered. However, listing only one treatment option is one factor that suggests the physician has performed only "straightforward" MDM, and it also obscures, rather than illuminates, the physician's thought process.

Challenge 4: Complex Coding Calculations

The conventional approach to E/M coding confronts physicians with a series of complex calculations at the conclusion of a patient visit, and the most complicated set of computations involves the MDM component. As noted, there are three subcomponents that contribute to determining the level of MDM, but each of these subcomponents is composed of two, three, or four separate subcategories, or elements. Physicians are first instructed to compare and calculate the levels of the subcategories to determine the complexity of each of the three subcomponents. They must follow this task with a second calculation to determine the two most complex of the three documented subcomponents. Furthermore, the calculations lead to different levels of MDM complexity for each different type of service. It has proven unreasonable for physicians to memorize the rules needed to perform these calculations and impractical for them to attempt to carry them out while caring for patients.

EHR DESIGN AND FUNCTIONALITY PRINCIPLES TO ADDRESS THE MDM CHALLENGES

Effective EHR designs, when combined with the application of the *Practical EHR* method, can successfully address these MDM challenges to create a user-friendly and efficient documentation environment that not only fulfills the criteria for E/M compliance, but also accurately reflects the complexity of decision making performed. EHR vendors need to provide these capabilities, not only to meet the needs of physicians and medical practices, but also to fulfill the Certification Commission for Health Information Technology's (CCHIT) certification requirement that "The system shall provide the ability to select an appropriate CPT Evaluation and Management code based on data found in a clinical encounter."[5]

Addressing Challenge 1: Providing Full MDM Documentation Capability

Effective H&P record designs can easily give physicians the ability to document all the subcategories of MDM by including graphic interface templates that address the commonly overlooked elements. Simply listing the choices for the levels of risk and for complexity of data, with check boxes adjacent to each possible choice, readily allows physicians to document these elements of decision making. The fact that each of these four elements depends on subjective judgment underscores the importance of physicians documenting these impressions in the medical record. By investing the minimal time and effort required to document these additional elements, physicians guarantee that the determination of complexity of decision making rests solely in their own judgment at the time of the visit, not in the assessment of a reviewer examining the chart months or years later.

The Documentation Guidelines provide the Table of Risk,[3] illustrated in Appendix C, which gives reasonable examples of the types of presenting problems, diagnostic procedures, and management options that correlate with the four levels of risk (minimal, low, moderate, and high). The software for EHRs should provide a pop-up window that shows this table of risk whenever a physician needs it as a reference while documenting MDM. There is no similar guidance available for assessing the level of complexity of data, so it remains the responsibility of each physician to be reasonable in this assessment. As a general guideline, most compliance experts agree that the review and interpretation of actual studies (eg, an electrocardiogram or computed tomography [CT] scan of the brain) usually involves moderate or high complexity, whereas simply reading a printed report of someone else's interpretation of the studies represents minimal or low complexity.

Figure 15.1 illustrates a sample design for the portion of an MDM interface that successfully addresses this challenge, including the presence of documentation prompts to advise physicians of the level of complexity that would appropriately correspond to the level of care selected for each visit based on the NPP.

FIGURE 15.1

Sample Portion of a Medical Decision Making (MDM) Form for Documenting Levels of Risk and Complexity of Data Reviewed. The documentation prompts in the shaded sections correlate with the MDM section for all three types of outpatient service: initial visit, established patient visit, and consultation. The letters b, b' and b" indicate that *risk* is the second of the three subcomponents of MDM and labels each of the three elements of risk; c" indicates the complexity of data and that this *data* is the third element of the three subcomponents of MDM.

Complexity of Data Reviewed or Ordered (c")			
1. Minimal (level 2)	2. Limited (level 3)	3. Moderate (level 4)	4. Extensive (level 5)
☐ Minimal	☐ Limited	☐ Moderate	☐ Extensive

Risk of Complications and/or Morbidity or Mortality (see Table of Risk[3])

	1. Minimal (level 2)	2. Low (level 3)	3. Moderate (level 4)	4. High (level 5)
Risk of presenting problem(s) (b):	☐ Minimal	☐ Low	☐ Moderate	☐ High
Risk of diagnostic procedure(s) (b'):	☐ Minimal	☐ Low	☐ Moderate	☐ High
Risk of management option(s) (b"):	☐ Minimal	☐ Low	☐ Moderate	☐ High

Addressing Challenge 2: Including Guidelines for Subjective MDM Elements

The terms *amount* of data and *number* of diagnoses or management options invite establishment of guidelines to provide quantitative values, which can assist physicians in compliant documentation and coding and can assist auditors in making reasonable and consistent determinations of the complexity of MDM. Based on many years of experience and extensive discussions with physicians, Medicare medical directors, insurance company medical directors, coders, auditors, and physician consultants, *Practical E/M*[4] suggested reasonable *quantitative* values for these *qualitative* MDM elements. Those recommendations, which are incorporated into *Practical EHR* documentation prompts for the corresponding sections of MDM documentation, are given in Figure 15.2.

FIGURE 15.2

Recommended Numeric Values for the "Number" of Diagnoses and Treatment Options and for the "Amount" of Data Ordered or Reviewed[4]

CPT Description of "Amount" or "Number"	Practical E/M Numeric Value
Minimal	1
Limited	2
Multiple or moderate	3
Extensive	4 or more

MDM and Compliant Documentation Guidelines

The Documentation Guidelines brought quantitative measures to the qualitative CPT descriptors related to the medical history and physical examination components of the H&P record. However, there continues to be a

continued

significant need for sanctioned quantitative guidelines for the MDM descriptions of *amount* of data and *number* of diagnoses and treatment options. To be acceptable to physicians and worthy of being sanctioned, guidelines for MDM documentation must have three characteristics that support the reliability and credibility of E/M principles:

■ An MDM guideline, when used correctly, must yield coding results that are consistent with the CPT E/M guidelines.

■ Such guidelines must be reasonable and easy for physicians and coders to understand.

■ Such guidelines must be sufficiently concise to incorporate into physicians' medical records (including electronic records) as documentation prompts that are compatible with quality care.

The numerical guidelines shown in Figure 15.2 meet these three requirements. They have also been used in physicians' paper charts since 1995, and none of those charts, when used as designed, has ever failed an E/M compliance audit.

Several unsanctioned quantitative guidelines for MDM documentation have been developed that do not meet all three requirements for an effective MDM guideline. The use of unsanctioned guidelines can result in noncompliance and inappropriate coding, audit "failures," and, subsequently, increased confusion and resistance among physicians and coders. Therefore, it is highly recommended that physicians and software developers conscientiously avoid unsanctioned and noncompliant approaches for assessing MDM.

Figure 15.3 illustrates a sample data-reviewed section for the H&P record, with inclusion of the quantitative definitions for *amount* of data reviewed in the documentation prompt. This appears on the second shaded line of the prompts, with the "number" of data elements indicated for each level of care being underlined for easy identification. Because data reviewed is the first element of MDM that physicians document and the first to appear on an MDM screen, this section also includes a passive documentation prompt on its first line that reminds physicians that E/M compliance specifies that only two of the three MDM subcomponents are required to meet or exceed the

FIGURE 15.3

Sample Data-Reviewed Section for Documenting Medical Decision Making (MDM) for Outpatient Office Services, With Documentation Prompts Based on Suggested Values in Figure 15.2. In the second line of the documentation prompt, the underlined values report the amount (number) of data appropriate for each level of care. The prompt in the top line advises physicians that documentation for at least two of the three MDM subcomponents must be compatible with the nature of the presenting problem and medically indicated level of care. a and a' are identifying labels used in the MDM section to indicate that the number of diagnoses and treatment options are one subcomponent of MDM; b, b' and b" indicate that the three types of risk are a second subcomponent; and c, c' and c" indicate that data ordered, data reviewed, and complexity of data together comprise the third subcomponent.

MDM	2 of 3 sections (a vs a', b vs b' vs b", c vs c' vs c") must meet or exceed indicated level of care			
	1. Minimal or none (level 2)	2. Limited (level 3)	3. Moderate (level 4)	4. Extensive (level 5)
Data reviewed (c):				

medically indicated level of care. This prompt also uses alphabetical indicators that will appear on the MDM screen as identifying labels to remind physicians of the elements of each of these three subcomponents:

- The two elements of number of diagnoses or management options are labeled a and a'
- The three elements of risk are labeled b, b', and b"
- The three elements of data are label c, c', and c"

Figure 15.4 similarly demonstrates a sample section for documenting diagnoses and plans/management options. It also includes documentation prompts based on these quantitative values. Because the CPT descriptors for levels of MDM are identical for outpatient initial visits, outpatient consultations, and established patient visits, the illustrated sections and prompts are valid for each of these types of service.

F I G U R E   15.4

Sample Sections for Documenting Impressions/Differential Diagnoses and Plans/ Management Options Subcomponents of Medical Decision Making (MDM) for Outpatient Office Services. The documentation prompts are based on suggested values in Figure 15.2; these numeric values are underlined. a and a' indicate the two elements for the MDM subcomponent "number of diagnoses and treatment options."

1. Minimal (level 2) 2. Limited (level 3) 3. Moderate (level 4) 4. Extensive (level 5)	
Impressions/Differential Diagnoses (a)	Plans/Management Options (a')
1) 2) 3) 4) 5)	1) 2) 3) 4) 5)

There are no reasonable means of creating quantitative measures for documentation of the four remaining subjective elements (complexity of data and the three types of risk). Physicians must apply their own judgment for these factors and document the conclusion, as discussed in the previous section and illustrated in Figure 15.1.

Addressing Challenge 3: Separately Documenting Data Ordered and Treatment Plans

The conventional teaching approach in medical school for documenting MDM is to first list the data reviewed followed by a section for impressions and then a list of plans. In this approach the plan reports both the diagnostic tests ordered and the treatments recommended. Although one of the goals for promoting usability of the electronic H&P record is to create designs that parallel physicians' familiar documentation patterns to the greatest extent possible, equally important goals of ensuring compliant documentation and error proofing compel a variation from this conventional design for this section of the record. Because E/M compliance lists data ordered and management options as elements of separate subcomponents of MDM, it seems wise for physicians to document them in separate sections of the chart rather than under a single heading of plans.

Partitioning these elements into separate compartments allows EHR designs to include reliable documentation prompts for both sections, facilitates compliant documentation for physicians, and avoids confusion for coders during an audit. Figure 15.5 demonstrates one design option for creating separate but adjacent sections for treatment options and data ordered, which are also attached to the section for documenting diagnoses. For increased efficiency, in addition to the areas for entry of free-text, the data-ordered section also contains check-boxes for rapid documentation of frequently ordered diagnostic tests. For physicians entering data by keyboard and mouse or by using a tablet PC, the design can also offer the option of supplementing the free-text entry area by clicking (or tapping with a stylus) on a drop-down menu to select the tests to be ordered from a physician's customized list of commonly ordered tests.

F i g u r e 15.5

Sample Record Design for Separate Documentation of Diagnostic Tests and Treatments Ordered. This example duplicates the template shown in Figure 15.4, with the addition of a separate section for documenting data ordered. This section also includes its own documentation prompt, with underlining of the numeric values that derive from the suggested values in Figure 15.2. CT, indicates computed tomography; EKG, electrocardiogram; a and a' indicate the number of diagnoses and treatment options; and c' indicates data reviewed.

Addressing Challenge 4: Eliminating Confusing and Time-Consuming Calculations

In the *Practical EHR* method, the need for complex coding calculations is replaced by software designs that include compliant documentation prompts. These prompts provide physicians with guidance to accurately document decision making to an extent that meets or exceeds the complexity warranted by the NPP. This guidance includes a reminder that meeting the documentation requirements for MDM requires satisfaction of any two of the three subcomponents of MDM as illustrated in Figure 15.3.

To assist physicians with correctly documenting the MDM component, in most cases, the challenge of MDM calculations can be significantly decreased or eliminated by avoiding the "two out of three" calculation. Instead, in all cases, physicians are advised to initially consider only the two subcomponents of MDM that are meaningful during every visit: (1) levels of risk and (2) number of diagnoses or treatment options. This is a logical approach because the amount and complexity of data may correlate poorly with the severity of a patient's illness during any particular visit—a visit for a healthy patient may include substantial data, and a visit for a very sick patient may include few data. The other two subcomponents, on the other hand, correlate extremely well with the NPP, and documenting them appropriately for the level of care warranted by the NPP ensures compliant MDM documentation. The templates in Figures 15.1 and 15.5 facilitate this documentation and remove the challenges and uncertainties that physicians and coders commonly associate with MDM documentation. Physicians continue to document the data they review and order, but they do so for purposes of providing quality care and good record keeping. In most cases, they will not need to spend time including consideration of the complexity of the data as part of E/M compliance.

Another advantage of this approach to MDM documentation is that the level of risk of the presenting problem(s) almost always reflects and confirms the NPP. Specifically, because the NPP is also a measure of risk (of morbidity, mortality, and/or functional impairment), the severity of the NPP correlates extremely well with the levels of risk of presenting problems shown in the Table of Risk.[3] For example, when a physician has determined that the NPP is of moderate severity (which warrants a maximum level 3 outpatient care), the risk of the presenting problem will almost always be found to be moderate, and this element of MDM supports the level 3 care. In fact, the moderate level of risk is also sufficient to support level 4 care that would be warranted by an NPP of moderate to high severity. The three levels of risk also provide the most reliable factor physicians have for documenting the difference between level 4 and level 5 care for outpatient office services. Because CPT descriptors indicate that the NPP is usually "moderate to high" for both level 4 and level 5 services, identifying at least one of the three levels of risk as high is the most reasonable way to document that a given service warrants level 5 care rather than level 4 care.

The advantage of fulfilling the second requirement for MDM by documenting the appropriate number of diagnoses and/or treatment options is that the more extensive documentation of this subcomponent encourages physicians to actively consider alternative diagnostic possibilities and to obtain additional testing to rule out contributory illnesses when medically indicated. This promotes a global rather than a linear approach to patient care. It also helps physicians recall their analytic processes during subsequent visits, which is particularly helpful if laboratory tests fail to confirm the primary diagnosis or if a patient's condition does not respond optimally to the initial treatment options.

Recording Differential Diagnoses and Comprehensive Care

Medical training emphasizes consideration and documentation of a differential diagnosis especially for patients with more severe or challenging problems. However, in practice, the economic pressures of needing to provide rapid and thorough care often lead physicians to document only the most probable diagnosis and the primary treatment option. For example, for a patient with recent onset of dizziness, an otolaryngologist might document "probable vestibular neuronitis" (a virally induced balance problem that generally resolves without intervention) but not document a list of rule-out diagnoses (eg, acoustic neuroma, Meniere disease, hypothyroidism, and diabetes).

If the patient returned for follow-up 1 month later, alternative diagnoses might then be considered if the symptoms had not resolved. However, compliance with E/M documentation requirements involves documenting differential diagnoses and, possibly, more actively considering the secondary options at the initial visit. As a result, the physician might order thyroid testing for a patient whose review of systems indicated fatigue, temperature intolerance, and/or skin and hair changes. Similarly, a patient with recent weight gain, frequent urination, and a family history of diabetes would likely receive an order for a glucose tolerance test. By proactively considering potential alternative diagnoses that are suggested by the patient's comprehensive medical history, physicians have the opportunity to promptly identify underlying and contributing medical problems and initiate appropriate treatment at the earliest opportunity. In this way, compliance with E/M documentation requirements can help provide more holistic care and improve quality of care by promoting early diagnosis and intervention.

Practical EHR Method for MDM Documentation Compliance, Quality, and Efficiency

In practical terms, the sequence of analysis and documentation steps involved in the *Practical EHR* approach to MDM adheres to the following straightforward sequence, with the MDM documentation compliance components shown in bold. After completing the comprehensive history and the extent of examination appropriate for the level of care warranted by the NPP, the physician documents the elements of the three subcomponents of MDM as follows:

1. Document all data reviewed.
2. Document the three levels of risk. It is important that **the risk of the presenting problem(s) should equal or exceed the severity of the NPP.** The physician should refer to the documentation prompt and the Table of Risk[3] to confirm this impression.
3. Document the diagnoses and treatment options. The physician should refer to the documentation prompt to ensure recording a *number* of realistic options appropriate for the medically indicated level of care.
4. Document any data ordered.

This compliant method is appropriate and effective for the MDM documentation component in the vast majority of patient visits. It facilitates compliance by requiring documentation of all subcomponents and elements of MDM. It eliminates the coding calculations by relying on the physician to provide appropriate and sufficient documentation of the subcomponents—levels of risk, diagnoses and treatment options—the two most relevant subcomponents in this approach.

DESIGN FEATURES FOR EACH SECTION OF MDM DOCUMENTATION

EHR Design Considerations for the Data-Reviewed Section

For medical data integrity, promoting quality care, improving patient safety, and providing medicolegal security, H&P documentation should contain a record of all data the physician reviews at the time of the visit, even though this information may appear in other sections of the medical record as well (eg, an electrocardiogram[EKG] report will also be saved in the "physiologic tests" section of the patient's record). For increased efficiency, many EHR designs permit physicians to actively copy and paste (or otherwise electronically copy) digital portions of these current reports from the data section of the record directly into the data-reviewed section of visit documentation. On the other hand, systems that include a passive (ie, automatic) transfer of data reports to the data-reviewed section of the H&P record must also add error-proofing functionality for compliance, quality, and patient safety. This software protection must require physicians to electronically sign the data-reviewed section to attest review of the reports at the time of the visit. In addition, the data-reviewed section must also allow entry of free-text narrative descriptions of test results. This capability permits and encourages physicians to review the actual tests (eg, CT scan images) by allowing them to document their personal interpretations in the record.

Paper forms used with a digital pen or as a data transfer medium can also gain a small amount of increased efficiency by including check boxes for tests physicians commonly review. Therefore, an internist who reviews many EKG, chest X-rays, and stress tests can request that labels for these studies be entered on the paper templates. Figure 15.6 shows a sample paper form incorporating these check boxes for convenience. Checking a box and then entering the results of the test saves the physician the time of writing "chest X-ray" many times per week. With this approach, the EHR screen needs to have a matching design for ease and reliability of data entry by a data entry operator or digital pen system. Similar use of check-boxes or drop-down menus are useful screen designs for physicians using direct keyboard entry or tablet PCs.

F IGURE 15.6

Sample Data-Reviewed Section of a Paper Form for Outpatient Services, With Check-Boxes for Increased Documentation Efficiency. (c) indicates data ordered.

Data reviewed (c):	1. Minimal or none (level 2)	2. Limited (level 3)	3. Moderate (level 4)	4. Extensive (level 5)
☐ Chest X-ray:				
☐ Electrocardiogram (EKG):				
☐ Stress test:				
☐ Laboratory test:				

EHR Design Considerations for Impressions, Plans, and Data Ordered

Although conventional H&P records commonly contain only two sections for recording clinical impressions and plans, for clarity and avoiding compliance errors, *Practical EHR* suggests including separate sections for the following: (1) impressions and differential diagnoses, (2) plans and management options, and (3) data ordered. Designs may include parallel columns, rows, or a combination of rows and columns, as shown in Figure 15.5.

Data Entry Design for the Impressions and Differential Diagnoses Subsection

The portion of MDM documentation in which physicians describe a patient's diagnoses requires only free-text entry to satisfy several complementary requirements for compliance and quality documentation. Even though straightforward listing of primary diagnoses could be accomplished by selecting from pick-list menus (a common design option found in many current EHRs for this section), the requirements for recording potential diagnoses extend significantly beyond this obvious requirement. In addition, physicians should include a complete list of differential diagnoses, including possible alternative and/or additional explanations for the patient's illness. One or more of these possibilities may subsequently prove to be valid following further testing or a suboptimal response to initial therapy. The need to categorize these alternative diagnoses on the basis of their relative likelihood, by using descriptions such as "rule-out," "probable," "possible," or "likely," mandates the need for narrative descriptions. Examples of brief narrative descriptions that convey the physician's depth of analysis include "cough, *probable* pneumonia" and "chest pain, *likely* secondary to reflux, must *rule out* myocardial disease."

A second benefit of free-text narrative entry is that it enables physicians to describe the relationships between possible diagnoses (eg, "chronic cough *secondary to* gastroesophageal reflux"). It also gives them the opportunity to insert descriptive adjectives that report the severity of a condition; for example, indicating that a patient has "*life-threatening* obstructive sleep apnea" conveys a distinctly different message from "*mild* obstructive sleep apnea." All of the descriptive details added in free-text narratives carry important qualitative information to the physician providing care during future visits, regardless of whether it is the same physician or another physician.

Challenges Created by Including Charge Entry and/or Data Mining Functions as Part of MDM Documentation

EHR software designers have faced strong temptation to integrate charge entry capability into the electronic H&P portion of the EHR. The goal of systems that provide this functionality is to save time and/or money for administrative staff. These EHRs require physicians to select International Classification of Diseases, Ninth Revision, Clinical Modification (ICD-9) diagnosis codes and their definitions from a drop-down menu in the diagnoses section of the MDM documentation rather than recording impressions in a free-text narrative interface. The selected codes then serve two functions: (1) recording the patient's primary diagnoses in the MDM section of the H&P record and (2) automatically transferring the primary diagnoses to the practice management system for billing purposes.

continued

In a similar fashion, restricting documentation to the use of lists of ICD-9 codes in the MDM diagnoses section enables it to be a datamining source. This approach allows the software to use this data field to identify patients who have specific diagnoses and then apply this information to disease management for appropriate groups of patients within a practice. In some programs, this pick-list documentation approach may also be used to prompt and activate a presentation of guidelines for clinical decision support (eg, picking a diagnosis for asthma could automatically activate the asthma management guideline).

Although the intent of using software capabilities to eliminate extra steps in the billing process or to search specified subpopulations in the practice for enhanced care sounds attractive, such benefits of technology should be implemented only when they do not also have the potential to disturb the physician's normal workflow and/or sacrifice E/M compliance and quality documentation. To prevent these problems, designers must apply the concept of error proofing before approving the use of potentially disruptive functionality. Unfortunately, introducing charge entry functionality into E/M documentation has intrinsic defects because *the requirements for compliant billing are incompatible with the requirements for compliant and effective E/M documentation.* The primary source of this incompatibility is the *prohibition,* by billing compliance standards, of the submission of claims that include rule-out diagnoses, whereas E/M compliance and medical standards for quality records require their inclusion in the H&P record. Furthermore, charge entry functionality requires replacing a narrative interface with selection of diagnoses from drop-down menus that provide no information other than a list of ICD-9 codes. The requirement for this restrictive vocabulary for charge entry, data mining, or to trigger the appearance of decision support tools unacceptably precludes the use of detailed, concept-rich descriptions needed to convey the relative probability and/or severity of the diagnoses described.

Acceptable designs for this element of MDM must respect the concept that there are separate and conflicting requirements for high-quality-compliant E/M documentation compared to the rules and requirements for charge entry or mining data. This leads to the conclusion that documentation of possible diagnoses in the H&P must be separate from the process of recording diagnoses (and procedures) for charge entry and mining data. A reasonable solution must require physicians to consider lists of diagnoses for charge entry data mining only after they have completed documentation of the H&P. As discussed in Chapter 16, it is acceptable for software designs to offer options for physicians performing charge entry, but only as a completely separate operation or as a secondary step that builds on the diagnoses listed in the MDM documentation section of the H&P record. Similarly, the listing of diagnoses through ICD-9 codes in the patient profile section of the EHR provides all the benefits of population management and simultaneously maintains the integrity of the information documented in the diagnoses section of the electronic H&P. Finally, there are multiple alternatives to activate clinical decision support, without relying on the reconfiguration of this critical element, for documenting high-quality differential diagnoses.

Data Entry Design for Management Options and Data-Ordered Sections

The management options and data-ordered sections of MDM documentation also need to provide physicians with narrative capability to describe an individualized blueprint for each patient's ongoing care, including contingencies for possible future treatments and diagnostic procedures. For example, after ordering a medication to control an acute problem, the physician may want to add a description of one or more alternative treatments to be considered if the patient's condition fails to respond to the initial choice within a specified time frame, if specific side effects develop in response to the initial choice, and/or for ongoing management after the acute problem is controlled. A physician may also want to describe one or more alternative treatment plans that would be contingent on specific laboratory results (eg, describing a particular thyroid medication and dosage to be started if laboratory results confirm a diagnosis of hypothyroidism).

Similarly, in the data-ordered section, physicians may want to include instructions for obtaining additional tests contingent on the results of an initial test battery. For example, a rheumatologist who orders a set of screening laboratory tests may also record instructions for obtaining an in-depth panel of immune tests if the result of one of the screening tests is positive. In the same way, a pulmonologist ordering chest X-rays and pulmonary function tests may document a plan to order a CT scan of the lungs if findings from the plain films are normal but the function tests show a significant degree of abnormality.

However, designs for these two sections can effectively combine graphic and narrative interface options. It is reasonable, for example, for an H&P screen to include an option for drop-down menus or a selection list with check-boxes that allows physicians to select initial treatments or indicate a set of diagnostic tests or procedures. The selection menus should list each physician's commonly used treatments for entry into the management options section and commonly ordered diagnostic tests for entry into the data-ordered section. An accompanying narrative area allows physicians the option of using free text to add further details. This combination design offers a versatile interface option for these two sections of MDM documentation, while also maintaining effective documentation and compliance. Figure 15.5 illustrates optional check-boxes in these two sections of an EHR screen (or a matching paper form).

DATA ENTRY TOOLS AVAILABLE FOR MDM

With its many subsections, the MDM documentation design offers the greatest opportunity in the H&P record for physicians to use a hybrid approach. The electronic H&P record design should permit physicians to select among a variety of data entry tools to find those that provide the greatest usability and efficiency for documenting each subsection of MDM.

Data-Reviewed Section

Design of the EHR should provide data entry tools for physicians who prefer to write (tools 1, 5, and 6, Chapter 11), to dictate (tools 2 and 3, Chapter 11), and to use keyboard and mouse entry (tool 7, Chapter 11). The additional feature that may be available for physicians working directly on a conventional computer or a tablet PC is the potential for copy-and-paste functionality. If transmitted reports have been entered digitally into the EHR, the design might offer the capability for physicians to copy and paste the conclusions of a report into this section of MDM documentation.

Impressions and Differential Diagnoses Section

For compliance and quality, this section requires a narrative interface. The design should provide one or more of the tools for physicians who prefer writing, dictating, or using direct keyboard entry.

Management Options and Data-Ordered Sections

These two sections provide the opportunity for physicians to use more than one format for entering information. Unless declined by individual physicians, designs can add a graphic interface for commonly ordered treatments and/or diagnostic tests to the required narrative-entry format needed to describe less frequently used options and to describe contingencies. The graphic interface possibilities include check-boxes for data entry on digital paper and by tablet PC (as shown in Figure 15.6) and a drop-down menu for direct data entry into a conventional computer or a tablet PC.

Complexity of Data, Levels of Risk, and NPP Sections

One of the critical features of *Practical EHR* design principles is providing physicians with the ability to document these generally overlooked E/M components, thereby ensuring compliance and providing audit protection. As illustrated in Figure 15.1 (for the complexity of data and levels of risk) and Figures 13.1 to 13.3 (for the NPP), a graphic interface with a single check-box next to each possible choice provides an ideal documentation tool that allows physicians to record their impressions for each of these components in only a few seconds. With the use of the graphic interface, there is no need to provide a dictation option. Physicians should have the alternatives of documenting directly into the software by mouse clicks on the computer, by touch-screen capability with a stylus on a tablet PC, or by writing on paper for entry directly via a digital pen or indirectly by a data entry operator.

FUNCTIONALITY OF MDM DOCUMENTATION AND THE NPP

Practical EHR Method

On completion of the physical examination, the physician should mentally conclude that the examination findings confirm the initial assessment of the severity of the NPP or that they call for a modification. The physician can then use this confirmed or revised level of NPP to guide documentation of MDM at levels appropriate for the severity of the patient's illness at the time of the visit. It is critical for the design to provide physicians with tools to document all elements of all three subcomponents of MDM.

The design for MDM documentation should include *passive* documentation prompts to provide guidance because it is unreasonable for physicians to memorize the myriad of complex coding and documentation rules intrinsic to this component of the H&P record. The first prompt, shown in the top line of Figure 15.3, reminds physicians that two of the three MDM elements must be documented as appropriate for the NPP. This prompt also provides identifying alpha symbols to identify all elements that constitute the three MDM subcomponents (a and a′ for the number of diagnoses and treatment options; b, b′, and b″ for the three types of risk; and c, c′, and c″ for data ordered, data reviewed, and complexity of data).

To facilitate a relatively easy-to-use approach to compliant MDM documentation, physicians should be instructed to concentrate on the documentation of the subcomponents for the levels of risk and the number of diagnoses and management options. When considering the three types of risk, physicians should compare the level of care they identified as appropriate for the NPP with the examples provided in the Table of Risk.[3] The CPT instructions regarding this subcomponent provide that the highest of the three documented levels of risk is considered the overall risk for the encounter. In particular, the level selected for "risk of the presenting problem(s)" is generally comparable to the severity of the NPP (which is also a measure of risk), and this level almost always equals or exceeds the level of care warranted by the NPP. The risk subcomponent can also help physicians achieve correct coding. When one of the three risk components is reasonably judged to be high, it can be a determinative factor for identifying patients with a "moderate to high" NPP who warrant level 5 rather than level 4 care. Finally, it is highly unlikely that a reasonable assessment of risk of the presenting problem will correlate with a lower level of care than warranted by the NPP. If this situation should arise, the physician should reassess the NPP and the indicated level of care.

Documentation prompts also assist physicians in understanding the extent of documentation warranted by medical necessity for the subcomponent of the number of diagnoses and/or the number of treatment options. This insight helps physicians document the diagnostic process applied throughout the visit and their blueprint for the best future care of each patient. Figures 15.4 and 15.5 illustrate the documentation prompt used for *passive* guidance of this element of MDM documentation. Designers may also include an interactive prompt to help physicians who enter data directly into the software (via regular computer or tablet PC). This type of prompt will show physicians' progress as they document each possible diagnosis and each potential management option. Figure 15.7 illustrates a sample *interactive* guidance prompt that could be used in addition to the passive prompt included in the template. This design displays the level of care as it is documented, showing whichever is the higher of the two elements of this subcomponent.

F IGURE 15.7

Sample Design for Interactive Guidance on the Number of Diagnoses or Management Options Shown in Figure 15.5. A horizontal bar graph with a moving indicator above helps a physician visualize the level of care supported by this documentation. For example, when the physician documents two diagnoses or two treatment options, the indicator shows that this supports the level 3 care that correlates with a moderate NPP. The box with the asterisk corresponds to the severity of nature of the presenting problem (NPP) identified at this point in the care.

Documentation of the final assessment of the NPP confirms the physician's impression of the severity of the patient's illnesses at the point of care. This step occurs at the conclusion of MDM, when the physician will have established a final impression of the appropriate NPP for the encounter. In addition, the method of NPP guidance will have facilitated the performance of medically indicated levels of care and corresponding documentation for all three key components. At this concluding stage of the patient visit, all that remains is for the physician to take a second or two to document the final impression of the level of the NPP by checking the appropriate box on the NPP template that appears at the end of the H&P record, samples of which are shown in Figures 13.1 to 13.3. This documentation ensures that

---

Documenting Thought Processes

A common physician objection, after negative results in an E/M compliance audit, is "I did the work, I just didn't document it." This statement often has significant merit for MDM documentation. Most physicians go through the medical diagnostic process while providing care. However, primarily owing to lack of effective medical record tools, most physicians go through this process on "automatic pilot." They mentally weigh the various diagnostic options and assess the severity of illness and relative need for urgent intervention, but, to save time, they document only the primary diagnosis and primary treatment recommendation. The *Practical EHR* method requires that software designs include effective tools and guidance for physicians to efficiently document the entire decision-making process.

---

the physician, not an auditor, is the person who determines the degree of medical necessity in case of a future compliance audit.

Error Proofing

With the use of sophisticated and comprehensive decision-making templates and documentation prompts, there is relatively limited need for error proofing in this section of the H&P record. The critical task of the software in error proofing the MDM component is to make certain that physicians have documented all required MDM elements—levels of risk, diagnoses, and management options in addition to the NPP. If a physician has failed to address any of these subcomponents, the software should require that this documentation be completed before permitting the physician to "sign off" on the record.

Compliant Code Selection

At the conclusion of the H&P record, there are two possible options for identifying the appropriate and compliantly documented E/M code. The first approach is passive, mirroring compliant E/M functionality in the paper world. The second calls for active code confirmation using additional EHR software functionality.

Passive Code Selection
Physicians who have followed the *Practical EHR* method throughout the care process should already know the appropriate code to submit. They will have:

- Performed a comprehensive history
- Selected and eventually confirmed a medically indicated NPP and *level of care* (ie, the appropriate E/M code)
- Performed and documented the medically indicated extent of physical examination based on this appropriate level of care
- Performed and documented the medically indicated complexity of MDM based on this appropriate level of care
- Documented the medically appropriate NPP confirmed at the conclusion of the care process

At this point, physicians can comfortably select the medically necessary and properly documented E/M code on a superbill or on a software entry screen. The documentation and coding will have been accomplished as an integral component of providing high-quality, medically indicated care.

Coding Engines for Compliance Confirmation and Interactive Guidance

An added benefit EHRs can offer is to supplement the passive coding guidance of documentation prompts with an active software coding engine to confirm that selected code levels are appropriate for medical necessity (NPP) and that the documentation fulfills the compliance requirements of CPT coding and the Documentation Guidelines. Achieving a reliable system requires that several benchmarks be met. First, EHRs must integrate a coding engine that accurately follows all CPT compliance principles and

---

Coding Parameters the Software Must Provide to the E/M Coding Engine

For active code confirmation, the EHR must communicate all of the necessary coding parameters to the coding engine, including:

- The type of service
- Medical history component
  - Initial visit services
    - For the past, family, and social history (PFSH), register whether or not there is a documented response to at least one question in the graphic interface section for the past history, the social history, and the family history
    - For the review of systems (ROS), register how many organ systems have a documented response to at least one question in the graphic interface section
  - Established visit services
    - Register whether or not there is a documented update to the PFSH
    - Register whether or not there is a documented update to the ROS
  - For the history of the present illness (HPI), the necessary use of a narrative interface will require physicians to actively select check boxes to indicate whether
    - The HPI provides a chronological description of the course of the patient's illness
    - The narrative includes one to three elements of the HPI
    - The narrative includes four to eight elements of the HPI
    - The narrative records the status of three or more chronic or inactive conditions
    - These check boxes could readily be integrated into the documentation prompt for this section, with an error-proofing function that requires their completion before moving forward
- Physical examination component
  - Indicate the type of examination template used (multisystem examination or a specified single organ system examination)

continued

- Register how many of the mandated elements of the examination are documented as normal or abnormal in the graphic interface section
- MDM component
  - Number of diagnoses and treatment options
    - Register the number of diagnoses documented (template design can facilitate this counting function)
    - Register the number of management options documented (template design can facilitate this counting function)
  - Three levels of risk
    - Register the documented level of risk for the patient's presenting problem(s)
    - Register the documented level of risk for diagnostic procedures
    - Register the documented level of risk for management options
  - Various components of data (software should inactivate calculating this component for most cases unless the physician decides to include this consideration in a specific case)
    - Amount of data reviewed
    - Amount of data ordered
    - Complexity of data ordered or reviewed
- NPP
  - Register the documented level of NPP
- Time, counseling, and coordination of care (described in detail in Chapter 16)
  - Register the documented amount of time involved in a visit
  - Register documentation that more than 50% of the time of the visit was involved in counseling and coordination of care
  - Register that a narrative description of the counseling was documented

excludes all noncompliant coding shortcut tools. The coding engine must also incorporate and process all the elements of the E/M system, including all subcomponents of decision making, and especially including the NPP.

With proper functionality, all of this information can be forwarded automatically to the E/M coding engine as it is documented into the H&P record, with the one additional step for physicians to check one or two documentation boxes associated with the HPI. The coding software should compile all of these data and properly apply the CPT E/M descriptors to calculate three separate codes and present them back to the physician: (1) a level of care based on the three key components, (2) a level of care based on the NPP, and (3) a level of care based on time (when time requirements have been met). This report should also advise the physician how to base final code selection. These instructions should be based on the following prioritization principles:

- In conventional visits (not based on time), CPT instructions indicate that medical necessity determines the appropriate level of care, so the code derived from the NPP should set the upper limit for the E/M code selected.

- The code determined by the three key components should be the code submitted unless it is higher than the code determined by the NPP, in which case the NPP-based code will be appropriate in most cases.

- CPT guidelines indicate that valid time-based visits (those that meet CPT guidelines) can supersede the level of care based on the three key components and NPP.

Figure 15.8 illustrates one design for a pop-up screen that integrates these three aspects of compliant E/M coding, with an added level of error proofing that should be available to ensure that the code warranted by medical necessity is the maximum level of service submitted for documentation-based coding.

FIGURE 15.8

Sample Pop-up Screen for E/M Coding. This screen shows the code level appropriate for the documented NPP and whether this level of care was documented. It also activates a section for time-based coding, as described in Chapter 16, when this has been documented. The first example illustrates a case in which the documentation is sufficient to fulfill requirements for the level of care warranted by the NPP. The second example illustrates a case in which the documentation is insufficient to fulfill requirements for the level of care warranted by the NPP. The final example illustrates a case in which time considerations yield a higher level of service. The use of larger and bold type indicates the most appropriate evaluation and management (E/M) code to submit.

Example 1

E/M Code Determination
1) E/M coding based on chart documentation
a) E/M care warranted by documented NPP: **99204**
b) Documentation of history, examination, and/or decision making DOES support **99204**
2) E/M coding based on time
a) Time-based coding is not appropriately documented in this record.

Example 2

E/M Code Determination
1) E/M coding based on chart documentation
a) E/M care warranted by documented NPP: 99204
b) Documentation of history, examination, and/or decision making DOES NOT support 99204
Appropriate code to submit based on these key components is: **99203**
2) E/M coding based on time
a) Time-based coding is documented, and supports code: 99202

Example 3

E/M Code Determination
1) E/M coding based on chart documentation
a) E/M care warranted by documented NPP: 99213
b) Documentation of history, examination, and/or decision making DOES support 99213
2) E/M coding based on time
a) Time-based coding is documented and supports code: **99214**

An integrated coding engine should also be able to support interactive documentation prompts, such as illustrated in Figure 15.7. This type of prompt can provide physicians with immediate feedback to confirm that the level of care is appropriate for the NPP.

Physicians using asynchronous data entry with a transcriptionist or other data entry professional will have to rely on passive guidance at the point of care to ensure adequate documentation appropriate for the NPP because the coding engine would not receive input at the time of the visit.

SUMMARY

Achieving compliant documentation in the MDM component of the H&P record has traditionally posed significant challenges for physicians and software developers. These challenges arise from four problems inherent to conventional MDM approaches: (1) unconventional documentation components, (2) subjective measures for amounts of data and number of diagnoses and treatment options, (3) failure to separately document treatment options and data ordered, and (4) complex coding calculations.

Solving these four problems leads to a logical approach to MDM documentation that can be integrated into EHR software and works easily for physicians. First, designs for the MDM documentation component must incorporate the capability to document all elements of MDM, including those not commonly included in conventional medical record structures (the severity of the three types of risk and the complexity of data reviewed). Next, the CPT subjective measures can be addressed with documentation prompts based on reasonable published guidelines that quantify the subjective terms for *amount* of data and *number* of diagnoses and treatment options. The third issue is readily addressed by providing separate areas of the chart for documentation of treatment options and data ordered. Finally, the *Practical EHR* method replaces complex MDM calculations with guidance to appropriately document the two most relevant subcomponents of MDM: (1) the levels of risk and (2) lists of all relevant potential diagnoses and treatment options that physicians generally consider in their diagnostic process but commonly fail to document. Incorporating these solutions allows a well-designed electronic H&P record to guide compliant documentation of MDM as a natural component of physicians' normal workflow and the diagnostic process.

The design features for documentation of MDM and NPP complete the process of integrating compliant E/M documentation and coding principles into the electronic H&P record and the patient care process. At the conclusion of each patient visit, physicians have determined the appropriate level of care (ie, E/M code) based on their determination of the nature of the patient's problems. They can also feel secure that the documentation prompts provided by their EHR system have guided appropriate amounts of care and documentation to support that code. They can simply enter this necessity-based E/M code into their billing document (paper or electronic) and proceed to the next patient.

Effective EHRs can assist and confirm physicians' documentation and coding compliance by integrating a *compliant* E/M software coding system, which must receive information about all documented E/M elements, including the NPP. This system should derive three code levels (based on NPP, level of documentation, and time) and guide physicians on which of the three is most appropriate to submit. Finally, this same coding software can also be programmed to provide interactive documentation prompts that can assist physicians who are using direct documentation tools.

References

1.   American Medical Association. *Current Procedural Terminology (CPT®).* Chicago, IL: American Medical Association; 2007.

2.   Department of Health & Human Services; Centers for Medicare & Medicaid Services. "Examples of Situations in Which Physician is Liable." In: *Medicare Claims Processing Manual.* Part 3, Section 7103.1(I). Available at: www.cms.hhs.gov/Transmittals/Downloads/R1826B3.pdf. Accessed July 1, 2007.

3.   Health Care Financing Administration. *Documentation Guidelines for Evaluation and Management Services.* Washington, DC: Health Care Financing Administration; 1997:47.

4.   Levinson SR. Documenting medical decision making. In: *Practical E/M: Documentation and Coding Solutions for Quality Patient Care.* Chicago, IL: AMA Press; 2005:139.

5.   Certification Commission for Healthcare Information Technology. Ambulatory Functionality Criteria 2007. Available at www.cchit.org/files/Ambulatory_Domain/CCHIT_Ambulatory_FUNCTIONALITY_Criteria_2007. Accessed July 1, 2007.

chapter 16

Additional Design Features for the Electronic H&P

Following the completion of a blueprint for an electronic history and physical examination (H&P) record that meets physicians' documentation needs for every type of service that is primarily based on the three key components and medical necessity, EHR designers can turn their attention to a variety of complementary design features that can further enhance the information available to physicians to provide and document quality care. All of the following medical record components will add value to every software system:

- Ability to document and code time-based E/M services based on time, counseling, and coordination of care
  - Documentation templates for preventive care and critical care services
  - Documentation templates for physicians working with residents and nonphysician practitioners
  - Ability to document patient educational materials provided to patients
- Translational consultation reports
- A "prior encounter summary screen" to access essential information from previous visits at the beginning of each established patient visit
- A "patient profile section," which maintains an inventory of patient health status information, valuable for ongoing management. Subsections of the profile may include a list of active and resolved problems, a medication list, lists of environmental and medication allergies, a record of positive elements of the family history, and a record of the social history
- Report functionality
- Preventive care protocols and disease management protocols
- Charge entry capabilities

This chapter presents an overview of each of these complementary features, including a review of physicians' requirements and sample templates that designers can use as starting points for developing individual customizations.

Sample Forms as a Starting Point

The sample forms in this chapter present hypothetical working solutions to important physician issues that EHRs should be able to address. They are presented as starting points, defining one potential design solution out of many possibilities. It is hoped that various EHR designers and developers will offer creative variations on these themes and that feedback from physicians will determine which designs are most effective.

TIME-BASED E/M CARE (COUNSELING VISITS)

The *Current Procedural Terminology* (*CPT®*) manual identifies time as one of the seven components of E/M services. It provides values for "typical" time of service as one of the descriptors for most types of E/M services, and it further states that these times are presented as "averages," provided specifically "to assist physicians in selecting the most appropriate level of E/M services."[1(p4)] The definitions for time are also related to different types of service. For outpatient care, the *CPT* manual specifies that this measure applies only to face-to-face time that the physician actually spends with the patient. Time is not counted when the physician is out of the examination room, even if a nurse or other staff member is interacting with the patient. For hospital and nursing facility care, including observation services, the *CPT* manual defines time as "unit/floor time." This concept includes face-to-face time and "the time in which the physician establishes and/or reviews the patient's chart, examines the patient, writes notes, and communicates with other professionals and the patient's family."[1(p5)] Even though the *CPT* manual includes time as one of the seven E/M components and describes it as a guideline, in most cases physicians are instructed not to consider time as a factor in determining compliant levels of documentation and coding.

However, under the special circumstance "when counseling and/or coordination of care dominates (more than 50%) the physician/patient and/or family encounter (face-to-face time in the office or other outpatient setting or floor/unit time in the hospital or nursing facility), then time may be considered the key or controlling factor to qualify for a particular level of E/M services."[1(p8)] In practical terms, when more than half of a visit involves counseling and/or coordination of care, as defined in the *CPT* manual, the physician has the option of basing the level of care and E/M code submitted on the conventional E/M components (history, examination, medical decision making, and nature of the presenting problem) or making the determination solely on the basis of the amount of time spent, depending on which approach produces the higher level of service. Time-based code determination is also valid for counseling visits, in which 100% of the visit is devoted to counseling and coordination of care, without inclusion of the key components.

How Reviewers Interpret Code Thresholds Based on Time

Even though CPT descriptors for time are defined as "average times" associated with each CPT code, consultants, auditors, and medical directors conventionally treat these values as *threshold* times for the selection of the proper code. For example, the CPT description of E/M service 99214 includes the statement "physicians typically spend 25 minutes face-to-face with the patient and/or family."[1(p10)] Even though this time value is presented in the *CPT* manual as an average, it is interpreted to mean that 25 minutes or more supports 99214, but less than 25 minutes does not. This analysis does not appear in the *CPT* manual[1] or Documentation Guidelines.[2] However, it is my observation of how time and code levels are consistently taught and applied by Medicare carriers, insurers, and compliance experts.

There are three documentation elements defined by the Documentation Guidelines that must be included in design requirements for time-based services: (1) The physician must document that more than 50% of the encounter involved counseling and/or coordination of care. The EHR can meet this requirement by allowing physicians to document the actual time involved in counseling or by providing a design with a check-box for physicians to attest that counseling comprised more than 50% of the visit. (2) The "total length of time of the encounter (face-to-face or floor time, as appropriate) should be documented."[2(p48)] (3) The "record should describe the counseling and/or activities to coordinate care."[2(p48)] This should include documentation of the discussion of written materials and/or pamphlets provided to patients during the visit. Figure 16.1 illustrates a sample design containing these three required elements for documentation of time-based services. It also includes a documentation-prompt, shown in the shaded section, that advises physicians of the CPT requirements for consideration of time as the basis for determining the level of an E/M service. This template can be incorporated as a final section of the electronic H&P form or as a pop-up window. It can also be added to a paper form that is used with a digital pen or as a data transfer medium.

FIGURE 16.1

Sample Documentation Template for Time-based E/M Services. This template includes a documentation prompt confirming the requirements for using time as the basis for determining an evaluation and management (E/M) code. It also includes a reminder for outpatient services that the total time includes only face-to-face time. For inpatient services, this statement changes to read "floor/unit." In the narrative section below the prompts, the physician must describe the gist of the counseling and/or care coordination activities. The design shown allows documentation of total time and a check-box to attest that counseling dominated the visit. Another option would be to list the total counseling and consultation time and the total visit time (eg, counseling time/visit time = 17/25 mins).

Complete this section only if documented below "> 50% of visit time" involved counseling and/or coordinating care
Time(face to face):_____ minutes   ☐ > 50% of visit time involved counseling and/or coordination of care

For maximum flexibility, the EHR design should offer physicians multiple options for completing this form:

- Direct entry via keyboard
- Writing on a paper template with a digital pen or for delayed indirect entry
- Hybrid of keyboard for entering the amount of time and a mouse click to check the box attesting that time-based services dominated the visit, combined with dictation of a narrative summary of the counseling and care coordination topics

Time Prompts

For time-based visits, EHR designs should include documentation prompts showing the correlation, for each type of service, between the total amount of time of the visit and the appropriate level of care. This should likely be available as a pop-up window for physicians to enter the type of service (or the first four digits of the E/M code), and include a screen with the information shown in Figure 16.2, which shows the time prompts for an outpatient established visit.

Similar tables should be available for each type of service that permits consideration of time for code determination under the appropriate circumstances.

F IGURE   16.2

Evaluation and Management (E/M) Codes and Time for Counseling and Coordination
of Care (Outpatient Established Visits)

Type of service	9921___			
Face-to-face time with patient (min)*	10	15	25	40
E/M Code	99212	99213	99214	99215

*Total time of the visit, with more than 50% of that time devoted to counseling and/or coordination of care.

UNCONVENTIONAL E/M SERVICES

Although the overwhelming majority of attention to E/M services is generally
directed at the types of service that are based on the seven components, there
are other important E/M services that do not consider these conventional
components but follow different sets of criteria.

- Preventive Medicine Services for new patients (CPT codes 99381-99387)
  and established patients (99391-99397) are based on "age and gender
  appropriate history, examination, counseling/anticipatory guidance/risk
  factor reduction interventions, and the ordering of appropriate
  immunization(s) laboratory/diagnostic procedures"[1(p31)]

- ***Critical Care Services (CPT codes 99291-99292), Inpatient Pediatric
  Critical Care (99293-99294), and Inpatient Neonatal Critical Care
  (99298-99300) are defined in *CPT* by the critical nature of the patient's
  illness or injury, the complexity of the decision making, and the amount
  of time involved. In addition, this care includes provision of a significant
  number of diagnostic and therapeutic procedures that would otherwise
  be coded separately[1(p19)]

Even though these services don't follow the documentation and coding paradigms of typical outpatient, inpatient, and nursing home services, they are
governed by a complex set of CPT rules that physicians should not be
required to memorize. By incorporating all these rules into usable, efficient,
and compliant screens, EHR designs can provide physicians with effective
medical record tools[3] that facilitate care, save time, and ensure compliance.

DOCUMENTATION TOOLS TO HELP PHYSICIANS WORKING WITH OTHER CLINICIANS

Additional Medicare documentation and coding rules also apply when
physicians submit claims for E/M services they perform in conjunction
with resident physicians in teaching facilities or with nurse practitioners
and physicians' assistants in the practice setting.

E/M documentation and coding criteria for physicians working with residents in teaching hospitals are governed by a set of Centers for Medicare &
Medicaid Services (CMS) rules referred to as "Physician Presence." Based on a
Health Care Financing Administration (HCFA) document from the early
1990s titled "Internal Letter 372" (IL-372), these rules have been further
defined in the Medicare Final Rule For Teaching Physicians dated May
30,1996, and have undergone subsequent refinements as well. The physician
presence concept addresses the circumstances under which physicians can

include some of the care performed and documented in the resident's clinical record and have it contribute to the level of care provided.

CMS provides another set of rules determining the circumstances under which care provided by "nonphysician practitioners" can be billed "incident to" the physician's involvement—allowing the physician to charge for this care at higher fee levels than the nurse practitioner or physician's assistant would be reimbursed.

EHRs that incorporate these specialized "physician presence" rules and "incident to" rules into data capture tools[3] can assist physicians by facilitating efficient and compliant documentation and coding as an integral element of normal physician workflow during patient care.

PATIENT EDUCATIONAL MATERIALS

Many electronic records have the capability of storing patient educational materials that the physician can print by clicking an instruction box to provide the patient with these relevant documents, which may include explanations of illnesses, instructions regarding medications, surgical information sheets (including preoperative and postoperative instructions), and disease management protocols. Physicians can also give out preprinted informational booklets as well. The electronic H&P record should include a section to document the materials provided, which should occur automatically when the physician selects the appropriate material for a given patient. This documentation can be augmented by having a section on the MDM-screen with check-boxes to record the selected information that was given directly to patients.

"TRANSLATIONAL" CONSULTATION REPORTS

One of the primary foci of the enthusiasm for adoption of EHRs is the establishment of a national health information network. One of the major benefits of this electronic interconnectivity is to enable multiple physicians caring for a specific person to share patient-specific information about medical findings, treatments, and the patient's response to care. This capability is intended to correct what health policy advocates commonly refer to as physicians practicing in "silos" to illustrate the prevalent lack of access to data. This electronic interconnectivity will build on and enhance, but not replace, the traditional approach to sharing patient information, which is communication among physicians by consultation letters.

The *CPT* manual formally defines the consultation as a type of E/M service "provided by a physician whose opinion or advice regarding evaluation and/or management of a specific problem is requested by another physician or other appropriate source."[1(p14)] It further notes that three requirements must be fulfilled for physicians to submit claims for this type of service[1(p14)]:

1. The physician must document the written or verbal request for the consultation in the patient's medical record.
2. The consultant must document his or her opinion and any services ordered or performed in the medical record.
3. The consultant must communicate, by written report to the requesting physician or other appropriate source, his or her opinion and any services ordered or performed in the medical record.

As EHRs facilitate electronic interconnectivity, consultation services will continue to require this defined written communication to convey the consultant's impressions and thought processes concisely to the requesting physician. This communication will simply be delivered electronically rather than by mail or fax transmission.

Why a Consultation E/M Service Has Greater Value Than an Initial Visit

When the "value" assigned to an outpatient *consultation service* is compared with the value of an outpatient *initial visit*, depending on the medically indicated level of care provided, the consultation is assigned between 0.37 and 1.29 more relative value units (RVUs) than the comparable initial visit service. In the resource-based relative value system (RBRVS), these value units are based on vignettes, which describe the details of every element included in that service.

Scrutinizing comparable levels of outpatient initial visits and consultations reveals that both types of service consistently reflect identical levels of medical history, levels of physical examination, complexity of medical decision making, and nature of the presenting problem. The obvious question is "What accounts for the increased RVUs assigned to consultation services?" The answer appears to be that the sole difference between these two services is the written report the consultant sends to the requesting physician or other appropriate source. The additional RVUs are, therefore, included to reimburse the physician for the costs and work value involved in creating this report.

What must consultants include in this report? The CPT definition provides sufficient insight into these requirements, which are summarized as follows:

1. The consultation letter should include the physician's clinical impressions and recommendations for treatment and/or further diagnostic studies and procedures.
2. The consultation letter should include a synopsis of the services performed during the consultation, ie, the medical history, physical examination, and any diagnostic or therapeutic procedures.
3. A photocopy of the H&P report from the medical chart does not satisfy the requirement of a written report.

One of the benefits of having an EHR is that it records all patient-specific information digitally. With the added benefit of a well-structured H&P record, these data can be mined and transposed into an original, patient-specific consultation letter without significant additional effort. A well-designed EHR should include the capacity to "translate" the already documented unique patient information from the E/M visit into an appropriate and compliant consultation letter format. Figure 16.3 illustrates a sample framework for a consultation letter that provides structure, but has no preloaded clinical information. To send a consultation letter to a requesting physician (or other appropriate source), the consulting physician should be able to instruct the software to access all relevant individualized clinical information from that visit and import it into the consultation framework, creating an original consultation letter specific to the patient and the encounter that satisfies all requirements for quality information and compliance.

SUBSEQUENT CARE: SUMMARY SCREEN FOR PRIOR ENCOUNTER

The medical record collects and stores a variety of clinical information during and after each patient visit. In addition to the E/M care documented during the visit, this information may include laboratory studies, radiologic tests, physiologic tests, and outside medical records from other physicians.

F I G U R E 16.3

Sample Consultation Letter Framework. With a preloaded consultation template containing structure but not preloaded clinical information, software should have the capability to "translate" clinical information specific to an individual patient and specific visit into a customized consultation letter. The italicized sections explain the information that the designer must program the software to import from the history and physical examination (H&P) record to create the consultation letter.

Letterhead Containing Practice Demographic Information

Date (imported from date of visit)

Physician name, MD   }
Address   }   *(imported from database of requesting physicians)*
Address   }

Re: *Patient name* (imported from patient's medical record)

Diagnoses: 1)   *(software imports "Impressions" section of H&P record)*
                                           2)
                                           3)
                                           4)

Recommendations: 1)   *(software imports "Management Options" and*
                                           2)   *"Data Ordered" sections of the H&P record)*
                                           3)
                                           4)

Dear *physician's name:* (imported from identification of requesting physician)

At your request, today I had the opportunity to evaluate *patient's name,* a *age*-year-old patient who arrived with the following primary concern(s): *Listing of primary symptoms: (software imports the entire history of present illness section narrative)*

Assessment of the patient's past medical history and review of symptoms indicates the following additional significant concerns: *Listing of secondary symptoms (software imports following additional significant concerns: Listing of secondary symptoms (software imports the narrative sections of past, family, and social history and review of systems, which lists details of "yes" responses)*

Relevant physical examination findings include *list of examination findings (software imports narrative section of examination record, which lists details of "abnormal" findings)*

I have reviewed my impressions with the patient. The symptoms and findings are compatible with the diagnoses listed above. Appropriate recommendations at this time are also listed above. Thank you for requesting my evaluation of this patient.

Sincerely,

Name of consultant, MD   *(software imports name of consulting physician)*

It may also include correspondence, documentation of phone conversations, and other notes a physician makes about the patient's care.

When a patient returns for a follow-up visit, before starting the encounter, the physician's first priority is to review the impressions and recommendations from the previous visit, plus all information entered into the record between encounters. When accessing the patient's EHR, the physician should first see a summary screen that concisely summarizes this information and offers direct access to the original documents if the physician wants to view them. This screen should provide a list of all of the patient's prior visits, in reverse chronologic order, with the most recent visit highlighted and at the top of the list. For the highlighted visit, it should next show the clinical details of three subsections of the medical decision making record:

- Impressions and differential diagnoses
- Management options
- Data ordered

These three sections provide a comprehensive overview of the physician's thought processes and plans during the previous visit. An additional field on this screen should indicate when clinical notes have been entered in the record since the previous visit. For physicians who create meaningful documentation, reviewing this summary screen and reading the interim notes will quickly allow them to begin the current visit smoothly, greeting the patient with a full understanding of the conclusions and recommendations from the previous visit. When physicians use the mouse to click on the date of any other visit on the list, the software should immediately populate the fields for the three medical decision making subsections and for the added notes with the information recorded from the selected visit.

The summary screen should also provide a series of radio buttons that will directly connect the physician to different areas of the chart to visualize more detailed information, including access to the complete H&P record of the selected visit and to the sections of the EHR that contain selected reports, documents, and the patient profile (discussed subsequently). Because this screen should be the same initial screen a physician would access when entering notations between visits, it should also provide a radio button for creating new notes. Figure 16.4 offers a potential design for such a central information screen, although it should be modified for consistency with different software systems.

The Benefits of Simplification

Many vendors currently provide physicians with comprehensive summary screens that show all the details of clinical, laboratory, and radiologic information on one screen. However, summary screens that present too many details on one page can result in too much information in one location and a cluttered image. Physicians are accustomed to seeing the "big picture" first, as illustrated in Figure 16.4, and then reviewing source material secondarily for greater detail. Vendors could consider offering physicians the choice between this focused summary screen combined with effective navigation and a comprehensive summary screen showing extensive details.

In the medical notes section, clicking with the mouse on a note in the left column will highlight that note and show part of the message on the right side. Most often, the medical notes the physician entered as test results arrived in the office will provide sufficient information to start the current visit. It will also guide the physician to other sections of the record for greater detail.

Clicking on the *View H&P* button will access the entire H&P record from the highlighted date (in the *Visit Date* box at the top of the form). The *View Notes* button will navigate to a listing of the complete notes entered since the previous visit. Clicking on the *View Tests* button will access the section of the medical record containing four (or more) categories: laboratory test results, radiology reports, physiologic test results, and other tests. For ease of access and reading, the tests should be listed by date, in reverse chronologic order, and this section should have the capability of listing all tests or listing them by category; when a physician clicks on a listed test, the actual test result page or images should open in a window for direct access.

Clicking on the *View Documents* button should lead to a section of the record that functions similarly to the *View Tests* section. All documents should be listed by date, in reverse chronologic order, and the software should allow the practice to set up categories for the documents (eg, consultation letters received, consultation letters sent, procedure reports, workers' compensation notices, and legal documents). A physician could then choose to see the listing for all documents or a listing by category.

F I G U R E   16.4

Sample Summary Screen. This screen contains information that should be immediately available to physicians when they access a patient's record, at the start of a follow-up visit or to view the chart and enter notes between visits. It includes the critical decision-making components from previous visits (opening to the most recent visit) and notes made between visits. It also provides one-click access to other major portions of the record so that physicians can view more detailed information when desired. Each section of the screen should have scrolling capability.

Central Information Center			Visit Date	Physician Seen
Name:	Jones, Joan		6/1/2007	Dr A
Record No.: 123456			4/14/2007	Dr C
DOB:	1/23/1945		3/3/2007	Dr C

Impressions and Differential Diagnoses

1) Acute right lower lobe pneumonia
2) Chronic bronchitis
3) Osteoarthritis, right knee, stable
4) Hypothyroidism, controlled with medication

Management Options

1) Amoxicillin/clavulanate potassium, 875 mg bid for 10 days
2) D/C all smoking
3) Continue Ibuprofen prn pain
4) Taking levothyroxine

Data Ordered

1) Chest X-ray, 1 week
2) Chest CT scan in 6 weeks
3) Pulmonary function tests in 6 weeks
4) Fiberoptic bronchoscopy in 2-3 months

Medical Notes

Date	Type of Note	Selected Message
6/2/2007	X-ray report	Chest X-ray shows right lower lobe pneumonia
6/7/2007	Phone call from patient	

View H&P	View Notes	View Tests	View Documents	View Patient Profile	Add Notes

The *View Patient Profile* button will access the portion of the record discussed subsequently. The *Add Notes* button should open a window designed for physicians to add dated notes about patient-related information between visits. These notes may include phone conversations, review of laboratory test results, review of documents, and recording any other information relevant to patient care.

PATIENT PROFILE SECTION

The EHR can provide a section to organize and store a summary of patients' important medical information. There should be enough flexibility in the EHR design for physicians to select the various types of information to store in these profiles. As a starting point, most physicians want to have lists of the their patients' medical problems, medications, allergies, pertinent social history, and pertinent family history.

The first design question that must be addressed is whether these profiles should be managed passively or actively. In other words, should the software automatically transfer the diagnoses listed at the conclusion of each visit into the problem list? Or should the software require physicians to perform active input to enter or delete information in the profiles? It is most reasonable for the profile sections to require active management to modify the information because a passive system would rapidly become oversaturated with nonprioritized and disorganized information that would reduce its usefulness for medical care. Figure 16.5 shows a sample design for a patient profile screen that includes the most commonly used patient information.

FIGURE 16.5

Sample Patient Profile Screen. This illustrates a possible design for the five subsections listed in the text, including descriptions that enhance the benefits of an actively managed and dynamic repository of essential patient information (eg, separating medical problems into an active section and a resolved section for ease of use). Each section should have a scroll bar.

Patient Profile

Name: Jones, Joan   Record No.: 123456   DOB: 1/23/1945

Problem List

Problem	Date Identified	Date Resolved
Active		
1)		
2)		
3)		
4)		
Resolved		
1)		
2)		
3)		

List of Medications

Medication	Dose	Frequency	Date Started	Date Ended
Active				
1)				
2)				
3)				
4)				
Discontinued				
1)				
2)				
3)				

List of Allergies

Medication Allergies	Date Identified
1)	
2)	
3)	

Environmental Allergies	Date Identified
1)	
2)	
3)	

Social History

	Yes	No	
Do you use tobacco?	☐	☐	Type and amount:
If no, did you use it previously?	☐	☐	Type and amount: ___ When quit:
Do you use recreational drugs?	☐	☐	Type and amount:
Do you drink alcohol?	☐	☐	Type and amount:
What is your occupation?			
Other:			

Family History

	Yes	No	
Heart problems / murmurs	☐	☐	
Allergy	☐	☐	
Diabetes	☐	☐	
Cancer	☐	☐	
Bleeding disorder	☐	☐	
Anesthesia problems	☐	☐	
Other	☐	☐	

Patient Problem List

Physicians managing patients with chronic illness or multiple medical issues frequently benefit from having an actively managed problem list, which provides a precise summary of current and resolved medical issues. Physicians may refer to this section at the start of a visit for orientation purposes. As new problems are identified, they should be actively added to the problem list, which the EHR design could facilitate by a variety of mechanisms to transfer a diagnosis entered in the "Impressions" section of a visit to the active problem list. The software should also permit physicians to prioritize the list of active problems in an order progressing from the most significant, located at the top of the list, to the least significant. While working in the list, by entering a date into the "Date Resolved" column, the software should move a listed diagnosis or problem from the active list to the resolved list at the bottom of the section (which may also be shaded, marked by a colored background, or changed to a different font for easy identification).

List of Medications

During an initial visit, the software should permit automatic duplication of the medication list from the past medical history section of the H&P record directly into this portion of the patient profile. A physician or staff member could embellish this initial information by adding the starting date for each treatment. At each subsequent visit, the staff or physician can review the medication list as part of the update of the past medical history. Any changes in medication can be listed in the profile section and on the H&P record. In addition, the software should facilitate a mechanism for the new medications ordered (and previously prescribed medications discontinued) during a visit to be easily transferred to the profile. Functionality might also allow the software to move the new treatments that include an ending date (eg, a 2-week course of an antibiotic) from the active list to the discontinued list automatically at the end of the treatment period. It should also offer the capability of moving all discontinued medications to the bottom of the list, where they can be identified by shading, colors, or a different font.

Allergies, Social History, and Family History

The software should be able to duplicate the list of medication allergies and environmental allergies automatically from the past history section of the initial visit. It should also duplicate the social history and family history to eliminate extra time and effort. During the update of the past, family, and social history in follow-up visits, the physician or staff can enter any changes into the patient profile.

REPORT DESIGN AND PROTOCOL FUNCTIONALITY

Different specialists should be seeking a variety of reports to assist them with identifying trends in the management of their patients, and EHR software designers should be able to meet their needs. There are two fundamental reports that benefit most primary specialists and other physicians managing chronic or ongoing conditions.

Laboratory Value Flow Sheet

The first report is a straightforward flow sheet that records quantitative results from clinical laboratory studies or certain physiologic studies (eg, the components of pulmonary function testing) over time. By charting the result for a specific test over time, physicians can identify trends in a patient's health status, and the software should be able to convert numeric values into a graphic representation that more easily illustrates trends. Figure 16.6 shows a straightforward spreadsheet data entry screen for laboratory values of a single type of test over time. Figure 16.7 illustrates a line graph derived from those data. The screen should be able to record and graph the results and dates for multiple laboratory tests. A physician might, for example, include high- and low-density lipoprotein and

FIGURE 16.6

Sample Data Entry Design for Laboratory Values Over Time. Each row provides for a different laboratory study, and each column records the date of a test. This example shows one laboratory value, total cholesterol, over time.

Test	1/1/2006	4/1/2006	7/1/2006	10/1/2006	1/1/2007	4/1/2007	7/1/2007
Cholesterol	201	222	210	236	228	235	248

FIGURE 16.7

Sample Graph of Laboratory Values Over Time. Line graph showing laboratory values for cholesterol over time, based on the values recorded in Figure 16.6. Multiple additional tests could be shown on the same graph, using different colors for each laboratory test.

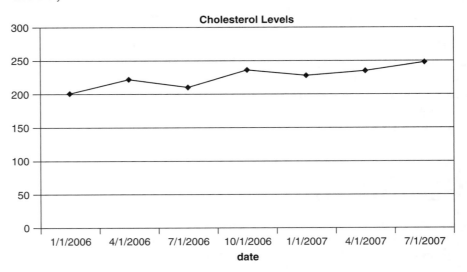

triglyceride values on this chart, while using one or more additional charts to monitor the progress of glucose, serum urea nitrogen, creatinine, and/or other chemistry tests.

Combined Laboratory and Treatment Flow Sheet

Management of certain chronic conditions, such as hypertension and diabetes, calls for obtaining laboratory studies at regular intervals, with the results of the tests leading to possible modification of medical therapy. Under these circumstances, software can readily provide a more sophisticated flow sheet, recording the medication dosage and associated laboratory results over time. Figure 16.8 shows a spreadsheet-type data entry screen that records the laboratory values and the medication dosages on specific dates. Figure 16.9 illustrates a line graph derived from those data including the dosage and the date on the X-axis. This type of graph helps physicians monitor the results of treatment over time.

FIGURE 16.8

Sample Data Entry Form Design for Combined Laboratory and Treatment Data Over Time. Each spreadsheet of this type addresses the laboratory values for one type of study. It will, however, accommodate more than one medication by adding columns or by listing two dosages together, separated by a slash (eg, 1500/25). (*This is a hypothetical spreadsheet for illustration purposes only. It is not intended to be a realistic representation of diabetes management.*)

Patient Name: Jones, Joan   Record No. 123456

Name of Medication: Xxxxxxxx

Start Date: January 1, 2006

Laboratory test: Hemoglobin A_{1c}

Date	Current Medication Dose	Laboratory Result	Revised Medication Dose
1/1/2006	1000 mg	8.7	1500 mg
4/1/2006	1500 mg	7.5	1500 mg
7/1/2006	1500 mg	6.6	1500 mg
10/1/2006	1500 mg	7.2	2000 mg
1/1/2007	2000 mg	6.1	2000 mg
4/1/2007	2000 mg	5.8	2000 mg
7/1/2007	2000 mg	6.2	2000 mg

Protocol Functionality

The EHR software should be able to provide designs that effectively integrate two types of medical protocols at the point of care so that clinical decision support is timely and interactive. Preventive care guidelines promise to promote early diagnosis and intervention by ensuring that patients receive medically indicated diagnostic services (eg, mammogram and colonoscopy)

FIGURE 16.9

Sample Graph of Laboratory and Treatment Data Over Time. Line graph showing laboratory values for hemoglobin A_{1c} (HbA_{1c}) related to changes in medication dosing over time, based on values in Figure 16.8.

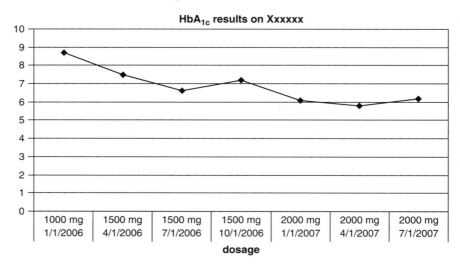

at the appropriate time. Presenting disease management guidelines at the point of care is proven to promote health and reduce the frequency of serious consequences from chronic illnesses. The design and functionality requirements are different for integrating each category of protocols into EHRs.

Design for Preventive Care Protocols

Preventive care protocols require a formatted screen that centralizes scheduling for each type of screening test. When a physician identifies a patient who should be enrolled for screening, the software should offer access to a pop-up window available directly from the patient's chart, and the physician should be able to select the desired type of testing from a drop-down menu. When the test is selected, the screen should provide the usual predetermined frequency of testing, which the physician may accept or modify based on clinical judgment. For example, it may be appropriate to increase the frequency of screening mammography on the basis of a positive family history and/or certain physical examination or radiographic findings. The physician must also enter a date for the first test to be performed.

Many current software systems already offer this functionality for preventive care protocols, and many screen designs are possible. Figure 16.10 illustrates a sample design for enrolling patients in one or more preventive care protocols.

The remaining functionality of preventive care protocols determines how the software will make the staff aware of the need to contact patients and schedule the appropriate tests. One reasonable approach is to use a monthly scheduling practice. On the first day of each month, the software should automatically generate a list of all patients who should be scheduled for preventive care examinations during that month. It should also automatically provide for a standard notice to be sent to all of the patients, advising them to schedule the appropriate testing. Finally, for error proofing, the system should coordinate the scheduling information with the test results as they are entered into the software. One month later, it should print a list of patients who did not have the recommended examination performed or visit scheduled so that the practice can contact them.

F IGURE 16.10

Sample Data Entry Design Screen for Preventive Care Protocols. The physician accesses a drop-down menu of preventive protocols, which should be accessible from any portion of the patient's chart, and selects the procedure to be scheduled. After selecting a protocol, the scheduling screen would open with the patient's name and medical record number already entered. The screen should appear with a default frequency in place, which the physician must confirm or change as medically indicated, followed by indicating the starting date for the first test.

Patient Name: Jones, Joan

Record No.:   123456

Screening Examination	Frequency	Start Date
Mammography	q _24_ mo	_12/1/2007_
	q____mo	__/__/__
	q____mo	__/__/__

Disease Management Protocols

A variety of protocols are available for assisting in the management of chronic illnesses, such as diabetes, asthma, hypertension, and congestive heart failure. The clinical decision support features of EHRs help medical groups incorporate these protocols to promote optimal care. Software should allow these protocols to be loaded and made available for appropriate patients at the point of care, likely through the use of alerting messages and/or pop-up windows.

As discussed in detail in Chapter 4, protocols should be designed and implemented as a platform or starting point for care, not as a restrictive box that limits care. Therefore, these protocols must permit flexibility because physicians may want to add their own modifications and because protocols will evolve over time. It is also important that the software provides data entry capability so that a physician can explain the circumstances that make a particular protocol inappropriate for a particular patient. This documentation explains the basis for the physician's judgment and provides potential support if medical liability becomes an issue.

Designs that integrate disease management protocols into patient care should provide an option to activate associated coding under so-called Pay for Reporting or Pay for Performance (P4P) programs. This option, if activated, must also allow for documentation of reasons (standard or individualized to the patient) for which it would be inappropriate to follow a given protocol for a specific patient or during a specific visit. Furthermore, such modifications should be coordinated with P4P coding and modifier requirements for the practice management system.

CHARGE ENTRY OPTIONS

As noted, it is critically important that the impressions and differential diagnoses section of the H&P record be dedicated to documenting detailed descriptions of physicians' clinical impressions, relative severity of illnesses, relative probability of the possible diagnoses, and the medical diagnostic process. Identifying specific diagnoses or symptoms appropriate for submission of insurance claims *must be a separate process*.

Before presenting design options for charge entry directly into the EHR, it is worthwhile to examine how charge entry forms work for physicians in the paper environment. Some practices may decide to continue using paper forms if the electronic version proves not to be as fast or as accurate. Two other related options are to use the design of a paper form with a digital pen and digital paper or to use the template of a paper form with a tablet PC. The advantage of using direct data entry into the computer is that it should save time for billing personnel, but this savings must not be allowed to come at the expense of increased physician time.

Charge Entry Design in Paper Format

For physicians using a paper format, the traditional superbill (or charge entry slip) has proven, when well designed, to be reasonably accurate and reasonably efficient. Examining the problems that physicians encounter in using the paper superbill provides insight into the additional solutions that must be provided by electronic formats. One section of the superbill form includes a list of the medical practice's most commonly performed procedures, along with associated CPT codes. In a second section, the form lists the practice's most commonly used diagnoses. Figure 16.11 provides an illustration of a limited portion of a conventional superbill, which, in complete form, usually fills an entire 8.5 × 11-inch page to contain as many codes as a practice commonly uses.

In certain cases, the paper superbill presents several challenges in selecting the correct diagnosis codes. One problem is that, at times, the precise International Classification of Diseases, Ninth Revision, Clinical Modification (ICD-9) code that best describes a patient's diagnosis is not listed on the form, and the physician or staff must search the codebook for the correct code. Two situations result in this problem: (1) A patient has an unusual diagnosis. (2) There are multiple code variations for a common diagnosis. Coding for diabetes mellitus is a prime example of this latter challenge: there are more than 40 ICD-9 code variations listed in this category, including a broad list of associated or complicating factors related to diabetes.

Another challenge occurs when a physician has selected multiple CPT codes and multiple ICD-9 codes for the same visit. To convey correct billing information to the charge entry staff, the physician must match appropriate diagnoses (in the optimal order) for each of the selected CPT codes. With a paper form, as illustrated in Figure 16.11, the physician can identify each selected (circled) diagnosis with a number and, next to each CPT code, place the number(s) for each appropriate diagnosis code, with the diagnosis of greatest significance listed first to meet billing requirements.

Charge Entry in Electronic Format

Accurate charge entry is a four-step process:

1. The physician selects the correct CPT code(s) that accurately describes the services, E/M *and* procedure services, performed during a visit.
2. The physician must select any procedure modifiers that are appropriate for billing purposes.

FIGURE 16.11

Sample Conventional Superbill Design. For brevity, this sample of a paper superbill form designed for an ear, nose, and throat practice omits the detailed practice and patient demographic information at the top of the page. It also shows only a partial (representative) collection of procedure codes in the top half of the coding section and a limited number of diagnosis codes in the bottom half. An asterisk next to a code indicates that there are multiple similar codes related to this diagnosis. A plus sign next to the code indicates that the listed code is considered nonspecific by the International Classification of Diseases, Ninth Revision, Clinical Modification (ICD-9). The superimposed bold numbers show how physicians can use paper forms to match diagnosis code(s) to each procedure code. CPT indicates Current Procedural Terminology; diag, diagnostic; E/M, evaluation and management; neopl, neoplasm; Post-Op, postoperative; Resp insuff, respiratory insufficiency; S/N, sensori-neural; surg, surgery; Unilat, unilateral; and URI, upper respiratory infection.

Patient and Practice Demographics

OFFICE VISITS	CPT	MODIFIER		PROCEDURES		AUDIOMETRY	
New patient or initial visit	9920_	Prolonged E/M Service	21	Nasal endoscopy, diagnostic	31231	Screening	92551
Consultation	9924_	Unrelated Post-Op Service	24	Nasal endo w debride/polyp	3123	Air conduction	92552
Established patient	9921_	E/M Service with Procedure	25	Nasal endo w control epistaxis	31238	Air and bone	92553
		Decision to Perform Surg	57	Nasopharyngoscopy, diag	92511	Comprehensive	92557
HOSPITAL CARE				Polypectomy, simple	30110	Tympanometry	92567
Initial Admission	9922_	MISCELLANEOUS SERVICES	CPT	Polypectomy, complex	30115	Acoustic reflex	92568
Subsequent Care	9923_	Post-Operative Visit	99204			Reflex decay	92569
Consultation	9925_	Office Visit, No Charge	99210				
		Emerg service, after hours	99050				
LEVEL OF CARE		Emerg service,10PM-8AM	99052				
1 2 3 4 5		Emerg svce, Sun & holiday	99054				

DIAGNOSIS ICD-9 if not below:

Nasopharyngitis, Acute (URI)	460	Pharyngitis, Acute	462	Reflux Esophagitis	530.11	Otitis Externa, Acute	380.12
Rhinitis, Chronic	472	Tonsillitis Acute	463	Acute Esophagitis	530.12	Otitis Externa, Fungal	380.15
Rhinitis, Allergic	477	Pharyngitis, Chronic	472.1	Other Esophagitis	530.19	Otitis Externa, Chronic	380.23
Deviated Nasal Septum	470	Tonsillitis Chronic	474.00*	Esophageal Reflux	530.81	Serous Otitis, Acute	355.9+
Turbinate Hypertrophy	478	Tonsil-Adenoid Hypertrophy	474.1	Dysphagia	787.2	Serous Otitis, Chronic	780.4
Other Diseases Nose/Sinus	478.1	Peritonsillar Abscess	475	Cervical Adenopathy	785.6	Dizziness	345.9
Nasal Polyp	471	Hoarseness	784.49+	Cervical Adenitis	683.0	Otosclerosis, Oval Window	387
Sinusitis, Acute Maxillary	461	Laryngitis, Acute	464.0	Thyroid Mass, Benign	226	Presbycusis	388.01
Sinusitis, Chronic Maxillary	473.0	Laryngitis, Chronic	476.0	Neck Mass	784.2	Noise-Induced Hearing Loss	388.12
Sinusitis, Acute Ethmoid	461	Vocal Cord Paralysis, Unilat	478.32*	Salivary gland neopl, Benign	210.2	Sudden S/N Hearing Loss	388.2
Sinusitis, Chronic Ethmoid	473.2	Vocal Cord Polyp	478.4			Tinnitus, Subjective	388.31
Sinusitis, Acute Pan-	461.8	Other Vocal Cord Disease	478.5+	Cellulitis, Face	682.0	Hearing Disorder, Conductive	389.03*
Sinusitis, Chronic Pan-	473.8+	Esophagitis	530.10+	Cough	786.2	Hearing Disorder, Neural	389.12
Epistaxis	784.7			Asthma, Extrinsic	493.00	Hearing Disorder, Mixed	389.2
Sleep Apnea / Hypersomnia	780.53						
Resp Insuff/Apnea/Snoring	786.09+						

* = Multiple ICD-9   + = Non-Specific ICD-9

3. The physician selects the appropriate ICD-9 diagnosis codes that support the services performed. These codes may be codes representing diagnoses and/or codes representing symptoms.

4. Each selected CPT code must be matched with the appropriate ICD-9 code(s), and these ICD-9 codes must be listed in their order of medical significance.

Physicians using EHR systems that facilitate the *Practical EHR* method, with passive or active coding guidance, will know the appropriate E/M code at the conclusion of an encounter. They must then carry out all the other charge entry steps, starting with selection of additional CPT codes for diagnostic or therapeutic procedures performed during the visit.

The initial decision EHR developers face in designing effective charge entry programs is how to present the code selection choices described in the first three steps. Many current systems use drop-down menus that provide an extensive list of procedure codes, often in numeric or alphabetical order. Modifiers may appear on a second drop-down menu, and a third drop-down menu lists ICD-9 diagnosis codes. However, searching through extensive drop-down menus at the conclusion of each visit is time-consuming and tedious. When selection of multiple codes is indicated, making selections from drop-down lists takes significantly more time than completing a paper superbill.

Therefore, *Practical EHR* suggests a hybrid approach, introducing a screen version of the customized superbill for ease of code selection in most cases. In most cases, physicians will be able to select the desired CPT codes, modifiers, and ICD-9 codes simply by clicking on the codes that appear on the screen. Drop-down menus can provide supplemental assistance for cases in which a service is missing from the template or, more commonly, when a code has an attached plus sign to indicate multiple related codes. It should also be possible to program the software so that when physicians use the mouse button to click on a plus sign next to one of the codes, the software will open a drop-down list showing all the related codes. This programming will allow physicians to quickly identify and click the most appropriate related diagnosis code.

The final charge entry step is to help physicians match the correct modifiers and diagnosis codes with each procedure code. Figure 16.12 illustrates a possible design for accomplishing this task relatively efficiently for physicians performing direct entry using the mouse. This coding matrix form would appear as a smaller pop-up window over a portion of the superbill and indicate a step-by-step protocol to correctly complete the charge entry process:

1. Select CPT (procedure) codes for each service provided: As the physician uses the mouse to check the box for each selected CPT code, beginning with the E/M service and followed by other procedures in the order of priority, each selected code should automatically appear (in the order selected) in the left column of the coding matrix.

FIGURE 16.12

Possible Design for Charge Entry Screen. Current Procedural Terminology (CPT) codes selected by clicking on the superbill (and/or drop-down menu) will appear in the left column of the larger coding matrix. Similarly selected International Classification of Diseases, Ninth Revision, Clinical Modification (ICD-9) codes will populate the smaller horizontal coding matrix in the top row. By a series of mouse clicks, the physician will choose a CPT code and then fill one or more of the following boxes in the same row, first with a modifier (if indicated) and then with one or more ICD-9 codes selected in the proper order. The codes shown correlate with those circled in Figure 16.11.

ICD-9 Codes:	473.2	473.0	471	389.12			

CPT Code	Modifier	----------------------Diagnosis Codes (ICD-9)--------------------			
99203	25	473.2	473.0	471	389.12
31231		473.2	473.0	471	
92557		389.12			

Submit

2. Select all appropriate ICD-9 (diagnosis) codes: The physician uses the mouse to double click on each appropriate diagnosis code on the screen, and each selected code automatically appears in the smaller (horizontal) coding matrix.

3. With all codes selected, the physician must match each CPT code with any appropriate modifier and each appropriate diagnosis code. By using the mouse in the CPT portion of the coding matrix, the physician will begin by clicking in the first row to highlight the first CPT code. Next, clicking on a modifier on the superbill screen should cause that modifier to appear in the column adjacent to the first CPT code. Finally, the physician will double click on one or more ICD-9 codes in the horizontal coding matrix, selecting the most relevant diagnosis first. Each selected code will appear in order in the remaining boxes in the first row.

4. The physician completes each row, in turn, in an identical manner until all CPT codes have been provided with appropriate diagnoses (and modifiers when indicated).

5. Clicking the *Submit* button will send this coding matrix to the practice management system or other appropriate location.

SUMMARY

Although the electronic H&P record provides the primary focus of *Practical EHR,* a number of additional medical record designs and functions can be considered, which will help physicians provide optimal patient care and fulfill administrative requirements. This chapter initiates discussion of a number of these features and presents a number of designs that can provide starting points for EHR developers to meet these needs.

References

1. American Medical Association. *Current Procedural Terminology* (*CPT®*). Chicago, IL: American Medical Association; 2007.

2. Health Care Financing Administration. *Documentation Guidelines for Evaluation and Management Services.* Washington, DC: Health Care Financing Administration; 1997.

3. Levinson, SR. *Practical E/M: Documentation and Coding Solutions for Quality Patient Care*, 2nd Ed. Chicago, IL: American Medical Association. In press.

PART 4

Practice Transformation and Health Information Transformation

This section presents an effective process for medical practices to plan a successful transition from paper medical records to an electronic health record (EHR) environment from the perspective of the history and physical examination (H&P) component of the EHR. It begins with a review of the concerns encountered using current approaches to transformation. It then explores, step-by-step, a protocol designed to put the medical practice in control of the process, including selecting the right team, setting criteria and benchmarks for electronic H&P software designs, system selection and modification, and testing the designs while training physicians to use the new system before implementation. This strategy is designed to minimize mistakes, avoid compromises to quality care, and bring about success.

chapter 17

Roadmap for Successful Practice Transformation: Avoiding the Electronic Chasm

"HIT is an element of patient care, not an add-on that provides [additional] work."[1]

Carolyn Clancy, MD, director of Agency for Healthcare Research and Quality[1]

When listening to physicians, compliance specialists, and medical practice administrators discuss electronic health records (EHRs), it becomes clear that most physician leaders and administrators of medical practices and academic institutions believe they lack sufficient information and criteria to make informed and knowledgeable decisions about evaluation, selection, preparation, and successful implementation of EHRs. The virtues advocated by vendors, policy makers, insurance companies, the Centers for Medicare & Medicaid Services, and informatics experts are counterbalanced by the high rate of system failures, physicians who report dissatisfaction with their own electronic systems, and high costs. These concerns are further compounded by reports from some practices and institutions of the introduction of EHRs causing decreased productivity, increased time to care for patients, and significant concerns about nonindividualized records and lack of compliance. In addition, although physicians and administrators can appreciate the "big picture" benefits of interconnectivity, interoperability, and a national health information network, they are highly concerned about being forced to be responsible for bearing the preponderance of the costs to achieve these advantages, when it has been shown that the financial rewards of EHR implementation accrue almost exclusively to payers (insurers and employers).

Practical EHR begins its approach to this planning phase with the axiom that physicians and their medical standards must dictate the direction and ultimate goals of a medical practice's transition to EHRs. It is only when this process meets physicians' standards that EHRs can prove to be a consistently positive factor for patient care; and only then will physicians be certain that the clinical information in EHRs will be sufficiently valuable and reliable to help promote system-wide improvement in health care quality and patient safety (ie, "cross the quality chasm").

Where Physicians Want Electronic Evolution to Take Them

Recent correspondence from an experienced internist, who is also an experienced EHR user, reported his impression of EHR strengths and weaknesses:

- Strengths: "My EHR is wonderful for my staff. They don't have to pick up charts all day. I love having some of the information available from anywhere in my office."
- Weaknesses: "I must tell you that I have become a slave to the screen and there are many nights when I am stuck here just typing away. . . . For primary care, the EHR is a disaster, a very costly disaster. . . . One of the concepts that I have had a real tough time getting across is the distinction between claims data and clinical data."

This physician is trapped in a dilemma already identified in this book. Software systems, as currently designed, do a superior job of data storage and retrieval. It is with data entry that they fall short of physician expectations and needs.

This physician's message of conflicting benefits and drawbacks concluded with an insightful analysis of how he believes that EHR design and functionality must progress to meet physicians' needs and achieve their promise: "a legitimate effort to get back to what the medical record is supposed to do, be a chronological representation of a multitude of systems, morphing and interacting over time with each other, the environment, and any number of other interfaces; to be a consistent means of communication with ourselves and each other, for the benefit of better and more predictable medical decision making."

The acknowledged EHR benefits of storing and accessing data do not preclude attaining the additional goals of having a usable, high-quality electronic H&P that helps physicians promote quality care. On the contrary, these additional goals underscore the message that not just any data entry design will suffice, rather that EHR vendors must give a high priority to meeting all the clinical criteria that physicians require for the features included in their electronic H&P.

THE MEDICAL PRACTICE TRANSFORMATION PROCESS

In this book, the term *practice transformation* is used to describe the entire EHR journey, from initial evaluation through implementation and on to future evolution. Medical practices clearly need a roadmap to guide them on this journey and allow them to plot a course for success. Although a number of different routes might lead to successful transformation, physicians and administrators prefer a direct course that avoids as many obstacles and potholes as possible. To accomplish this, the roadmap must first set a direction that avoids the problems of the "electronic chasm," which can confront practices with inconsistent and incompatible goals, nonaligned incentives such as speed vs quality care and/or speed vs data integrity, and failure to address some of physicians' primary requirements. It should lead instead to a path that is marked with well-defined objectives at each stage of the journey. Successful transformation from a paper storage environment to an electronic record requires that these objectives be completely achieved at each phase of the journey before moving to the next phase.

Health Information Transformation

Practical EHR introduces a new intermediate step in this overall process, identified as *health information transformation* (HITr). This phase should occur after a medical organization makes a (tentative) decision to purchase a particular EHR system but before actual implementation of the EHR as an adjunct to patient care.

The current approach to preparing medical practices for EHR implementation concentrates almost exclusively on "workflow transformation" for the nonphysician staff, which involves analyzing existing office workflow practices and then introducing improved protocols and information-handling procedures that will facilitate the workflow benefits of EHRs. The importance of introducing these workflow-transforming protocols for the support staff has been well recognized by medical practices, vendors, and health policy advocates; it has also been stressed in a number of excellent publications. There is even government-funded assistance available to provide medical practices with workflow transformation guidance. Quality improvement organizations (QIOs), which are funded by the Agency for Healthcare Research and Quality (AHRQ), provide expertise to help practices accomplish these changes efficiently and effectively.

Although the present approach to workflow transformation seeks to address most of the information processes that occur in a medical practice, it generally fails to consider the interaction among physicians, patients, and the EHR at the point of care. Vendors may demonstrate to physicians how to access different sections of the software, but most are not prepared to assist with achieving compliance, quality, usability, efficiency, and data integrity benchmarks during patient visits. There is rarely, if ever, training with actual patients (or patient surrogates) before implementation. This training deficit deprives physicians the chance to identify and correct problems with the electronic H&P or with their ability to use it properly before implementation. The current absence of a structured HITr protocol is responsible for a substantial part of the electronic chasm, contributing significantly to the problems many practices experience during and after implementation.

The HITr process revolutionizes this second phase of the overall practice transformation process. It takes on the responsibility of addressing this overlooked component of practice preparation, achieving compatibility of the software design and physician training to ensure a smooth transition and a successful implementation. It provides three pillars of preparation for effective use of the electronic history and physical examination (H&P) record. The first phase involves an in-depth analysis of the current medical records and clinical workflow, identifying flaws in the critical elements of compliance, efficiency, and quality of the documentation. Physicians and compliance staff must work together to eliminate weaknesses in these areas by implementing an effective workflow method (as described in the "*Practical EHR* Method" section of Chapter 11) and introducing the type of tools that will be incorporated into the electronic H&P record to facilitate this method.

The second phase of HITr calls for compliance staff and physicians who have completed the first transformation phase to carry out a thorough review of the EHR designs and customizations. Working with existing medical charts as a source for entry of clinical information, they must evaluate the electronic H&P record and all other components of the EHR to ensure that the designs and functionality meet the practice's criteria and benchmarks (discussed in

Chapter 18), requesting modifications that correct or eliminate design elements that have the potential to interfere with achieving these goals.

The final phase of HITr involves bringing trained physicians together with the approved EHR software system for validation trials that involve physicians performing "test drives" of the software in situations that provide a realistic simulation of patient encounters. Physicians, coders, and software designers should review these trials by measuring the success of the software in meeting the practice's benchmarks under actual patient care conditions. The team must identify the cause of any failure to meet a benchmark and then determine the appropriate corrective measures. This step will create an ongoing, iterative process for successful resolution of any potential problems. Problem correction may involve modifying the training protocol for physicians, further modification of the H&P software, or a combination of both. The validation trials conclude when all benchmarks for success are met with 100% satisfaction. This goal must be achieved before final implementation of the selected EHR system for patient care.

Results of the HITr Process

If the trial runs identify problems in meeting one or more of the practice's criteria and benchmarks, implementation must be deferred until the transformation team and software designers can determine the source of the problem(s) and develop effective remedies. This should involve an iterative process of modifying software design and/or physician workflow to overcome the obstacles. When trial runs prove successful, the practice can move forward to phase 3 with the assurance that implementation will be successful, with no decrease in efficiency or productivity and with physicians who are pleased and satisfied with the outcome.

When practices have achieved success at level 3 of the HITr pyramid (see Figure 17.2), they can plan for introducing the advances in levels 4 and 5, when these systems become available. Medical organizations must be certain that these advanced systems will meet their needs before they proceed with implementation. They should, therefore, follow a protocol similar to HITr for each successive system improvement so that any modifications, upgrades, and/or further training should be completed and confirmed before moving forward with implementation.

Understanding these components of HITr will also provide the members of the medical practice's transition team with important insights during the preliminary stages of investigating EHRs, empowering team members to ask appropriate questions, set forth practice requirements, and make proper decisions that will facilitate meaningful screening during the selection process and create a foundation for success. The HITr process effectively brings the principles of error proofing to the overall practice transformation process, thereby providing benefits for all who participate.

The medical practice gains by knowing, before final acceptance of a system and before "going live," that its physicians have been successfully trained and that the chosen system will work for them and their patients. The HITr process is further designed to eliminate the danger of reduced productivity following implementation and to significantly diminish the risk of a failed implementation.

Software vendors also realize significant advantages. Customizations will be completed before implementation, at a time when it is more efficient and more cost-effective to make modifications. Furthermore, most of the customizations that meet the high standards of one practice should prove to meet similar goals of other practices, improving the quality of the software system and saving costs over time. There is also a significant benefit from a practice having developed an effective internal training team and implemented a reliable and successful training protocol. Vendors' trainees will also need to acquire similar compliance and quality care assessment skills to coordinate with the transformation team of a large practice and to directly assist physicians in small practices in achieving these same levels of accomplishment. Finally, the best outcome for any vendor will be having medical practices that are enthusiastic about the success of their EHR.

The advantages of establishing a training and evaluation program based on physicians' standards for quality medical records should have a direct positive impact on the broader national goals for improving quality care and patient safety. "Quality data in" is a prerequisite for "quality data out," and using the HITr process correctly ensures that practices will implement EHR systems only after they have validated that the software facilitates care and helps physicians record high-quality clinical information. Ensuring the availability of high-quality data will increase the benefits of information exchange and the reliability of evidence-based medicine studies derived from data mined from EHRs. Finally, when systems are proven to meet physicians' needs at the point of care, more medical practices will be encouraged to begin their own transformation efforts.

HITr and the Electronic Chasm

The electronic chasm has resulted in large part from failure of EHRs to meet physicians' requirements and expectations for an effective H&P record at the point of care. The HITr process provides a missing link in the conventional EHR training process. Before a practice accepts or implements a software system, it will have already certified that the software H&P record design— and the physician training required to implement that design—can combine to achieve compliance, usability, efficiency, quality care, and data integrity.

When considering buying a highly sophisticated and technologically advanced (ie, expensive) automobile, buyers first want to make sure that the vehicle is equipped to meet all of their goals for buying that car. Similarly, to be sure that buyers are equipped to operate the car correctly and safely, the dealer wants to train them to properly use the car's various special features. Finally, buyers will test drive the car to make sure it fulfills all their expectations and that they know how to drive it correctly.

The HITr process brings this same process for quality, safety, and satisfaction to the purchase of an EHR system. The HITr process should provide the roadmap that guides each medical practice to avoid the electronic chasm and achieve successful EHR implementation and practice transformation.

THE PRACTICE TRANSFORMATION PYRAMID

The transformation pyramid provides a graphic image of the organization and timing of the various stages of the overall process of investigating, purchasing, and implementing an EHR. By first examining the conventional transformation process illustrated in Figure 17.1, physicians and administrators can note the absence of the HITr components that has resulted in significant difficulties as practices convert from paper to EHRs. The *Practical EHR* pyramid in Figure 17.2 completes the missing sections with the addition of the three pillars (or phases) of HITr to level 2.

F IGURE 17.1

Conventional Practice Transformation Pyramid. Representation of the conventional approach to practice transformation. The right column marks the levels of the pyramid (ie, stages of the overall transition process)

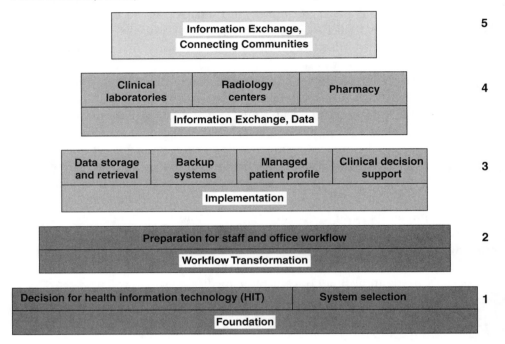

The Conventional Transformation Pyramid

Figure 17.1 illustrates how physicians usually perceive the overall process of converting to EHRs. In this approach, information technology advocates concentrate almost exclusively on the potential EHR benefits listed in the top three levels of the pyramid. The formal preparation in the second level addresses the changes in workflow and modifications of individual tasks for nonphysician staff members. However, it fails to include formal physician training or EHR customization. In addition, in this model, the guidance available to assist practices in making the critical selection and contracting decisions in the foundation level generally considers only the data storage and retrieval benefits of electronic systems. It commonly fails to address physicians' medical record criteria for the H&P record, data entry challenges, and short- and long-term financial consequences to help practices make informed decisions.

Most physicians understand that the government has issued an executive order for them to invest in EHRs by the year 2014.[2] However, under the conventional approach to practice transformation, most physicians cannot be certain whether the conversion to EHRs will bring benefits or greater hardship to their practice of medicine. Most are also left with the impression that they do not have the tools to control this process and that they must rely on EHR vendors to tell them what they need.

Practical EHR Transformation Pyramid

In contrast with the conventional pyramid, *Practical EHR* requires that physicians' medical record needs must guide this process determining how EHRs should function for physicians during patient care. Figure 17.2 illustrates how this approach expands and concentrates on the first two levels of the pyramid. Medical practices must attain success with the

FIGURE 17.2

Practical EHR Practice Transformation Pyramid. Representation of the *Practical EHR* approach to practice transformation. The right column marks the levels of the pyramid. PM refers to EHRs that have an integrated practice management system. Local Area Network (LAN) and Application Service Provider (ASP) models are determined by whether the practice or the software system "hosts" the central processing unit. E/M indicates evaluation and management.

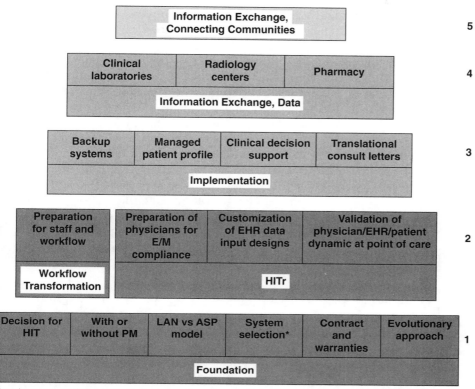

*Practices may prefer to delay final confirmation of a potential software system until completion of the health information transformation (HITr) process in phase 2.

foundation and transformation stages to achieve the successful support structure required for the upper three stages to work properly.

TIMING

In the *Practical EHR* paradigm for EHR transition, medical practices approach the foundation phase with a set of practice-specific decision tools that will evolve and become further refined as the investigation proceeds. These tools give each practice the power to be in control of the decision, selection, and contracting processes in their entireties. They allow each medical practice to set its own criteria for evaluating software systems and weighing the rewards and risks involved in commitment to EHRs in general, followed by establishing the professional standards that any specific EHR system must meet to receive consideration for possible purchase.

If the trial runs that conclude the HITr process fail to fulfill physicians' goals for their medical record in the day-to-day practice of medicine, the system should not be implemented. The practice leadership must determine the source of the problems and work with physicians and software designers in an iterative process to develop effective remedies. When these trial runs meet the established criteria, the practice can proceed with physicians' support to the third stage of the practice transformation, with confidence that the implementation will be successful and without a decrease in efficiency or productivity.

Do Physicians Have the Time to Invest in Proper System Selection and in HITr?

Physicians and administrators readily acknowledge two potential hurdles to implementing this effective strategy for practice transformation:

1. **Physicians do not have extra time to invest in this investigation and preparation.** A careful assessment of the benefits of following this paradigm will show that it actually saves physician time and practice costs. In conventional approaches, vendors commonly advise practices to reduce the number of patients seen per day by up to 50% (which amount to the equivalent of 80 hours of lost time per month) to enable physicians to adapt to the new electronic H&P at the time of implementation. In contrast, the preparation and validation phases of HITr should only require less than 10% of that amount of time to train the physicians and to ensure that the system meets their clinical and administrative requirements

2. **Physicians prefer to concentrate on patient care rather than on administrative duties.** While this is certainly true for most physicians, a failed conversion can be devastating to an entire practice. The electronic record will be each practice's future platform for quality patient care and efficiency. The time invested in proper planning will be recovered and rewarded in the time saved and the increased quality care and documentation achieved by a successful EHR transition and implementation.

In group practices, those clinicians who invest their time as members of the transformation team will relinquish some patient care time, and so they must be appropriately appreciated and compensated for the critical work they are doing to benefit the entire practice. For solo and small group practices, the physicians will have to invest some pro bono time. Regardless of the size of the practice, ensuring success and maintaining productivity is worth the effort.*

Contractual Guarantees?

Practices should involve a health care attorney who has information technology expertise throughout the entire EHR selection and implementation process. In the traditional approach to EHR adoption, practices receive, and are asked to sign, the vendor's contract during stage one of the HITr process, committing to the software system before physicians begin training and before determining whether the selected software system will meet the physicians' medical record requirements. This approach places a significant financial burden on the practice before it has enough information to know whether the system will meet its needs.

Adding the HITr steps to the selection and preparation processes is intended to allow practices to confirm, within reason, that the software will be functional and acceptable before they commit to implementation. This change in preparation and insight may also allow a practice's attorneys to rethink the timing of contract signing, if possible delaying until the HITr process is complete. Alternatively, the approach should permit attorneys to incorporate the practice's criteria and benchmarks into the contracts, with specific remedies available if the training and validation phases of HITr reveal that the software design and functionality fail to meet these specifications.

---

*A physician member of a prestigious academic-based practice recently shared with me his practice's experience of implementing and using an EHR. Fifteen months after the initial implementation (and, despite many hours of conventional training) all the physicians find the electronic H&P unusable for documenting their clinical care.

Future Software Modifications

After successful implementation of the basic components of an EHR, practices can look forward to introducing the information exchange features in level 4 (and, eventually, in level 5 of the practice transformation pyramid when these features becomes available). The transformation team should go through a similar transformation protocol to test and approve these features and to introduce each successive version or improvement provided by the software vendor. The software should be assessed, physicians should be trained, and trial runs should be successful before incorporating changes.

Upgrade vs Downgrade

The medical director of a large multispecialty group described his practice's experience following the changeover to the next version of the established EHR system. After listing the new problems the group experienced with decreased usability, decreased efficiency, and less meaningful documentation, the physician concluded, "I call our new upgrade a downgrade."

This observation underscores the importance of medical organizations maintaining the same level of control over all future software additions and modifications that they exercised in the initial selection, training, and implementation processes.

The Partially Inverted Transformation Pyramid

A significant number of organizations, particularly hospitals, have preferred to invert the upper four levels of the transformation pyramid. After creating individual patient records with appropriate demographic information, they decide to implement the EHR in somewhat the opposite order from that shown in Figure 17.2. Their implementation begins with electronic connectivity between the patient care areas and the pharmacy, clinical laboratory, and radiology departments (level 4). In some cases, this early implementation may also include sharing of clinical information with community physicians who have systems that can accept these electronic data (level 5). Nurses' notes, including documentation of patient vital signs, will be brought online quickly as well. Throughout this portion of the project, however, physicians' clinical documentation often continues to be recorded on paper and stored in traditional charts. The transition to using the electronic H&P component of the software is projected to occur after most or all of the other portions of the EHR have been successfully implemented.

What Happens If It Doesn't Work?

During a consultation at a significant Southwestern hospital, I attended a presentation by the director of the organization's electronic record project. The hospital had already launched the early phases of their implementation, which included establishing patient records and activating computerized physician order entry (CPOE) for medical orders, including pharmacy. The director outlined the hospital's five-year project for stepwise implementation, concluding with the statement that "physicians' clinical records will come last, because *they haven't figured that part out yet.*" When I spoke with the director afterwards, he indicated that his organization remains concerned that physicians are faced with too many usability and compliance problems with the H&P component of currently available systems.

When I asked, "What happens in five years if they still haven't figured it out?" he could only respond, "For our sake, I certainly hope that is not the case."

After purchasing a particular software system and committing to its implementation, there is understandable logic in the approach of starting with the proven parts of the system and delaying attention to the more challenging portions. On the other hand, when medical organizations acknowledge the medical priority that an EHR must first work well as a clinical health record, it becomes troubling to consider that it will take years of significant time, effort, and expense to learn whether the software will, in fact, fulfill its first priority. Understanding that the tools described in this text are available to meet physicians' medical record goals means that before making a final software decision, medical practices can (and should) verify that the systems they purchase will meet their physicians' needs for the H&P record. Once this is ensured, each practice can develop an implementation schedule based on its own preferences, not on concerns that critical portions of the system might fail to meet its needs.

SUMMARY

To reach health system goals of an interconnected and interoperable health system, individual practices must first have a reliable roadmap for the transition from paper record documentation and storage to electronic systems. Currently, this transformation has proven to be daunting for most medical practices. Overcoming these challenges requires implementation of a reliable protocol for HITr. This process begins with recognition that physicians' medical standards must dictate the direction and ultimate goals of medical practice transition to EHRs.

The HITr pyramid in Figure 17.2 offers a graphic representation of the overall process for practices to make the transition to EHRs. It starts with the medical organization making a decision to investigate information technology followed by going through multiple stages of evaluation and preparation, which ultimately leads to implementation and health information exchange. Considerable effort is being expended nationally on how EHRs can mobilize and share their stored data. The concept of health information transformation brings similar attention and creativity to the first two stages of this process, including the need to train physicians in effective workflow processes and to validate EHR capabilities that physicians can use efffectively before implementing a system. This new approach ensures that a practice knows how to select and evaluate an appropriate EHR, in order to be certain it will have the capability of meeting all physicians' medical record requirements while they work with their patients at the point of care.

References

1.   Connecting Communities National Conference. Director of AHRQ, Carolyn Clancy, MD, Keynote Address. Washington, DC. April 11, 2006.

2.   The White House. News and Policies. First Executive Order On Health Information Technology. Published April 27, 2004. www.whitehouse. gov/news/releases/2004/04/20040427-4.html. Accessed June 10, 2007.

Preparation for Practice Transformation

"Adopting IT [information technology] is one part technology and two parts work flow and culture change."

Carolyn Clancy, MD, director, Agency for Healthcare Research and Quality[1]

Each medical practice must go through several preliminary steps before deciding to purchase an electronic health record (EHR) system. This chapter offers a general framework for starting this process, while once again focusing on the concepts that relate to the history and physical examination (H&P) component of EHRs. Each practice should also expand its research and criteria beyond these core elements to include consideration of the other important features of EHRs that are not encompassed in the present focus, such as security, compliance with the Health Information Portability and Accountability Act (HIPAA), interconnectivity, interoperability, and staffing requirements.

BUILDING A TRANSFORMATION TEAM

The first preparatory step is creating a transformation team that will be responsible for the entire practice transformation process. Regardless of the size or number of physicians in a particular practice, the goals for successful transformation should be essentially the same. However, it is obvious that a small, one- to three-physician medical practice will have far fewer staff members with less varied job descriptions than a large multispecialty or single-specialty medical practice. Large practices will likely already have employees on staff who are qualified to fill most or all of the required positions. It is unlikely, on the other hand, that small- to medium-sized practices will have full- or even part-time employees with the qualifications to address a number of the required positions; these are marked with an asterisk in the list following the next paragraph. Some of the possible alternatives for meeting these needs will be examined at the end of this section.

In selecting the transformation team, it is important to include representatives of each section of the practice that may be affected by EHRs. Because the medical record is central to medical practice workflow, most departments should have a representative on the team. The members of the team who will be working with the H&P component of the EHR should ideally include the following:

1. Clinical staff: physicians, nurses, therapists, opticians, etc
2. Administrative staff: practice administration, billing staff, posting staff, reception staff, etc
3. *Compliance staff: coders, information management staff, compliance staff, etc
4. *Financial staff: chief financial officer or staff
5. *Legal staff: health care attorney with information technology expertise
6. *IT staff (for practices that choose to purchase an in-house system rather than an Internet-based system)

All members of the transformation team need to be involved in every aspect of the practice transformation. Effective communication and shared goals are critical to achieving the smoothest possible practice transition and avoiding conflicts between the goals, plans, and timetables of the various components of the project. However, within this cooperative framework, the primary responsibility for meeting various practice goals for the electronic H&P will logically fall to the most appropriate staff members. Physicians need to concentrate on the *usability* of the system and its ability to promote individualized *quality* health care. The compliance staff should concentrate on compliance features, particularly with respect to evaluation and management (E/M) services. They should also work together with physicians on ensuring that this compliance is maintained while encouraging optimal *efficiency* and ensuring *data integrity*. Finally, the administrative and financial staffs will focus on the impact of the H&P component on practice *productivity*. The IT staff may need to assist with ensuring the usability features while it focuses on support and maintenance of the hardware and software.

The Pivotal Role for Specialists in Coding, Compliance, and Information Management

Multiple medical practices have reported that some vendors strongly encourage the exclusion of coding, compliance, and information management specialists from the practice's transformation team. Although several reasons have been advanced in an attempt to justify this request, experience demonstrates that the vendors' major concern may be the likelihood that these experts could raise significant objections to software designs that they identify as having noncompliant documentation and coding features.

Medical practices must resist such requests by vendors and reiterate that compliance is one of the top priorities for EHRs. Their coding and compliance specialists are pivotal members of the transformation team, collaborating with physicians for proper software selection, physician training, and verification of effectiveness of a system in the practice setting.

As software companies realize that practices require compliant documentation and coding as a qualification for purchase, they should welcome a collaborative effort with these specialists. They will help verify that the software designs satisfy physicians' needs, and they assist in the design of training programs to prepare physicians to use the software for documentation of patient records that are clinically meaningful and compliant.

Meeting the Needs of Small Practices

Even though smaller practices do not have experts in several of these areas on their staff, the transformation team needs to be aware of the importance of addressing all these elements of practice transformation as they go through the process. This will help them identify critical issues and recognize when they require assistance from outside sources; eg, they will want their existing legal and accounting firms to contribute their expertise at the appropriate time and to recommend input from specialists if appropriate.

There are a number of reasonable options that practices can explore to find qualified assistance with the compliance and IT requirements. Although small practices are appropriately sensitive to the cost of hiring consultants for the required expertise, they must be equally cognizant of the costs of purchasing a system that fails to meet physicians' goals, compromises physicians' productivity, and/or leads to an unsuccessful implementation.

For obtaining support in documentation compliance, an obvious solution would be hiring a consultant with expertise in coding and software systems. The practice needs to work with an expert who appreciates its goals and can assist throughout this process. References for qualified consultants may be available from state or county medical associations, a national specialty society, the regional chapter of the American Academy of Professional Coders, the regional chapter of the American Health Information Management Association, or other medical practices that have used a coding consultant. Another option would be to cooperate with several other groups exploring EHRs by working with the same coding consultant and coordinating their scheduled activities to maximize cost-effectiveness. For physicians in a community exploring the development of a regional health information organization (RHIO) or health information exchange (HIE), that organization should be able to provide an expert who can assist physicians in selecting an EHR system that will work for the practices and be compatible with the central system for the RHIO or HIE.

For practices needing technical support for a system in their own facility, it is critical to identify an IT specialist who will eventually be contracted with the practice to support the new EHR. This individual should also assist at appropriate times with the transformation team. Appropriate references may be available from the regional chapter of the Health Information and Management Systems Society (HIMSS) and from IT specialists working at other practices or medical centers. Once again, referrals from other medical groups may lead to finding a business that will contract to provide technical support or share the costs of an individual support specialist. Community-based RHIOs may also be able to refer businesses or individuals who can assist with technical service.

ESTABLISHING CRITERIA FOR THE ELECTRONIC H&P

Importance of Identifying Practice Priorities

In her keynote address, quoted at the beginning of this chapter, Clancy also emphasized the importance of establishing practice priorities so that these could guide the IT transition process: "It takes a culture to raise a technology. What does it take to create a culture?"[1]

continued

> A reasonable answer might be that creating a culture requires defining practice goals, principles, and ethics and applying them as criteria and benchmarks for all actions that affect the practice.

One of the transformation team's initial tasks will be development of formal criteria for the electronic H&P record. These criteria should include a broad range of requirements that begin with general principles of patient care and proceed to specific design features that are needed for each component of the H&P record. Figure 18.1 gives a list of sample criteria for the H&P issues discussed in Parts 2 and 3 of this book. This list can provide a starting point for each practice to determine which features are most important for its particular needs. This template can also provide a model for creating similar lists of practice criteria for each of the other components of EHR systems (eg, interconnectivity and interoperability, security, and HIPAA compliance etc). Practices must also be aware that many of these features are not yet standardized in EHRs, even though they are frequently cited by IT advocates as benefits of using EHRs. During the selection process, the transformation team will need to learn which required features are available, which are in development, and which are not being considered for development by each vendor that is under evaluation. Eventually, it will be important for contracts to specify the lists of existing features and future upgrades that are to be included in the cost of the software purchase.

Creating formal sets of EHR criteria will allow medical practices to clearly define their EHR requirements and priorities. This exercise should provide a valuable foundation for investigating EHR systems and determining whether available systems meet the practice needs sufficiently to warrant pursuing implementation of an EHR system. The criteria will subsequently assist in selecting an appropriate system and will allow the practice to provide vendors with a list of features or modifications required before acceptance.

Special Considerations for Evaluating Medical Decision Making Functionality

The medical decision making (MDM) component of E/M documentation and coding has created several compliance challenges for electronic coding and electronic auditing software systems. As reviewed in detail in Chapter 15, these obstacles derive from multiple complexities of the MDM component and have significant potential to interrupt physicians' normal patient care workflow:

- Nontraditional documentation categories defined in the *Current Procedural Terminology* (*CPT®*) manual[2]
- MDM elements that call for physicians to make *quantitative* assessments, but CPT and Documentation Guidelines provide only *qualitative* descriptions
- Traditional H&P records guide physicians to document treatment options and data ordered in the same category, which is commonly labeled as "plans." However, CPT's E/M guidelines place these two elements into different subcomponents of MDM
- As traditionally taught and applied, the determination of the complexity of MDM requires several burdensome sequential calculation steps that require comparing or combining both quantitative and subjective elements.

F IGURE 18.1

Electronic History and Physical Examination (H&P) Record Criteria. Sample worksheet for evaluating design features of electronic health record (EHR) systems. Practices may use this list as a starting point for developing their own criteria. For illustration purposes, a high level of priority has been entered for a few essential elements. CPOE indicates computerized physician order entry; CPT, Current Procedural Terminology; E/M, evaluation and management; HPI, history of present illness; ICD-9, International Classification of Diseases, Ninth Revision, Clinical Modification; MDM, medical decision making; P4P/PQRI, pay for performance/physician quality reporting initiatives; PFSH, past, family, and social history; RHIOs, regional health information organizations; and ROS, review of systems.

Criteria	Priority		
Physician Priorities	**High**	**Medium**	**Low**
Immediate access to medical records	☒	☐	☐
Savings on cost of paper records (estimated = $ _____ per month)	☒	☐	☐
E/M compliance and audit protection	☒	☐	☐
☐ Passive guidance prompts only			
☐ Passive and active guidance prompts			
High-quality, functional medical records	☒	☐	☐
Improved practice productivity	☐	☐	☐
Contract to consider "evolutionary" approach	☐	☐	☐
☐ Maintenance payments include upgrades			
☐ Must incorporate new upgrades to stay current as EHR standards and capabilities evolve			
EHR Features			
CPOE for pharmacy (interconnectivity and interoperability)	☐	☐	☐
CPOE for clinical laboratories (interconnectivity and interoperability)	☐	☐	☐
CPOE for radiology services (interconnectivity and interoperability)	☐	☐	☐
Connectivity capability for communities (RHIOs)	☐	☐	☐
Connectivity capability for national health information network	☐	☐	☐
Clinical decision support: preventive care services, external programs	☐	☐	☐
Clinical decision support: preventive care services, practice generated	☐	☐	☐
Clinical decision support: disease management protocols, external	☐	☐	☐
Clinical decision support: disease management protocols, by practice	☐	☐	☐
All decision support should have recall capability with monitoring.	☐	☐	☐
Clinical decision support: P4P/PQRI protocols	☐	☐	☐
Data mining: identification of patients with specified features, single	☐	☐	☐
Data mining: identification of patients with specified features, multiple	☐	☐	☐
Data mining: report writing capability, preloaded	☐	☐	☐
Data mining: report writing capability, by practice (with ease)	☐	☐	☐
Connectivity to existing practice management system	☐	☐	☐
Single entry for: ☐ Patient demographics ☐ Patient recalls			
☐ Scheduling information ☐ P4P/PQRI reporting			
☐ Referring physician list			
☐ CPT codes ☐ ICD-9 codes			
Integrated practice management system ☐ Direct charge entry?	☐	☐	☐
Data Entry Options			
Asynchronous data entry permitted, on-site or off-site	☐	☐	☐
Patient data entry via secure Web site	☐	☐	☐

continued

Patient data entry at kiosk in office	☐	☐	☐
Patient data entry via digital pen in office	☐	☐	☐
Physician data entry by keyboard and mouse ☐ Active mouse entry	☐	☐	☐
Physician data entry by dictation and transcription	☐	☐	☐
Physician data entry by dictation and voice recognition software	☐	☐	☐
Physician data entry by tablet PC	☐	☐	☐
Physician data entry by digital pen	☐	☐	☐
Document scanning capabilities to appropriate sections of patient charts	☐	☐	☐
Medical History Features			
Physician entry for initial visit PFSH and ROS	☐	☐	☐
Staff entry for initial and follow-up visit PFSH and ROS	☐	☐	☐
Yes and No check boxes for patient entry on graphic elements	☐	☐	☐
Free-text narrative for entering details of PFSH and ROS	☐	☐	☐
HPI record has only narrative interface; no preloaded clinical macros	☐	☐	☐
HPI record has documentation prompts based on medical necessity	☐	☐	☐
Physical Examination Features	☐	☐	☐
Graphic interface with Normal and Abnormal check boxes	☐	☐	☐
Graphic interface allows inclusion of explanations of "normal" finding	☐	☐	☐
Free-text narrative interface for entering details of abnormal findings	☐	☐	☐
Examinations section includes documentation prompts based on medical necessity.	☐	☐	☐
MDM Features			
Inclusion of all elements of MDM	☐	☐	☐
Separate documentation of management options and data ordered	☐	☐	☐
Drop-down menus or check boxes + free text for management options	☐	☐	☐
Drop-down menus or check boxes + free text for data ordered	☐	☐	☐
Separate (graphic) documentation of complexity of data	☐	☐	☐
Separate (graphic) documentation of three subcomponents of risk	☐	☐	☐
Documentation prompts based on medical necessity	☐	☐	☐
Documentation of nature of the presenting problem (NPP)	☐	☐	☐
Documentation of time-based visits			
Inclusion of all three doumentation elements	☐	☐	☐
Documentation prompts based on CPT guidelines	☐	☐	☐
Documentation of information sheets provided to patients	☐	☐	☐
H&P Functionality Features			
Documentation prompts for passive guidance based on medical necessity	☐	☐	☐
Documentation prompts plus active guidance based on medical necessity	☐	☐	☐
Error-proofing functionality to ensure compliant documentation	☐	☐	☐
Security Features			
++++ Transformation team to define	☐	☐	☐
HIPAA Features			
++++ Transformation team to define	☐	☐	☐

As a consequence of this complexity, most existing E/M software calculation programs found in EHRs have incorporated calculation shortcuts to "simplify" the determination of the complexity of MDM. Unfortunately, these shortcuts fail to match CPT coding and documentation compliance requirements; ie, when used as designed, they can result in selecting MDM levels that are too high (particularly for relatively minor problems that are new to the patient) or too low (particularly for relatively major problems that are already established for a patient). Primary requirements for software coding systems must be that they accurately adhere to CPT guidelines, without additions or subtractions, and that they derive compliant E/M codes.

Coders can most readily identify such noncompliant software when they encounter coding systems that assign different values (or "points") for new problems, established problems, further evaluations, and/or different types of diagnostic studies. Such systems usually total these different artificial and noncompliant points to assign a complexity for MDM. When members of a transformation team find this type of noncompliant MDM functionality, they should present the problem to the vendor's management. The practice can emphasize that it cannot afford to purchase software that automates noncompliant coding due to the possibility of loss of revenue from undercoding and the risk, in the event of a compliance audit, of severe financial consequences including the potential for false claims damages. It is important to determine whether the vendor will agree (preferably in writing) to rectify the problematic software and replace it with compliant MDM design and functionality as a condition for consideration of the EHR. The transformation team should also decide whether final acceptance of the software (including payment) should be contingent on a compliant solution to this problem.

Special Considerations for Evaluating NPP Functionality

When evaluating an EHR system, it is critical for the transformation team, especially the coders, to investigate whether the software has the ability to accept documentation of the nature of the presenting problem (NPP) and to evaluate how it integrates this E/M component for guiding levels of care and for code assignment. If the software fails to take NPP into account, the system will be incapable of weighing the critical element of medical necessity and the Centers for Medicare & Medicaid Services (CMS) overarching criterion for compliance and payment of services in code determinations. In addition, the vendor will be unable to make available design features that guide physicians in the provision of medically indicated levels of care and documentation. As with the issue of MDM noncompliance, once this deficit is identified, the team should address it with the vendor's leadership and determine whether the vendor will commit (in writing) to providing compliant NPP functionality as a condition of consideration of the EHR. Similarly, the transformation team should also decide whether final acceptance of the software (including payment) should be contingent on a compliant solution to this critical issue.

If the software being evaluated provides NPP functionality and guidance, it is important to verify that the program includes all levels of severity of NPP and also has the capability of providing this information for all types of service. The NPP descriptors vary for nearly every type of E/M service that builds its documentation on the three key components. Appendix H has consolidated all E/M descriptors from the *CPT* manual into a table that looks at each type of service and reports the maximum level of service that is medically indicated for each level of NPP severity. This table provides a straightforward and effective means to review an EHR's functionality for NPP and determine whether it is compliant. Once again, if the practice identifies noncompliant programming for the NPP, this issue must be addressed with the vendor so that it can be corrected as a condition for acceptance of the software.

ESTABLISHING BENCHMARKS

In addition to defining the criteria for design features desired in an electronic H&P record, the transformation team should establish a list of benchmarks that any system must meet to achieve a "passing grade" for acceptability to the practice. Benchmarks will assist the practice during two critical stages of the health information transformation (HITr) process:

- Stage 1: Preliminary evaluation of systems being reviewed. Physicians should test the software by entering actual clinical information from their own medical records and thereby determine whether the system performs well enough to attain the required levels of performance for quality, compliance, efficiency, etc.

- Stage 2: The HITr process culminates in validation trials, which will determine whether the program of physician training combined with optimized software design will meet the standards set by the medical practice. If one or more benchmarks are not met, the practice can work with the vendor in an iterative process to further refine designs and/or training and meet the required goals.

Figure 18.2 lists many of the benchmarks considered earlier in this book. Each transformation team should develop its own list of benchmarks, customized to its own practice's EHR needs.

SETTING ECONOMIC PARAMETERS

Medical practices cannot afford to overlook the costs involved in committing to the purchase of an EHR system. As noted initially, increased overall productivity is one of physicians' primary goals and calls for careful examination of the potential savings, potential costs, and potential income gains from implementing EHRs to help establish budget guidelines. The net financial effect of IT adoption will be certain cost savings plus any increased income on one side of the equation, compared with IT purchase and maintenance costs plus any decreased income on the other side. Although the top economic priority is assessing the "bottom line," or net cost or gain of implementing health IT, practices need to be aware that some of the cost savings and productivity gains from using EHRs could also be attainable through the use of other alternatives.

Potential Cost Savings With EHRs

Savings generated from eliminating existing practice expenses may offset some of the costs of EHRs. The most obvious savings result from eliminating the costs of managing a paper-based system and thereby improving office workflow. It is interesting that many smaller practices are unaware of the expense involved in supporting paper records. Appendix A provides worksheets to help administrators perform a straightforward cost analysis of this expense. The minor expenses involve the costs of paper, chart jackets, and labeling supplies, plus the cost of space for storing current and older records.

FIGURE 18.2

Benchmarks for H&P Success. List of some of the suggested benchmarks for ensuring that an electronic history and physical examination (H&P) record is capable of meeting physicians' standards.

Benchmark for Compliance: When used as designed, the system guides compliant documentation and coding for every visit, including consideration of medical necessity.

Benchmark for Usability: (1) Design is compatible with physicians' diagnostic process; (2) Design permits all modes of data entry: (legible) writing, dictation, and/or direct computer entry (keyboard and mouse)

Benchmark for Efficiency: Design must facilitate physician's completion of patient care and compliant evaluation and management documentation (including consideration of medical necessity) for a typical comprehensive new patient visit in not more than _____ minutes of physician time (use time considered by the practice to be appropriate for the specialty)

Benchmark for Quality: Documentation prompts that guide level of care appropriate for nature of the presenting problem(s)

Benchmarks for Data Integrity: (1) Documentation is individualized and specific to each patient and to each visit; (2) Another physician (or an attorney) can review a record and find it to be appropriate for the patient and to make medical sense.

Benchmark for Productivity: There should be no decrease in practice productivity on implementation of an effective electronic health record (EHR).

Benchmark for Training Success: Training and customization time for effective and efficient use of the data input component of the H&P record is expected to require no more than _____ hours of physician time. (*Practical EHR* suggests that a maximum of 8 hours of training should be sufficient for this component.)

Benchmark for Transformation: The medical practice should be certain that a system will be successful before making a final commitment for purchase.

There are also intermittent expenses for the destruction of outdated records in compliance with privacy requirements. However, the major cost of supporting paper records is for the personnel time involved with pulling charts, filing charts, and finding misplaced charts. Each practice should perform its own analysis because of significant variations based on practice location, size, and individual workflow processes. However, a reasonable estimate is that this cost will, for many typical practices, fall into the range of $1,500 to $2,500 per physician per month. In a larger practice, the financial savings (cost of supporting paper records) of introducing an EHR will be directly demonstrated when the practice is able to reduce the number of its filing personnel. In a group of only one to three physicians, it is likely that size of the staff will need to be maintained, but staff energies can be devoted to more productive tasks. These new efforts may be valuable to the practice, but they may not translate into actual dollar savings.

Another cost reduction that is commonly attributed to the introduction of EHRs is elimination of some or all expenses for medical transcription, which can be substantial. These savings must, however, be accomplished by use of a compliant alternative, such as voice recognition software, typing narrative text into the software, or writing legibly with a digital pen. As noted, compliance and quality care criteria require the continued use of free-text narrative descriptions in multiple sections of the H&P record. For physicians who dictate these portions of the record, savings would require the substitution of voice recognition software for transcription. Even if physicians want to continue transcription because they find it more accurate, the total cost may be reduced through the use of patients for recording portions of the clinical documentation and through the use of compliant graphic interfaces with check boxes to reduce the total amount of information a physician dictates.

Potential Costs of EHRs

Before examining the actual costs of EHR system purchase and operation, practices must address the two significant potential losses of income related to the transformation process itself:

1. Decreased efficiency and productivity during and after implementation
2. Failed implementation. Several conditions can be interpreted as a failed implementation.

  - Terminate usage of the EHR system.
  - The practice may decide to stop utilizing the entire EHR system or just the electronic H&P portion. In either case, failed implementation indicates that the practice has made a decision to store its patients' H&P records in a paper system or a document management system.
  - The decision to terminate may occur as early as during an attempt at implementation, or at any time thereafter. The practice's effort may prove unsuccessful for a variety of possible reasons. As noted previously, challenges physicians encounter in using the electronic H&P is one common cause of failure.
  - In most cases, the investment in the EHR system is not recovered.

One intent of the HITr protocol is to establish a cooperative environment between the medical practice and the software vendor to prevent both of these negative outcomes through a shared goal of effective preparation leading to successful implementation. It advocates that physician training and design modification must be completed and successfully tested before implementation, thereby certifying an operable and effective system before any attempt at implementation.

LAN vs ASP Model for EHR Systems

Medical practices should consider both the local area network (LAN) and the application service provider (ASP) options for the configuration of an EHR system. The more traditional approach utilizes a LAN model. In this model, the medical practice purchases and owns EHR software and all required networking hardware, which may come from the same vendor or a different supplier. In LAN systems, the practice generally needs to have one or more IT experts on staff, although a small practice may rely on an independent IT support consultant or organization for this support.

Some newer software companies have offered physicians the alternative ASP approach, and a number of the established EHR companies are offering this option as well. In the ASP model, the software company owns and maintains the server (central processing unit) that stores the data and provides data backup services. The medical practice accesses the server through secure Internet connections, for which it pays monthly licensing or access fees. This approach may prove particularly attractive to smaller medical practices because the costs for equipment purchase are significantly lower in this model and there are usually no additional costs for maintenance and support. Users pay a monthly fee that includes access, support, and future upgrades. Figure 18.3 lists some of the issues practices should consider in setting their cost and data protection criteria when investigating EHRs, allowing for a comparison between LAN and ASP models.

FIGURE 18.3

Electronic Health Record Cost Issues. List of some of the cost considerations allowing practices to enter their own financial criteria for the evaluation and selection processes. The check-boxes in the left column are to be checked when a vendor satisfactorily addresses this requirement. ASP indicates application service provider; IT, information technology; and LAN, local area network.

Financial Criteria		Priority	
Cost Features	**High**	**Medium**	**Low**
LAN model system	☐	☐	☐
Initial cost Goal: < $_____ total			
Hardware cost $_____ Software cost $_____			
Maintenance cost Goal: < $_____ per annum			
Upgrades cost Goal: ☐ included in maintenance cost			
IT personnel cost Goal: < $_____ per annum			
Insurance cost Goal: < $_____ per annum			
Obsolescence cost Goal: > _____ years of usefulness			
☐ Data backup arrangements			
☐ Contingency for vendor problems			
ASP model system	☐	☐	☐
Initial cost Goal: < $_____ total			
Monthly cost Goal: < $_____ per physician per month			
or: < $_____ per practice per month			
☒ Practice owns all data ☐ Adequate data backup by vendor			
☐ Option of backup on site ☐ Contingency for vendor problems			
Features that promote return on investment			
No loss of productivity on implementation	☐	☐	☐

Practices considering the ASP model are usually advised to carefully evaluate the system's data-access speed and the transition from one screen display to the next (ie, "click speed"). Because a slow transition from one screen to another can disrupt physicians' workflow and, therefore, affect patient care and productivity, the criteria for acceptable click speed should be included in the practice's criteria list. The practice's contract with the vendor should also specify the maximum allowable click speed time for all navigation between different screens within the EHR program, and it should include a full range of notifications and remedies (including termination of the contract) if the program fails to achieve this performance. Another high priority item is the inclusion of contractual provisions that a practice owns all its data and that the vendor cannot withhold or obstruct access to this data, either overtly (through obstructing electronic access) or covertly (through inordinate increases in monthly fees that must be paid or access will be denied).

Legal and Contracting Issues

Regardless of the EHR model selected (LAN or ASP), medical practices should retain expert legal assistance during the contract negotiation phase. Although the elements of the contractual process go beyond the scope of this book, some of the issues of concern that must be analyzed and negotiated for both the LAN and ASP approaches include ownership of data, protection against excessive cost inflation over time, training, and support. Contracts must also create provisions to deal with meeting practice criteria and benchmarks (as discussed in Chapter 17) and policies for data recovery and/or data transfer if the software ultimately fails to fulfill a practice's requirements, the vendor is sold, or the vendor goes out of business.

Potential Income Gains With EHRs

Some practices may reap financial benefits with the implementation of an EHR system that meets standards for guiding compliant E/M documentation and coding. However, this economic potential will depend on the existing coding practices of the physicians. Providing tools and E/M compliance training to physicians who are currently undercoding (ie, performing documentation and coding at levels below the extent of care warranted by the NPP) should result in correct coding, which will have a significant positive effect on income. On the other hand, if physicians in a practice are generally overcoding (submitting codes higher than indicated by medical necessity), introducing correct coding practices will likely decrease income, even though it will provide audit protection.

Because an important element of investigating the possibility of implementing an EHR system is performing a cost-benefit analysis, most practices will want to analyze the economic effect of compliant coding practices on income. To obtain this assessment, the coding and compliance members of the transition team should perform a "current status" audit of the physicians' E/M documentation and coding practices, including a comparison of the code levels submitted relative to the NPP in each case. A small sample audit of 5 to 10 charts for each of a representative number of physicians will provide an overall picture of the current coding practices. In general, physicians who are not significantly overcoding (ie, the physicians are not consistently submitting level 4 and 5 E/M codes for patients with low- or moderate-level NPPs) should anticipate a significant financial boost from training physicians to use *Practical EHR* protocol and tools during the HITr process. The administrative staff can use results of this audit to approximate the productivity effects of compliant documentation and coding; eg, if 50% of the charts have been submitted with codes one level below the level of care warranted by the NPP, the anticipated gains will be at least the value of one additional code level for half of the patient visits.

How the *Practical EHR* Method Can Improve Income

A number of factors contribute to the productivity benefits realized by most physicians who employ the *Practical EHR* approach with EHRs, that provide the documentation and coding tools required. Foremost among these is the confidence that the documentation and coding are compliant that in turn allows physicians to be comfortable submitting medically indicated level 3, 4, and 5 codes. Another productivity gain results from the time physicians save as a result of patients and staff directly documenting medical history information, particularly during initial patient visits and consultation visits. In addition, reviewing a comprehensive history during every visit frequently leads physicians to identify additional and sometimes more complex illnesses that deserve higher levels of care than indicated by the patient's presenting condition. These additional health issues may also lead to an increased number of

continued

medically indicated diagnostic tests, some of which may be performed in the practice's office, and an increased number of medically indicated visits until all problems resolve.

All of these factors can justifiably increase the level of care provided, documented, and submitted. In addition, obtaining the comprehensive medical history and providing medically indicated levels of care promote preventive care, early diagnosis, and effective medical intervention. All of these consequences of providing compliant care promote increased quality of care and patient safety, which are the desired goals for introducing IT.

SUMMARY

Medical practices should use a systematic protocol when evaluating the possibility of purchasing of an EHR system and initiating a formal practice transformation process. The first step is to identify enthusiastic and committed staff members, drawn from all the departments of the practice that will be involved with the electronic clinical record, to form an official transformation team. The team members who will focus on the electronic H&P record should include physicians, coding staff, compliance staff, information management staff, and administrators. The compliance staff and others (such as IT staff) will address the other components of EHRs as well. Everyone involved in this team should be motivated to identify an EHR system that promotes quality care and meets all of the organization's medical record standards.

One of the transformation team's initial tasks should be to create a table of medical record criteria that includes features and capabilities that EHR designs must include to meet the practice's medical record needs. This table can be used for preliminary evaluation of the merit of purchasing an EHR and as a future assessment tool for comparing EHR systems, for obtaining a request for proposals (RFP), for creating contract provisions, and, eventually, for certifying that a system is capable of fulfilling practice goals. A related task, which can be performed simultaneously, is the creation of a set of clinical benchmarks that the electronic H&P record must be capable of achieving. These clinical measures will also serve multiple purposes, which include aiding in preliminary assessment of EHR systems, evaluating the success of physician training, and identifying customizations that may be needed for the software designs to be effective for the practice. A third task will be collecting financial data and selecting cost and productivity criteria that the practice can use to determine the feasibility of a purchase (a cost-benefit analysis) to ensure an economical implementation.

Once a team is assembled and has created its preliminary evaluation tools, the practice will have a solid foundation to begin investigating practice transformation. Following this approach should empower medical practices to be in control of the transformation process. This process itself should continuously evolve as the team obtains more information and receives feedback during its investigations. The H&P record criteria, benchmarks for success, and cost criteria should also continue to evolve during the HITr phase as physicians are trained, systems are tested, and team members continue to gain experience and insight.

References

1.   Clancy C, MD. Keynote Address. Presented at: Third Annual Connecting Communities Learning Forum and Exhibition. April 11, 2006; Washington, DC.

2.   *American Medical Association. Current Procedural Terminology (CPT®).* Professional Edition. Chicago, IL: American Medical Association; 2007.

chapter 19

Practice Transformation: Foundation Level

"It's not just about the technology. It's about the people who use the technology and what it takes to make it work."

Carolyn Clancy, MD, director, Agency for Healthcare Research and Quality

The practice transformation pyramid presented in Figure 17.2 presents a useful graphic framework that medical practices can expand and modify to meet their individual specifications when planning a practical transformation program. Although it demonstrates a linear progression through various levels of this process, in reality, transformation should develop as more of a three-dimensional model. Several steps may be occurring during the same time frame, including steps from different stages of the pyramid. For example, physicians on the transformation team may undergo early training for compliant documentation as a means of helping them in the system evaluation and selection steps. The system selection process in the first phase also has obvious overlap with the refinement of design features in the second stage, which is health information transformation (HITr). Practice transformation should also be an evolutionary and iterative process, with lessons learned during one particular step leading to ongoing modifications of the criteria and goals established at the outset.

The purpose of presenting a formal approach to practice transformation is to provide medical practices with insights and tools they can use to put themselves in control of this complex process of making informed and successful decisions for their individual practices. It should enable practices to appropriately establish physicians' quality care and practice requirements as the standards for electronic health record (EHR) selection, preparation, and implementation. Finally, moving to an environment in which EHR software designs must evolve to support physicians' recognized standards of quality care and meaningful documentation should encourage software developers to work with physicians and medical practices to achieve their well-defined goals.

Paradigm Shift

Physicians, coders, information management specialists, and administrators have indicated that many medical practices have struggled to define criteria for EHR selection and/or to establish satisfactory benchmarks for success. This

continued

---

leads to the subtle message from physicians that "*we need someone to tell us the 'right' electronic record to buy, and we expect that the 'right' EHR will (automatically) solve all our problems.*"

The paradigm that results from this approach is that a medical practice will purchase an established EHR product and then try to customize physician workflow to fit the requirements of the software design. It has been well demonstrated that this approach is not a blueprint for success.

The *Practical EHR* paradigm calls for medical practices to identify a set of H&P record goals that EHRs must meet in order to be an effective and valuable asset for the practice. These goals should be built on the established principles of the medical diagnostic process that physicians rely on for quality care and compliance. It is essential that physicians recognize and acknowledge these goals and then find vendors whose software is able to incorporate them. Physicians cannot achieve their aspirations for high-quality documentation and resolution of the evaluation and management (E/M) compliance challenge if their software lacks the capacity to record all components of compliant care and lacks compliant coding software. Similarly, EHR companies and their software developers require guidance and motivation from medical practices to appreciate the necessity of incorporating this functionality. Physicians and EHR developers can benefit from this new paradigm, which calls for physicians to specify critical design criteria for the electronic H&P record and then identify software programs capable of providing these features.

The *foundation* level of the HITr pyramid moves a practice forward into active investigation and decision making for an EHR. The components of this stage include the following:

- Making a decision to investigate the purchase of an EHR system
- Researching various EHR systems to initiate a selection process
- Weighing the advantages and disadvantages of local area network (LAN) and application service provider (ASP) models
- Defining requirements and goals for vendor relationship, including the goal of agreeing on an "evolutionary approach" to practice transformation
- Negotiating the contract, including warranties

These general subdivisions of the foundation stage are interdependent, with the decision to commit to a specific software system being the result of evaluating the features of a variety of systems and determining how they fit with practice needs.

INITIAL INVESTIGATIONS

After completing the preparatory phase, practices must begin to investigate the available EHR systems and evaluate whether the features of the systems will meet their requirements. It is often convenient to perform initial investigations at meetings or trade shows, where multiple systems can be evaluated in a relatively short time. It will be important for physicians to focus on the H&P component and to actually attempt to enter data as if they were documenting a patient visit. It will be equally important for coding and compliance specialists to be certain that the systems provide only compliant designs, including consideration of medical necessity and a compliant coding engine.

Practices may also evaluate systems that have been endorsed by colleagues. This circumstance often offers an opportunity for early on-site visits to observe how the software works for physicians and staff. Preliminary review of these systems can be followed by more in-depth demonstrations of selected systems at the practice's office. In addition to the focus on clinical perspectives, as shown in Figures 18.1 and 18.2, practices will need to investigate other administrative and clinical features related to functionality and interoperability, benefits of LAN and ASP models, and costs related to purchase and maintenance (partially outlined in Figure 18.3).

Guidelines for Features Peripheral to the H&P Record

The Web site for the Certification Commission on Health Information Technology (www.CCHIT.org) provides separate tables of "functionality" and "interoperability" criteria that CCHIT uses for evaluating and certifying EHRs. These criteria can help a practice establish its own table of administrative guidelines that complement the clinical standards addressed herein. Each practice should do its own reviews because meeting CCHIT criteria indicates a general level of design accomplishment but does not guarantee that systems will meet the needs of a particular practice. These standards are also continuing to evolve as CCHIT receives feedback.

In earlier chapters, compliance and quality issues were identified related to CCHIT's "encounter" standards for the H&P component. It is interesting that only 6 of CCHIT's more than 300 total ambulatory EHR criteria are related to what CCHIT labels as the "encounter," ie, the H&P. In contrast, the table presented in Figure 18.1 contains 64 more encounter criteria than the CCHIT's list, and this is suggested as a starting point for practices. This degree of detail illustrates the need for practices to build on CCHIT's base of general requirements to develop more extensive and specific criteria of their own.

The transformation team should view its investigations as a dynamic process, refining the criteria as team members learn from evaluating different systems and from other practices using them. Going through this effort will give team members the added confidence in their criteria and in their ability to evaluate different systems accurately, allowing them to develop the customizations or weigh the compromises that may be required to meet the practice's medical record needs.

OVERVIEW OF SOFTWARE EVALUATION

Identifying a number of basic system features will help practices categorize the type(s) of EHR systems to investigate. Practices can then focus on the critical area of the H&P component.

Relationship to the Practice Management System

In some ways, the practice management software transformation of the early- and mid-1980s parallels the health system's time course for adoption of EHRs. At the outset, developers promised to reduce paper and administrative costs, connect different areas within a medical office, and electronically connect different offices. Initial systems presented some challenges, and some failures occurred. However, as the means of overcoming these challenges were identified, practice management systems became an essential component of operating a successful medical business office.

At present, some EHR systems address only the clinical record, whereas others are designed with integrated practice management systems. However, EHRs that do not include practice management software should be able to establish effective electronic communication to send and receive the shared elements with most recognized practice management systems. There are several major attractions of an integrated system. It facilitates seamless sharing of data between the two components, allowing all demographic and coding information to be entered only once. Most important, it can be supported by a single vendor and information technology (IT) team, thereby avoiding the issues of finger-pointing that can occur when the support teams for separate systems blame each other if a communication error occurs.

There are also several potential drawbacks to an integrated system. The most obvious is that an integrated system costs proportionately more than a comparable free-standing EHR system. This significant additional investment may seem unnecessary if the practice is pleased with an existing successful practice management system, as long as duplicate entry of significant amounts of data can be avoided. Purchasing an integrated system calls for two transformation teams that must carefully evaluate both parts of the system and ensure that each one meets practice standards. If one of the two parts proves to be less than optimal, the system cannot be purchased. Finally, the transition to the new system will require increased training time and training cost. Commonly, the conversion to the new system will occur in two stages. However, if the second part of the system were to fail to measure up to requirements, all the implementation effort of the first phase was likely wasted. This underscores the importance of using the same process as HITr for the practice management component as well; it provides a thorough evaluation and verification prior to purchase and implementation.

Considering the amount of attention that has been directed toward this decision by vendors, consultants, HIT advocates, and medical groups, there are surprisingly few data that need to be shared between an EHR and the practice management system. The essential shared element is patient demographic information. No practice will want to separately enter this information into two separate software systems. Additional elements of shared information can include the electronic appointment scheduling system, although this could be kept solely in the EHR system, and a list of referring physicians. Finally, systems that have physicians perform charge entry (coding) at the point of care must be able to share *Current Procedural Terminology* (*CPT*®) codes and International Classification of Diseases, Ninth Revision, Clinical Modification codes. (As pointed out in Chapter 16, EHR systems providing this feature need to include a separate charge entry step because correct billing functionality must not be permitted to interfere with E/M compliance and quality in the medical decision making portion of the clinical record.

Each practice should weigh the advantages and costs of an integrated system and determine the approach that best suits its current needs and budget. For many practices, the most compelling rationale for choosing an integrated system vs a pure EHR system will depend on their satisfaction with the existing practice management system. If it is functioning well and fulfilling their needs, the practice has a reasonable right to expect that it should be possible to establish connectivity between the two systems to share the appropriate electronic information. For practices choosing to establish an interface between a new EHR and the existing practice management system, the transformation team must, prior to final acceptance of the EHR, carefully test and confirm the ability of the two systems to share the appropriate information. Also, satisfactory arrangements must be made and contractually confirmed regarding technical support and maintenance of the two systems. Parenthetically, because EHRs are touted as the medical system's answer to interconnectivity and interoperability, it is reasonable to expect (and require) a well-designed EHR to interconnect and be interoperable with sophisticated practice management software. However, at this time, a national standard for this functionality has yet to be established; therefore, practices must test the communications between the two specific systems and confirm for themselves that it is satisfactory for their needs.

LAN vs ASP System

Several decisions center around whether the practice decides to host its own hardware system or purchases less extensive hardware and accesses its data through a Web-based application with the network server (Intranet), technical support, and maintenance all hosted by the EHR vendor. The issues involved in this choice include cost, reliability, speed, availability of technical support, and, most important, data security and backup. Many practices, especially larger practices that already maintain an IT department for support, may be more secure in having hardware and data storage on their own premises. However, Web-based (Internet) applications have become widely accepted in many areas of business and are becoming more common in medicine as well. A number of national practice management systems have successfully employed the ASP approach. The monthly fees for this model usually have the advantage of including all support and upgrades. Furthermore, the ASP approach eliminates most of the costs of obsolescence for the hardware.

Under the LAN or ASP approach, the medical practice must be certain that its contract specifies that the practice owns all data and has guaranteed access to it. Provisions should also be included to cover the transfer or conversion of medical data if a vendor sells its business or goes out of business. Finally, long-term pricing protections should be included contractually to protect against unreasonable financial increases or surcharges and prohibit restriction of access in the event of a dispute. These and other issues warrant the use of a health care attorney who understands medical record and privacy issues and also has experience with IT procurement for guidance.

Holding Data Hostage

Under all circumstances, the integrity and reliability of the software vendor are of paramount importance. Although physicians' focus is on clinical matters, there have been rare anecdotal reports for both practice management and EHR systems of serious concerns related to data access, data maintenance, and/or data conversion if problems occur for the vendor. These have included loss of support or severely increased fees for access to data. Contractual protections should, therefore, be an integral part of the relationship with a vendor.

SOFTWARE EVALUATION TOOLS

Transformation teams have three important evaluation tools they can use in their initial software evaluations: their own software tests, assessments from existing users, and reviews of medical records obtained from the existing users.

Testing Software With Sample Forms

Physicians and coders should work together on trial runs to analyze whether a software system is capable of meeting practice needs. An H&P record criteria form, such as the one shown in Figure 18.1, provides a checklist of each practice's assessment of the design elements that software must provide for achieving usability, efficiency, compliance, and meaningful documentation. This same form can be modified for use as a scoring sheet by relabeling the three check-boxes on the form to indicate whether a specific feature is present or absent, or to indicate that the vendor has agreed to add or correct a missing or unsatisfactory feature.

It will also be extremely helpful for the team to have a set of sample medical records that physicians can use for conducting trial runs by entering clinical information into the H&P record of software systems under review. These samples can be in the form of deidentified patient records from the practice that have been approved by coders as representing compliant documentation and by physicians as representing realistic and meaningful clinical data. As an alternative, the team can create its own standardized sample records to meet these same criteria (such as the forms shown in Appendix G). By having physicians enter information directly from the forms into an EHR's H&P record, the members of the team should quickly gain insight into the usability and flexibility of that system, its efficiency for entering data, and its ability to record meaningful data. The data entry trials can be timed to provide efficiency comparisons among different systems.

Coders who are aware of the appropriate E/M code levels for the sample charts will be able to evaluate the coding compliance features of systems that indicate they have coding capability. Appendix G provides examples of an initial visit (documented for E/M code 99204) and an established visit of the same patient (documented for E/M code 99213), which can be used as sample test records. The established visit has intentionally been documented so that coding software will "count" a level 99214 visit based on two of three key components, but consideration of the nature of the presenting problem (NPP) should limit the coded level of care to 99213. This sample, therefore, will provide a test of the medical necessity function of a software system.

Using the practice's established criteria and benchmark forms as a scoring system to evaluate the success of entering standardized clinical charts will give the transformation team valuable data to determine which software systems have the potential to best meet their needs. It will also provide a thorough inventory of the features that need to be enhanced or redesigned to meet the practice's goals. These modifications can be reviewed with vendors to find out their ability and willingness to make the changes needed to meet the practice's needs. In some cases, it is likely that the EHRs capable of meeting most of a practice's requirements will have some features that they are unable to modify sufficiently to meet practice criteria. The transformation team will need to assess the importance of such deficiencies, and they should consider whether alternative solutions could fulfill their needs in the mean time until the vendor is able to meet this need at a future date. Chapter 21 presents some "temporizing measures" that practices can use to compensate for elements of EHR designs that do not meet their requirements.

Customizing Standardized Forms

The outpatient forms in Appendix G have a medical history section that is most appropriate for adult patients, and the physical examination graphic interface reflects the general multisystem examination appropriate for many specialties, including the specialty of family practice. Transformation teams are encouraged to use a photocopy of these forms as a template for inserting customizations appropriate to each physician. Pediatricians, for example, will want to modify the past, family, and social history and review of systems. Obstetricians and gynecologists will want to work with the specialty-specific examination for "genitourinary female."

Assessments From Existing Users

EHR vendors maintain a directory of customers using their software. It is unlikely that a vendor would provide statistics on the number of medical groups that have discontinued use of their software or expressed dissatisfaction. However, practices should request the names of at least three groups using the software who have indicated they are willing to discuss their experiences. The transformation team should begin with phone calls to physicians, coders, and administrators in each practice. Once again, the use of a standard list of questions will help evaluate the software's ability to perform required tasks and the customer's level of satisfaction. Figure 19.1 offers a sample list of questions designed to determine a practice's satisfaction with its EHR system. It utilizes check-boxes to record whether the various features meet that practice's expectations and, where appropriate, whether the vendor is working on rectifying identified problems, and at what additional cost if any. The team should also learn whether the vendor follows through on its promises to add features and resolve issues.

Compliance Audits

When the transition team asks a vendor for references from practices using its software, it is likely that the vendor will refer the team to medical practices that are generally pleased with the performance of their EHR system. Regardless of the practice's degree of satisfaction, this referral provides a superb opportunity for the transformation team to assess the quality of documentation and degree of compliance produced by the H&P component of the system being used. The team should request that the endorsing practice send charts of 15 deidentified individual medical visits for review, including an indication of the E/M code submitted.

Coders should audit these charts for documentation and coding compliance, including the selection of E/M code levels appropriate for the NPP (ie, not too high or too low). Physicians should review the charts to assess the quality of the documentation, including absence of "cloning" (charts that read essentially the same with only minor variations) and the record's ability to convey the patients' medical issues and the appropriateness of physicians' recommended evaluations and treatments. At the conclusion of this review, the transformation team should have a reliable impression of how well the

FIGURE 19.1

Sample Questionnaire for Obtaining Information From Practices Using a Vendor's Software. The first two columns of check boxes indicate whether a feature is present or absent in the design. For an absent feature, the next two columns indicate whether the feature has been promised and, if so, whether it is included at no additional cost. DEO indicates data entry operator; E/M, evaluation and management; H&P, history and physical examination; NHIN, national health information network; and P4P, pay for performance.

Inquiry	Response			
Benchmarks	**Yes**	**No**	**Correcting?**	**Cost?**
Satisfaction with all aspects of system is A⁺	☐	☐		
Physician satisfaction with H&P record Grade =	☐	☐		
Physician satisfaction with other features Grade =	☐	☐		
Coder satisfaction with compliance Grade =	☐	☐		
Administrator satisfaction with other features Grade =	☐	☐		
Design ensures E/M compliance, including medical necessity	☐	☐		
Pemits data entry				
By writing: ☐ DEO ☐ Tablet PC ☐ Digital pen	☐	☐		
By dictation: ☐ Transcription ☐ Voice recognition	☐	☐		
By keyboard and mouse	☐	☐		
Compliant level 5 care performed and documented in 15 minutes	☐	☐		
Maintain productivity following implementation	☐	☐		
< 8 hours of physician time for H&P record training	☐	☐		
EHR Features	**Yes**	**No**	**Future?**	**Cost?**
CPOE for pharmacy/laboratory/radiology	☐	☐	☐	
Connectivity for: communities/NHIN	☐	☐	☐	
Clinical decision support: prevention/management/P4P	☐	☐	☐	
Data mining: capability/ease of report creation	☐	☐	☐	
Connectivity to practice management system	☐	☐	☐	

software performs and its potential for meeting the practice's major requirements for the electronic H&P record. Team members will know whether the system, as currently designed, guides compliant documentation and coding. They will also appreciate whether it promotes creation of a high-quality H&P record that includes reliable clinical information, which is necessary to provide the best care for patients.

Practice Visits

At this point, the transformation team will have performed its own tests on the vendor's software, reviewed endorsements by practices that are using the software, and evaluated the records created in those practices. For systems that pass these reviews and remain under active consideration, it will be beneficial for the transformation team to visit one or more of the endorsing practices to observe how the software works in daily practice, for physicians, other clinicians, coders, billers, and administrators.

DEVELOPING AN ITERATIVE PROCESS

This preparatory effort at the foundation level serves several important purposes. First, it allows the leadership of a practice to clarify and refine its goals and requirements for moving forward with a transformation program.

It will gain the information to determine whether now is the time to move forward, learn whether a satisfactory software system is available, and establish the economic parameters needed to make this a financially supportable venture. In addition, it provides the opportunity to explore relationships with various software companies and determine which ones will prove to be good and responsive partners for customization, transformation, and ongoing relations.

It is probable that these evaluations will reveal a number of software companies whose software meets most of the practice's administrative criteria (eg, Health Information Portability and Accountability Act compliance, security capabilities, support, and training) and many of the H&P record criteria and benchmarks as well. The practice should, however, adhere to the highest standard of practice: to be acceptable, a software system needs to meet all of its baseline H&P record criteria for compliance, usability, efficiency, medical record quality, and, most important, promote quality patient care. If one or more critical features are missing, the team will need to establish a dialogue with the designers and leadership of the software companies being considered to have them make the modifications that will meet these standards. Once a company agrees to the changes and to make them within a reasonable time frame, the evaluation process can continue.

These initial discussions between the practice's representatives and the EHR company's leadership and designers should evolve into an ongoing dialogue, because at each stage of its evaluation, the transformation team will likely find specific design features that are missing or need improvement. This type of relationship should result in a continuing iterative process, with retesting and refining of the system after modifications have been completed to be certain that they correct the deficits and that the system meets specifications. Working with the software company in this manner will provide insight about that organization's responsiveness and willingness to continue to support improvements in the future.

Modifications will require the software company to invest time, personnel resources, and money. When only a single practice is bringing this degree of focus to the quality of the H&P component, vendors may resist making requested changes before having a signed contract. Under this circumstance, well-designed contracts will be required to protect the practice and the vendor in a cooperative effort toward optimal EHR design and functionality.

Transforming the Software Development Landscape

Until now, the primary demands on software developers have come from health policy advocates, government agencies, and payers. The focus of these groups has been almost exclusively on EHR features concerned with data storage and retrieval, ie, information exchange, data mining, and clinical decision support. Although these are all necessary and important benefits of EHRs, they are, as noted, insufficient to meet physicians' and patients' medical record requirements.

One of the highest priorities for *Practical EHR* is to help physicians develop and apply effective criteria that will compel an equally powerful focus on the EHR features related to the design and functionality of the H&P component of the electronic record as it affects physicians and patients at the point of care. These tools require EHR systems to function as effective medical records that

continued

assist in patient care, meet compliance requirements, and facilitate documentation of high-quality individualized clinical information. Physicians and health care advocates alike should hope that, ideally, EHR companies would be motivated to incorporate features that promote quality care and patient safety into their software designs. As increasing numbers of medical practices require that EHRs meet these standards as a condition for purchase, the software industry should also have a powerful economic incentive to respond and meet these requirements.

Contract Dynamics and an Evolutionary Approach

Despite the best efforts of the transformation team during its investigations in the foundation phase, a practice cannot be certain that a system's design will fulfill all requirements and meet all benchmarks until completion of the HITr phase, before actual implementation. Because practices must have a system that will succeed, contract provisions should be developed that require systems to meet specified goals before there is a final purchase commitment on the part of the practice. Such provisions should underscore the shared responsibility and the shared incentives for design and training that help meet practice criteria for success.

Traditional relationships between medical practices and EHR software companies have commonly approached medical record software as if it were a relatively static technology, with upgrades generated at the discretion of the vendor. However, a number of current HIT realities encourage the development of an "evolutionary" approach to this relationship. This can be achieved by having the customary annual *maintenance* costs include the updates required to keep the EHR's capabilities current with advances being promoted by external sources, including national policy initiatives and medical quality imperatives. Foremost among the reasons for introducing this concept is that many of the promised beneficial features of EHRs have not yet been standardized, and, therefore, have not been integrated into the software when a system is purchased. Currently, for example, there is no nationally approved standard for interconnectivity among physicians' offices and hospitals, laboratories, or radiology offices. Although active development of these features is in progress, the capacity to achieve such automatic connectivity without incurring significant additional customization costs will occur some time in the future. Because this functionality is one of the reasons advanced for purchasing an EHR, practices should expect it to be incorporated into their software, without additional cost, at the earliest possible time after standards are established. In addition, the capabilities and design requirements for HIT are evolving at a rapid pace, with major improvements commonly occurring every 5 to 10 months. In an evolutionary relationship, practices should have the expectation that these costly systems will incorporate these updates without additional cost to remain state of the art during the next 5 to 10 years.

Conventional contracts for LAN-type systems generally may require additional payments for all upgrades. However, in this rapidly changing electronic environment, practices might consider negotiating contract provisions that commit the EHR vendor to partner with the practice in an ongoing evolutionary process rather than just making the sale of a static, finished piece of software. This relationship should continue the cooperative efforts of software evaluation and system improvement that begin during the foundation and HITr phases of practice transformation.

Physicians and software companies both need to be responsive to a rapidly changing medical and technological environment. Resources traditionally paid for maintenance need to be re-assigned to covering the costs of upgrades, customization, and change. As a result of this changing dynamic, the traditional sale-and-purchase relationship should be replaced with a relationship of partnership between the providers of patient care and the providers of HIT, with the shared goal of continual improvement of patient care.

Lessons From the Past

More than 25 years ago, while I was practicing medicine in a relatively small, three-physician practice, the decision to purchase an electronic practice management system fell to the physicians. This was a major investment for the group in terms of both finances (involving a 5-year loan) and staff effort. Some of the lessons from that experience resonate as valuable guidance for practices incorporating EHRs today.

The first attempt at implementing a practice management system was in 1981. The vendor promised that a new operating system would overcome existing computer operating system limitations by allowing multiple terminals to operate from a single central processing unit. The vendor's demonstration worked well, and the practice looked forward to going ahead with the purchase and installation. It was at this point, before training or a trial period, that the software vendor required a signed contract. Fortunately, one of our advisors insisted on adding a list of benchmarks to the contract, based on the representations of the software company. During the training period, the new operating system failed to fulfill its promise of supporting operations on multiple terminals. Fortunately, the practice was protected by the guarantees added to the contract. The vendor removed the system and returned our practice's investment. Although the attempt failed, the physicians and staff had gained valuable experience without a painful economic setback.

We introduced a second computerized practice management system in 1983. Once again, during the training period, it was learned that the software could not meet the benchmarks the vendor had promised and agreed on in the contract. For a second time, incorporating specifications for the system's capabilities into the contract permitted terminating the experiment without financial harm.

Our third attempt in 1985 proved to be completely successful. The lessons learned from the two previous efforts refined our search criteria, and we found another software system that promised to be capable of meeting our needs while avoiding the problems of the first two systems. That practice management system met the practice's administrative needs for the next 8 years, until increasing complexity of Medicare and insurer practices eventually exceeded its capabilities.

INVESTING IN A SOLID FOUNDATION

In medical practices of all sizes, from solo practitioners to academic centers and multispecialty groups with hundreds of physicians, the introduction of an EHR has ramifications for all aspects of the practice of medicine. The effect on the clinical component of medicine is most apparent to physicians, potentially affecting their workflow, efficiency, interactions with patients, the quality of care they can deliver, and even the levels of satisfaction and enjoyment they derive from practicing medicine. However, all of the administrative functions are similarly affected, with implications that include workflow, billing and collections, income, expenses, compliance, technology interfaces, and the overall relationships among staff and the culture of the practice. The ultimate goal for all members of the medical practice should be for a successful transition that brings benefits to every part of the practice and to every member of the staff. As presented in Part 1, the current approach to practice transformation (illustrated in Figure 17.1) has resulted in unsatisfactory outcomes for an unacceptably high number of practices. Therefore, continuing to use the same approach to evaluating, purchasing, and implementing EHRs should not be an acceptable option.

Based on the *Practical EHR* approach to practice transformation (illustrated in Figure 17.2), the steps outlined in this and the previous chapter for preparation and for building the foundation involve a significant investment of time and effort, particularly on the part of the members of the transformation team. It is important for all members of the practice to appreciate the value of this investment, because it will pay significant dividends as the practice progresses through each level of the transformation pyramid. The higher the quality of this investment, the greater will be the dividends, which will be realized in time saved and better results. Good preparation and creating a solid foundation will provide the basis for increasing the efficiency and success of the administrative staff training and physicians' HITr at the next stage, and this will contribute to similarly improved outcomes for implementation, connectivity, and information exchange. These benefits will be compounded at each stage of the transition, and they should culminate in the ultimate payoff of a successful implementation that improves the quality of all aspects of the practice, especially those related to caring for patients.

Small Practice Perspectives on Investing in a Solid Foundation

In small practices, the efforts of preparation and the foundation stage usually fall on all the physicians and all the members of the staff. While their task may be no greater than that of the members of a larger practice's transformation team, the smaller practice is burdened with the reality that there is no one else to carry on the normal functions of the practice at full capacity while the team is taking the time to perform these transformation tasks. In addition, while the small practice can tap their internal resources for the clinical and administrative members of their transformation team, they will have to invite input from their usual legal and financial advisors or perhaps obtain advice from accountants and/or attorneys with greater expertise in the area of IT. Additionally, they also need to obtain assistance from experts in compliance and information technology. This will involve a cost, but the cost and consequences of not obtaining this guidance at the early stages of an EHR project can be far greater during the later stages.

In summary, the stakes for success and failure are just as high for a small practice as for a large one, and the benefits of good preparation and laying a solid foundation are just as great. Every hour invested in good preparation will be paid back in many hours of time saved during training, software verification, and implementation. Every dollar invested in obtaining expert guidance will see a compounded return by the preservation of full productivity, efficient and safe improvement of documentation and coding, and protection against an unsatisfactory or failed implementation. From this perspective, no practice, large or small, can afford *not* to invest in thorough and meticulous preparation.

SUMMARY

The foundation phase of practice transformation follows logically on the preparation stage of assessing practice needs and goals for changing a practice's medical record system from paper storage to electronic. It utilizes the tools employed to evaluate practice needs and goals as criteria for evaluating EHR software systems. The members of the evaluation team should gain new insights from examining each software system, allowing them to continually refine and improve their criteria.

At first, software developers are likely to find it unusual to have medical practices presenting design requirements for their EHRs, particularly for the data entry design and functionality features of the electronic H&P record. Until now, they have been receiving their guidance primarily from organizations other than medical practices, with the result that the primary focus of EHR development has centered on the collection, processing, and communication of data, not on the usability of the H&P record and the caliber of documented information. Similarly, current national certification standards for ambulatory EHRs devote less than 2% of their more than 300 criteria to the H&P component of these systems.

This new focus on the usability and functionality of the H&P component at the point of care creates a paradigm shift toward physicians' measures of quality medical records and quality patient care. It specifies that EHRs must provide H&P designs that require the input of high-quality clinical information. This level of input is necessary to achieve the integrity of clinical data needed to realize all of the promised benefits of electronic interconnectivity and interoperability. It is critical that EHR companies and software designers hear the voice of medical practitioners and bring the same high levels of creativity currently being applied to solving data storage, retrieval, and sharing challenges to the data entry features and quality of content recorded in the electronic H&P record.

chapter 20

Practice Transformation: Health Information Transformation (HITr)

"It's not just the knowledge or expertise; it's the soul of the enterprise, the fit between people and technology, the processes, and the relationships."

Carolyn Clancy, MD, director, Agency for Healthcare Research and Quality[1]

In the current approach to training for electronic health records (EHRs), physicians usually do not have the initial experience of creating documentation with the electronic history and physical examination (H&P) record in a realistic patient care environment until after EHR implementation. Furthermore, implementation occurs without prior evaluation to determine whether the design and functionality will meet practice needs and physician requirements for promoting quality care and compliance. Almost universally, at the time of implementation, vendors advise practices to significantly reduce the number of patient appointments scheduled so that physicians have time to learn to use the new system. However, physicians frequently experience this learning process without expert instruction or supervision, and, as previously discussed, the designs commonly alter their accustomed H&P workflow. Physicians often feel unprepared and uncomfortable with this approach to implementation, and if physicians are not comfortable with any part of the process or software, this discomfort creates a foundation for future problems.

Structuring a formal preimplementation phase, which provides realistic physician training for clinical use of the electronic H&P record and allows verification of its usability and effectiveness at the point of care is an important theme of health information transformation (HITr). While introducing any new system will always require an adjustment period, this training approach reduces the time and stress of learning. It also minimizes the impact of the transition on the delivery of medical services to patients.

WORKFLOW TRANSFORMATION

Workflow Transformation for Administrative Staff and Processes

Until now, the primary focus of preimplementation training has been on "workflow transformation" (level 2 in Figure 17.1). This training involves preparing the administrative staff to implement effective workflow practices that will enable them to help move patients and information smoothly through the practice environment because successful use of EHRs requires an efficient and effective professional environment.

> **Optimizing Office Workflow**
>
> There are multiple advantages of optimizing the administrative workflow policies and practices in a medical office. It increases administrative efficiency and may decrease costs. Even more important, when staff members are working smoothly toward clearly stated goals, office morale is positive, staff has more time for attention to patients, and physicians and patients benefit from the positive working environment. Several physicians have pointed out that improvements in the organization of the office and staff performance have been the most advantageous features of introducing an EHR.
>
> The transition to an EHR acts as a catalyst to promote positive changes because it is critical to accomplish these improvements before implementing an EHR. Transitioning to an EHR generally begins with an analysis of existing workflow patterns, followed by the process of identifying any possible bottlenecks in the existing flow of information and any other processes that may be effective and functional in a paper environment, but may have to be modified to optimize the workflow in an electronic setting. Just as an unpaved country road would need to be properly paved before one could expect a sophisticated race car to perform there to its full potential, the establishment of a smoothly running office and solid administrative support structure is a prerequisite for maximizing an EHR system's potential.

Workflow Transformation for Physicians

Just as the proper use of sophisticated EHR administrative tools demands effective staff training and workflow reengineering, the optimal use of well-designed clinical tools also calls for effective training and workflow reengineering for physicians. Vendors commonly provide physicians with proper instruction in the use of the EHR features related to the storage and retrieval functions that they highlight as the positive features of their software. These may include the following:

- Immediate access to existing clinical records
- Electronic availability of the office schedule
- Lists of tasks to be performed
- Review of laboratory test results and flow sheets
- Review of radiology reports and images
- Access to patient profile tables
- Electronic prescribing
- Electronic messaging
- Application of clinical decision support tools (such as disease management protocols and preventive care guidelines)

In contrast, the effect of EHRs' H&P component on physicians, patients, and the comprehensiveness of care has been underappreciated. Vendors have generally been unable to offer effective preimplementation training that provides physicians with the ability to enter meaningful data into the electronic H&P record easily and efficiently while working with patients in a manner that meets their primary goals for the electronic H&P record. This is the role to be filled by HITr. Effective transformation provides protocols that address these factors so that physicians are well prepared for a positive experience when using the EHR for documenting care while working with their patients.

As previewed in Chapter 17, HITr suggests three physician-centered and interrelated preparatory phases before implementation. First, it provides physicians with training in documentation and coding compliance as part of the preparation for using a well-designed electronic H&P record. Second, it presents the EHR software designers with feedback and guidance for improvements and/or modifications needed to achieve practice criteria and benchmarks. Third, the final verification step uses trial runs in realistic patient care situations to confirm that physicians can use the final software design effectively to achieve all of the practice's benchmarks. Successful verification is a condition for implementation.

Addressing the Issue of Creating "Macros"

Before implementation, many vendors ask physicians to modify or create "macros," which, as used in this text, are generic paragraphs that can be copied and pasted into various sections of the electronic H&P. The vendors instruct that the macros are intended for use in documenting multiple sections of the electronic H&P record that are usually documented using free-text in a narrative interface that should be used for as many "common" clinical circumstances as possible to maximize the speed of documentation. Once created and entered into the software, they are subsequently used repeatedly for documenting the medical history and/or the findings of the physical examination with the addition of minor modifications. This approach surmises that once the software can automatically copy and paste a pre-entered generic macro for every patient's history and examination, documentation will be done quickly and physicians will have no further concern for documenting the H&P record. However, as discussed in detail in Chapters 5 and 7, this approach fails to allow physicians to record the appropriate depth and breadth of clinical information required to create documentation of E/M services that is *individualized*, patient specific, and visit specific. H&P records compiled using this approach can effectively diminish the quality of care, compromise the integrity of the information recorded, and conflict with the principles of E/M codes.

Considering HITr Under Ideal Circumstances

To appreciate the value of the HITr stage of overall practice transformation, it is useful to consider how readily physicians would be able to migrate from using a paper record to an EHR if they already practiced in an ideal paper-based medical record environment, which would include the following:

1. *Standardized* H&P record designs built on the established E/M standard for documentation and coding that reinforce the diagnostic process physicians use to promote high-quality care

2. *Standardized* medical education for obtaining and documenting the H&P

    a) Medical students in their first and second years continue to learn the medical diagnostic process and proper documentation of a comprehensive history and physical (as they do today)

    b) Medical students would subsequently be trained to use compliant medical record tools that continue to promote comprehensive care while increasing efficiency

---

continued

c) Senior medical students and residents would receive further training in E/M compliance principles and the role of medical necessity in identifying appropriate levels of care and documentation

3. The physician's office has optimal workflow for its existing paper record environment

4. Physicians in the practice use paper records that are usable, efficient, and compliant and facilitate provision of high-quality care

5. The medical practice introduces a well-designed EHR constructed with a "common user interface" that is compatible with its existing paper forms

■ The medical record's data entry functionality accommodates each physician's preferred format (writing, dictating, and/or using keyboard and mouse)

In this idealized environment, in which all medical record documentation tools are built to meet the E/M documentation standard that reflects medical education in the diagnostic process, transition from a paper H&P record to a matched electronic H&P record should occur seamlessly and with minimal effort. The training period could then focus on the advanced decision support and reporting tools that are among the special benefits derived from EHRs.

HITr strives to create this type of optimal environment before "going live" with EHRs. With effective training plus effective tools, the resulting transition should be accomplished seamlessly and reliably.

COMPONENTS OF HEALTH INFORMATION TRANSFORMATION (HITr)

As illustrated in Figure 17.2, the HITr process includes three related components (or pillars): (1) physician training, (2) software design evaluation and modification, and (3) monitored patient care trials. It combines these elements into a sequential iterative process of assessment, training, design enhancement, and reassessment. This process continues until the physician and software components of the system are able to work well together to achieve the practice's medical record goals.

PILLAR 1: PHYSICIAN COMPLIANCE ASSESSMENT AND TRAINING

Nearly all medical students receive extensive training in obtaining a comprehensive H&P and in applying the medical diagnostic process. Unfortunately, time and economic constraints combine to provide physicians with perverse incentives to perform and document problem-focused care. Fortunately, however, physicians remember their medical record training very well. They can easily reinstitute the appropriate comprehensive H&P method as soon as they are given tools that permit them to do so in the time they have available. *Practical EHR* provides these tools for the EHR, and the HITr process prepares physicians to use them. This preparation program for physicians and clinical staff should logically occur at the same time the administrative staff undergoes training for the workflow transformation to prepare for the changes associated with EHRs.

Assessment of Current Medical Record Documentation

The transformation team's first step in this phase of the HITr should be to perform an initial analysis of physicians' current documentation success as a basis for physician training. The coders should perform "current status audits" of a small number of each physician's recent medical records. These should be educational audits, which go beyond merely comparing codes submitted with the level of care and documentation. The elements of educational audits should include the following[2]:

- Identifying whether code selection is in accord with medical necessity (ie, comparing the level of code submitted with the level of care warranted by the nature of the presenting problem [NPP])

- A conventional audit assessment of whether there is sufficiently extensive care and documentation to support the code levels submitted

- Noting whether a comprehensive medical history was obtained and documented for every visit (to allow effective assessment of the NPP)

- Analyzing if the records document all elements of medical decision making (MDM), including the three levels of risk and the complexity of data (to ensure compliant documentation)

- Determining if records document the NPP (to ensure compliance with medical necessity)

For each physician reviewed, these audit reports* should indicate whether the physician is documenting and coding correctly or, instead, is (1) under-coding, (2) overcoding, and/or (3) underdocumenting. If the audit identifies overcoding (selection of codes higher than warranted by medical necessity) or underdocumentation (documenting levels of care insufficient to support the codes submitted), the review can underscore the protection that compliant medical records will provide against potential financial penalties from a compliance audit. On the other hand, if the audit reveals undercoding (submission of codes and/or documentation of care at levels lower than warranted by the NPP), the report can emphasize the potential for legitimately increasing income by introducing compliant documentation and coding. This information should provide the practice's physicians with a powerful incentive to master medical record tools that, in addition to contributing to improved patient care, also ensure compliance and appropriate reimbursement.

Physician Training for the Compliant Electronic H&P Record

The protocol for training should provide one-step preparation for physicians to use the compliant medical record design that was modified by the EHR vendor to meet the practice's criteria. Ideally, the training should begin at the same time the software designers are programming the agreed upon customizations to the electronic H&P record. Training can begin before the modified software screens are available by using paper tools with interface designs that identically match the electronic screens for the EHR, ie, the paper interface should exactly reproduce the design planned for the EHR screens. These paper records should

---

*To ensure confidentiality of these reviews, all audit documents should be marked "peer review protected" or "for educational purposes" or with other pertinent explanations recommended by the practice's compliance or legal experts.

permit data entry by writing for the graphic (ie, check-box) portions of the H&P record and by writing and/or dictating for the narrative portions.

Learning on Paper vs Learning on the EHR

A veteran certified health information management specialist recently shared her experience with simultaneous compliance training and EHR implementation for physicians in a medium-sized internal medicine practice. She concluded that performing both training tasks simultaneously significantly increased the challenge for physicians. It also allowed physicians to (incorrectly) attribute coding and documentation errors to the use of the EHR, rather than to improper documentation methods. The specialist recommended that the most effective experience for physicians would be first to learn compliant documentation using a high-quality paper record by writing and dictating. After this step has been successfully completed, transitioning to identical electronic screens should be straightforward and require relatively little additional training. At that point, physicians should be able to concentrate their efforts on learning the additional features available in the EHR, without experiencing further challenges related to compliance.

For *Practical EHR* purposes, either approach should be successful. The physicians and coders on the transformation team can evaluate the simultaneous learning protocol and the two-stage protocol and identify the approach that provides the greatest ease, efficiency, and acceptance by physicians for their practice.

Physicians should work together with coders during the training phase so that physicians can receive feedback on their progress and immediate answers to their questions. This environment should provide maximum learning efficiency while also allowing for immediate consideration of any additional design modifications that could further increase medical record usability and effectiveness. The training period will also allow physicians to experiment with the data entry modalities available (writing, dictating, and direct computer entry) to learn which option(s) are most convenient for them for each part of the medical record. Using the *Practical EHR* approach with well-designed medical record tools should require no more than several hours of training with the forms for physicians to identify and be comfortable with the approaches that work best for each of them. The *Practical EHR* forms in Appendix F illustrate the type of content and structure these screens or forms should contain because all compliant records need to include the same E/M components.

Suggested Training Protocol

An effective training protocol should begin by first reviewing an effective method for compliant documentation that also duplicates physicians' customary diagnostic process. It should then provide a section-by-section review of each portion of the medical record, demonstrating how effective design integrates the concepts of medical necessity, compliant documentation, and quality patient care. A suggested training sequence is as follows:

1. Review of the medical diagnostic process and its use in compliant documentation
   a) Comprehensive medical history at the beginning of every visit
   b) At the conclusion of the history, assess the *probable* severity of the NPP and the medically indicated level of care for this NPP. (Guidance

is available from the NPP documentation prompts on the MDM screen of the electronic H&P.)

c) Perform and document the medically indicated extent of physical examination. (Guidance is available from the documentation prompts at the bottom of the examination section of the screens and forms.)

d) Perform and document the medically indicated extent of medical decision making (MDM). (Guidance is available from the documentation prompts in the MDM section of the screens and forms.)

e) Do a final reassessment and documentation of the medically appropriate level of the NPP.

2. Review how to use each section of the H&P optimally during patient care

a) Review the past, family, and social history (PFSH) and review of systems (ROS) medical history sections for initial patient visits

   i) Provide physicians with a sample form with all *Yes* and *No* check-boxes filled in for the PFSH and ROS, as if completed by a patient. Some details may also be completed on the PFSH sections. This completed form shows the first information a physician sees when evaluating a new patient

   ii) Working with these screens and forms, the physician would

   - Review patient responses.

   - Obtain and document indicated details for any positive PFSH responses.

   - Obtain and document appropriate medical history for all positive responses to signs and symptoms in the ROS.

   - Sign or initial indicated boxes at end of PFSH section and at end of ROS section.

b) Review the PFSH and ROS *Update* sections for established patient visits

   i) Review type of questions required to elicit meaningful patient responses.

   ii) If this information is obtained and documented by another member of the clinical staff, physician should review it, obtain and document further information when indicated, and initial indicated boxes at the end of each section.

c) Review the history of present illness (HPI) medical history section

   i) Chief complaint (CC) should be specifically identified or easily inferred. For initial visits, the patient will have entered the CC on the PFSH form or screen.

   ii) Obtain and document a valid history, ie, "a *chronological description* of the development of the patient's present illness from the first sign and/or symptom, or from the previous encounter, to the present."[3(p7)]

   iii) Review the eight elements that contribute to eliciting a meaningful HPI and the requirement to include at least four of those elements to document an extended HPI.

   - The eight elements should be listed in a documentation prompt on screen and on paper.

   - Consider the merit of including the elements *duration*, *timing*, and *severity* as portions of every medical history.

    d) Review preliminary assessment of the NPP

        i) Note the NPP documentation prompt at the end of the H&P form on screen/forms

        ii) Review Appendix C of the *Current Procedural Terminology* (*CPT®*) manual for accepted clinical examples of each level of care, which illustrate the levels of NPP severity included in the *CPT* E/M descriptors.

        iii) Working together with coders, have physicians conduct a "coding forum" to identify examples of the clinical cases they commonly encounter that would warrant each level of care.

    e) Review physical examination section of screens and forms

        i) Identify the most appropriate examination template for each physician, based on the 1997 Documentation Guidelines[3]

        ii) Review customization of templates

            ■ For general multisystem templates, consider eliminating organ systems that will never be examined and/or moving those organ systems that will rarely be examined to a separate screen (of the EHR) or page (of a matched paper form). No more than five organ systems should be segregated and/or eliminated in this manner.

            ■ Add additional *Optional* elements (identified by an asterisk or other symbol) for commonly used examination elements that are not included in the standard examination templates.

        iii) Review guidance by documentation prompts to ensure provision of extent of examination warranted by the NPP.

    f) Review MDM section on screens and forms

        i) Consider the three subcomponents (diagnoses and treatment options, data reviewed and ordered, three levels of risk), and total of nine elements that together constitute MDM.

        ii) Review compliant documentation of the MDM elements that generally are not documented in conventional medical records: risk of presenting problem(s), risk of diagnostic procedures, risk of management options, and complexity of data ordered and/or reviewed.

        iii) Review and practice an effective MDM documentation strategy, eg:

            ■ Focus on the two subcomponents of MDM not related to *data* (because addressing all three subcomponents requires cumbersome coding calculations; further, in a significant number of cases, the amount or complexity of data does not correlate with medically indicated levels of care).

            ■ *Document* the levels of risk; this is particularly valuable for the risk of presenting problem(s) (as illustrated in the Table of Risk[3(p31)]), which correlates well with the severity of NPP (as described in the CPT descriptors and clinical examples).

            ■ *Document* the numbers of diagnoses (including reasonable differential diagnoses) and/or management options warranted by the NPP.

    g) Review final assessment and documentation of the NPP, including final selection of the appropriate and medically indicated level of care

---

The Role of Coders in HITr and Physician/Coder's Symbiotic Relationship in *Practical EHR*

The training protocol discussed in the NPP section (2d, p. 330) previews the positive role coders play in the HITr and shows the initial and future possibilities of the symbiotic relationship between physicians and coders when an effective EHR that meets compliance and quality standards is adopted.

In an effective and compliant EHR environment, coders can significantly decrease their traditional role of identifying incorrect documentation and coding practices and admonishment of physicians to memorize and follow compliance rules. This is because EHR systems that are based on *Practical EHR* principles should already have all the compliance rules incorporated into the electronic H&P design and documentation prompts.

During the HITr process, coders can work closely with physicians to help demonstrate how to use the screens and electronic forms to facilitate both care and compliance. As physicians become more familiar and manage to achieve compliant and effective documentation, the coders' role can progress and evolve to one that is more of an ongoing and interactive process; ie, an ongoing reassessment of procedures and protocols: help maintain the successful documentation practices, evaluate issues related to medical necessity, and consider whether E/M codes selected were appropriate for the NPP and/or if any were undercoded or overcoded.

In summary, the effectiveness of *Practical EHR* principles and its recommended features in solving *conventional* compliance issues allow coders to continue to be educators and partners with physicians in advancing quality care through the use of compliance guidelines. From physicians' perspectives, this partnership is reinforced by the fact that coders not only assist them in removing conventional compliance concerns, they also provide an invaluable service of contributing to the overall effort toward the ongoing reinforcement and guidance for meaningful documentation and data integrity.

Although this HITr protocol should be used primarily to train groups of physicians as they prepare to implement a new EHR system, it may also initially be used during the foundation stage to prepare physicians for the transformation team to critically evaluate EHR systems.

Identify Data Entry Modality Preferences for Each Physician
During the training phase, each physician should experiment with the spectrum of data entry tools available, identifying those that seem most user-friendly, efficient, and compatible with his or her practice style while caring for patients. Some physicians may favor hybrid entry approaches, using combinations of writing, dictating, and direct keyboard entry for different portions of the H&P record.

Documentation Time Trials
During this training phase, the team will be able to gain further insight into the usability and efficiency of their system and of different data entry modalities by performing documentation time trials. For standardization, these trials should first be carried out during the early portions of physician training, when physicians are not working with patients but are copying check-boxes and narrative descriptions from a standardized H&P form that has been completed with representative clinical information, such as the forms illustrated in Appendix G. A particular advantage of the initial time trials (additional measures should be carried out during the verification phase) is that by being

performed in the absence of patients, they are able to convey an accurate picture of the absolute time physicians need to accurately document high levels of care using optimal medical record tools, independent of the time physicians require to perform care. These results provide powerful insight that the transformation team can apply to identify H&P design features that meet usability and efficiency requirements and those that need further enhancement.

Figure 20.1 provides a sample form for time trials that can be used to analyze the efficiency, accuracy, and usability of various data entry tools for each portion of the medical record. A separate form should be used for each data entry tool, allowing physicians and reviewers to compare the effectiveness of using the different tools for data entry.

F I G U R E **20.1**

Time Trials Form for Evaluating Data Entry. A separate sheet should be used for trials with each data entry tool, allowing the quantitative and qualitative results to be compared. This form includes tracking of the following: (1) the amount of time needed to document each element of the history and physical examination (H&P), (2) the accuracy of the documentation (recording a percentage of errors or a subjective ranking of accuracy), and (3) the physician's subjective assessment of ease of use (ie, usability). abnl indicates abnormal; HPI, history of present illness; MDM, medical decision making; nl, normal; PFSH, past, family, and social history; and ROS, review of systems.

Physician's Name _____   Chart No. _____   Data Entry Tool _____

Section of H&P Record	Time for Documentation	Accuracy of Documentation	Usability Assessment
PFSH check-boxes			
PFSH free-text details of positive responses			
ROS check-boxes			
ROS free-text details of positive responses			
Update of PFSH & ROS on established patient			
HPI			
Physical Exam check-boxes for nl/abnl			
Physical Exam, narrative for abnormals			
MDM			
Data reviewed			
No. of diagnoses and management options			
Data ordered			
Levels of risk and complexity of data			
NPP(s)			

Speed Is Not Efficiency

Practical EHR maintains a distinction between electronic H&P tools that promote efficiency and those that focus on speed. Most of the time, when information technology advocates, policy makers, insurers, and even EHR vendors tout that EHRs can promote "increased efficiency," they are referring to shortcut tools that increase only the *speed* of documentation, not *efficiency*. To be labeled as efficient, design tools that allow physicians to document faster must also continue to support the diagnostic process, ensure 100% E/M compliance, and permit only the recording of patient-specific and visit-specific clinical information. Designs that promote this type of efficiency are highly

continued

desirable. Designs that allow faster documentation but also introduce the potential for reducing the amount of care actually provided, impairing quality, failing to achieve compliance, and/or sacrificing data integrity are labeled as "speed tools" and are considered unacceptable.

The problem of using such speed tools is immediately spotlighted in the time trials, when physicians are entering patient-specific and visit-specific clinical information (as exemplified by the charts in Appendix G). Ironically, physicians attempting to record such *individualized* patient information, when handicapped by macros as a starting point, need much more time to accurately enter this meaningful information than they require to document it as free-text narrative.

PILLAR 2: CONFIRMATION OF EHR DESIGN AND FUNCTIONALITY CUSTOMIZATIONS

In stage 1 of HITr, a practice has control over the physician evaluation and training process, with more or less assistance from the vendor's trainers as the practice dictates. The practice will also have control of the verification process in stage 3. However, stage 2 involves a mutual and cooperative effort between the practice's transformation team and the vendor's leadership. In an ideal situation in which the vendor's existing software fulfills all or most of a practice's criteria except for minor modifications, stage 2 would include the reevaluation of the modified software, postimplementation of the requested modifications to the H&P design and functions that were specified during the foundation stage. The transformation team should analyze each modification to certify that it meets specified design requirements, as noted in the teams' electronic H&P record criteria. For any sections that fail to meet specifications, consultation with the EHR design team should lead to clarification and correction of problems. Physicians and coders will then evaluate the effectiveness of these designs for patient care during the verification process.

Identifying Missing Features and Imperfections

Realistically, in the current EHR marketplace, most developers have not been incentivized, either by medical practices or the current certification criteria, to change and develop the electronic H&P component of their systems to meet all the criteria described in this book. Although vendors should enthusiastically accommodate modifications that require only peripheral changes, such as eliminating the use of macros in various sections of the H&P, requests for changes in an application's intrinsic designs and features, as expected and *perhaps* understandable, would encounter more resistance. Although the potential for EHR purchase by a large medical practice may offer sufficient financial incentive to encourage vendors to invest in more complex enhancements or modifications, a small practice will be unable to exert such significant economic leverage. Nonetheless, it is hoped that as small and large practices alike continue to make requests for similar improvements, an increasing number of EHR companies will voluntarily initiate the much-needed design and functionality changes for the H&P component. Ideally, this will result in an ongoing cooperative and evolutionary relationship between practices and vendors, as described in chapter 19.

Nevertheless, practices exploring EHR adoption in today's environment will have to compromise in order to move forward with their EHR plans. The criteria illustrated in Figure 18.1's checklist should prove helpful in this endeavor, because it provides a systematic approach for a practice to rank its electronic H&P record criteria by priority (high, medium, or low). The criteria with the highest priority assume the greatest importance in identifying the most appropriate system(s) and where the most crucial modifications would be needed.

Temporizing Solutions and Long-Term Enhancements

When the transformation team identifies features that fail to meet requirements, the ideal solution would be an immediate modification by the vendor to meet the requested standard. However, when this is not possible, contractual agreement by the vendor to include the requested changes and improvements in future versions of the software will pave the way for optimal solutions in the long term.

For the short term, however, the transformation team should exercise creativity in discovering temporizing solutions to address the remaining problems. These can occur through the use of complementary paper forms or dictated text to create the required additional documentation, which can be saved in the document section of each patient's record. For example, many existing electronic H&P designs lack documentation prompts to guide physicians to the appropriate levels of care and documentation for the severity of a patient's illness. These prompts can be made available through the use of laminated reference cards that physicians can refer to during patient care. Chapter 21 gives additional examples of using portions of templates, as in the illustrated templates in *Practical EHR*, to give physicians the ability to separately document extra and/or missing information; this additional documentation is then scanned and uploaded into an existing electronic H&P. For example, a physician could rapidly complete a short paper form that records the missing documentation elements for complexity of data, the 3 levels of risk, and the NPP, and the form could be scanned into the appropriate section of the EHR. Other physicians may prefer to dictate this important compliance information and the transcribed document would be stored in the same fashion. This approach allows a practice to use all the required tools that promote quality care, usability, efficiency, and compliance even before they are fully integrated into the practice's selected EHR.

The transformation team should explore and develop the needed supplemental tools to be included in the testing and verification process before phase 3 of HITr. This will let physicians test the system realistically and to make sure that the supplemental tools as well as the EHR are usable, efficient, and meet physicians' needs.

PILLAR 3: VERIFICATION OF SUCCESSFUL TRANSFORMATION

The final phase of HITr is to combine trained physicians with the approved software product in clinical trials. These trials should verify that well-trained physicians using the final version of customized software are capable of meeting the practice's benchmarks for success in a patient-care environment.

There should be at least three levels of testing and verification trials, allowing physicians to increase comfort levels in using the electronic H&P record under conditions that are progressively more complex and more like the patient care environment.

The first level lets physicians experience data entry by copying information from some of the practice's existing *compliant* medical charts or from several standardized charts such as the examples in Appendix G. This step is similar to the time trials used during training. Physicians will enter all information from these charts into the appropriate data entry sections of the H&P record as if they were having a dialogue with a patient. For each section of the H&P record, the software should allow physicians to choose their preferred data entry tools, including all options for writing, dictating, and/or entering data directly with a keyboard and mouse. Other members of the team can observe the process and monitor the effectiveness of the final system by using the time trial form shown in Figure 20.1.

Second-level trials concentrate on the ease of entering medical history information during an actual patient encounter, with physicians eliciting history information from a person rather than copying from a chart. The physician and another member of the transformation team receive copies of the medical history section of a sample record. The other team member serves as the "patient," following the script and responding to the physician's inquiries. The physician will interview the patient to elicit details about the documented positive PFSH and ROS responses on the form and obtain the HPI.

For data entry by writing (with pen on paper, tablet PC, or digital pen), most physicians should be comfortable recording responses during the interaction. Physicians using dictation tools will dictate at the conclusion of the dialogue. This scenario can also provide physicians and their pseudo-patients with an opportunity to experience the pros and cons of attempting to use the keyboard to enter detailed information into the software during an encounter and/or at the conclusion of the interaction. The physician and the patient can report their impressions, feelings, and reactions to the data entry process using the various data entry tools. These reactions can be recorded on the more sophisticated time-trial form shown in Figure 20.2, which includes separate consideration of the time for performing the care and the time for entering the documentation. In addition, the results of the trial run should be compared with the practice's benchmarks for success.

The third-level trials allow physicians to use the system during several real patient encounters, without a script. Ideally, another member of the transformation team should monitor the encounter. Once again, objective and subjective evaluations should be recorded on the time-trials form, and the success of each encounter should be measured against practice benchmarks. Appointments for patients participating in these trials should be slightly prolonged. Although the care and documentation process may have already reached optimal efficiency at this stage of the verification process, it is important that the physician be allowed to continue his/her evaluation of the system should this be needed, without the pressure to stay on schedule. Because this trial with patients occurs at the conclusion of the HITr process, the need for prolonged appointments should require only a small number of patients and should not have a significant negative effect on the physicians' productivity.*

---

*This approach to *going live* is in marked contrast to conventional training approaches that lack a HITr stage. Under the conventional circumstances, physicians first learn how to use the electronic H&P after implementation, while they are seeing their regular patients. Vendors commonly recommend and physicians, in turn, commonly require prolonged appointments to complete their care and documentation for a period of weeks or even months, resulting in a significant negative impact on practice productivity.

FIGURE 20.2

Time Trials Form for Evaluating Time of Performing Care and Time of Data Entry. A separate sheet should be used for trials with each data entry tool, allowing the quantitative and qualitative results to be compared. This form includes tracking of the following: (1) the amount of time needed to perform the history and physical examination (H&P), and MDM elements, (2) the incremental additional time needed to document each element using the various tools, (3) the accuracy of the documentation (percentage of errors or a subjective ranking of accuracy), and (4) the physician's subjective assessment of ease of use (ie, usability). abnl indicates abnormal; HPI, history of present illness; MDM, medical decision making; nl, normal; PFSH, past, family, and social history; and ROS, review of systems

Physician's Name _____   Chart # _____   Data Entry Tool _____

Section of H&P Record	Time to Perform	Added Time for Documentation	Accuracy of Documentation	Usability Assessment
PFSH, check-boxes completed by patient				
PFSH, not completed by patient				
PFSH free-text details of positive responses				
ROS, check-boxes completed by patient				
ROS, check-boxes not completed by patient				
ROS free-text details of positive responses				
Update of PFSH & ROS on established patient				
HPI				
Physical Exam, check-boxes for nl/abnl				
Physical Exam, narrative for abnormals				
MDM				
Data reviewed				
Number of diagnoses and management options				
Data ordered				
Levels of risk and complexity of data				
NPP(s)				

In an ideal world, the verification process will proceed smoothly, physicians and patients will have 100% positive responses to the experience, and the transformation team and software vendor will agree that all contract conditions have been achieved. If, on the other hand, problems are detected during the verification process, their causes need to be identified and corrective measures applied to physician training and/or software design. Once success is achieved, the practice can schedule software implementation for the clinical H&P record with assurance of success and maintenance of optimal practice quality, compliance, efficiency, and productivity.

Time Trials During the Second- and Third-Level Trials

The second- and third-level trials add the complexity of providing care in addition to recording documentation rather than simply copying standardized forms. Gauging physicians' efficiency under these more sophisticated circumstances calls for observing the time for performing each component of care separately from the time required for documenting it. These two distinct components should be easily measurable for physicians who document the entire H&P after concluding their patient care and for physicians who dictate or document after each section of the H&P. Physicians who write at the time they are obtaining the medical history may require little or no additional time for documentation of this component. For physicians who type while obtaining the medical history, an observer may have to estimate the amount of additional time required for documentation. Figure 20.2 is a sample form for these more sophisticated time trials. When physicians want to try different modalities, observers should use a separate form for each data entry modality to allow comparison of the efficiency of the different data entry tools.

Comparing the results of time trials during the second- and third-level trials provides four important pieces of information. First, it should help physicians make optimal choices for themselves among the various data entry tools. Second, it should demonstrate the amount of time required to *perform* the medically indicated extent of care for different levels of service. Third, it should show that when using optimal tools for efficiency and compliance, the major portion of most E/M visits will be devoted to performing patient care, with significantly less time needed for documentation. Finally, this data should demonstrate how efficiently physicians are currently providing and documenting care. This information should help practices identify if further efficiencies can be achieved without sacrificing either quality care or data integrity. If physicians are found to be performing at optimal efficiency, the statistics from these time trials will support the message that any further efforts to increase the speed of care (eg, by further reductions in payment for services) will threaten to undermine and potentially destroy the goals—quality care, patient safety, and meaningful data—that are driving HIT adoption.*

STREAMLINING THE HITr PROCESS FOLLOWING INITIAL SUCCESS

After the initial group of physicians has successfully navigated the training process, HITr can be abbreviated to a one- or two-step training program for subsequent groups of physicians. The second stage of the HITr is eliminated because the transformation team will have approved the H&P software customization. As a result of the groundwork performed by the transformation team, physicians can then be trained using the actual EHR. Alternatively, practices may, as a first step, have their physicians train using simulated paper forms that replicate the EHR screens, allowing physicians to address compliance issues and learn an effective process first and thereby decreasing the time and effort required to learn how to use the EHR.† With either, each physician should still experiment with the various data entry tools to find his or her optimal approach, and there should be final verification trials to confirm that each physician is able to meet practice benchmarks and is comfortable with the system before using the EHR full time for patient care.

---

*Detailed discussion of the dangers of further efforts to increase speed of care appears in Chapter 10 in the sidebar entitled "Setting the Limits of Efficiency."

†The pros and cons of these two options were considered in greater detail earlier in this chapter in the sidebar entitled "Learning on Paper vs Learning on the EHR."

VALUE OF THE HITr PROCESS

As noted previously, numerous medical practices and their physicians have found the current approach to HIT adoption to be a challenging, uncomfortable, and often-disruptive experience. The existing environment generally requires practices to commit to purchasing and implementing an EHR system without allowing physicians to perform a thorough assessment of the electronic H&P—the information core of the EHR—to determine its ability to meet their medical record and point-of-care requirements. The current environment requires physicians to experience their initial EHR-enabled patient care under the pressures of their normal patient care schedule. In order to learn while providing care requires that physicians increase the scheduled time for appointments, which adds additional pressure to the entire process. Such an atmosphere creates a formula for suboptimal implementation with the potential for imperfect utilization of the EHR, physician dissatisfaction, patient inconvenience, and loss of productivity, all of which combine into a major obstacle to successful adoption and optimal application of the benefits of HIT.

The potential major obstacle described above is the target of HITr, which serves as an error-proofing stage before implementation. It provides a realistic test drive in a minimal-pressure environment for physicians to learn the electronic H&P record that they have to use in lieu of their existing medical chart. This approach speeds physicians' mastery of the electronic H&P, which helps ensure a seamless and successful implementation. After the electronic H&P record has been successfully incorporated into patient care, the additional EHR tools that positively affect patient care, such as clinical decision support and health information exchange, may be introduced and scheduled without disruption.

Just as effective preparation and building a solid foundation yields a high dividend in time and money, HITr multiplies these yields by reducing training time and minimizing and/or eliminating loss of productivity. Beyond the time and financial yields, it also greatly reduces the pressure, stress, and uncertainty of EHR implementation for physicians and administrators.

SUMMARY

Before they commit to the purchase and implementation of an electronic record, medical practices need to be certain that their physicians and their software can work together to meet all of the practice's medical record criteria and benchmarks. Practices can achieve this objective by adding a transformation stage after the initial decision to convert to an EHR and the selection of a software system. The potentially negative consequences of not having a HITr far exceed the effort of having one, especially one that is well undertaken in terms of the overall costs in time, money, staff morale, and the quality of care.

The HITr process involves a three-pronged approach that includes the following:

■   Assessment of physicians' present documentation habits followed by training for use of an electronic system that will help them to meet quality, efficiency, and compliance standards

- Evaluation of the final version of the EHR software following agreed upon design enhancements to ensure that all practice design criteria are met

- Verification trials by trained physicians using the enhanced software to ensure that the system enables them to meet all practice benchmarks

Temporizing documentation tools can be utilized to supplement electronic H&P features that currently fall short of meeting practice criteria in an otherwise desirable EHR.

Successful completion of HITr, combined with a successful workflow transformation process for the administrative staff, should result in a positive environment for a successful EHR implementation, satisfied physicians, optimal patient care efficiency, and continuation or enhancement of practice productivity. As the importance of achieving these goals is emphasized by all practices, large and small, it is hoped that EHR vendors will be enthusiastic partners in developing enhanced designs that meet the common criteria of most practices and offer sufficient flexibility for reasonable customization requests.

References

1.   Clancy C. Keynote Address. Presented at: Connecting Communities National Conference; April 11, 2006; Washington, DC.

2.   Levinson SR. Internal E/M audits for practice benefits. In: *Practical E/M: Documentation and Coding Solutions for Quality Patient Care*. Chicago, IL: AMA Press; 2005:215-230.

3.   Health Care Financing Administration. *Documentation Guidelines for Evaluation and Management Services*. American Medical Association; 1997.

4.   American Medical Association Council on Ethical and Judicial Affairs. *Code of Ethics of the American Medical Association*, 2006-2007 Edition. Chicago, IL: American Medical Association; 2006:section 8.13 (2) (g); p. 244.

chapter 21

Assessment and Transformation for Practices Already Using EHRs

The focus of Part 4 of *Practical EHR* to this point has been on the evaluation and transformation process for practices considering the adoption of an EHR. Based on current reports of implementation failures[2] and compliance challenges for those physicians using current H&P software designs,[3,4] it becomes equally important to recognize and address the potential concerns of medical practices that have purchased and implemented, or attempted to implement, an EHR system. A HITr analysis can help these practices reassess their software programs with the goals of enhancing the effectiveness of the H&P component of the systems they are using (or that they have attempted to use) and improving the ability of their physicians to use them.

It is important for practices and physicians who are EHR pioneers to help drive the medical community's transformation efforts by constructively sharing their experiences (both positive and negative) and their expectations for quality care and high-quality documentation through the use of an effective electronic H&P, with EHR developers and the medical community at large. The benefits of this reevaluation and communication also align with the incentives of health policy advocates, who not only want to encourage EHR adoption by medical practices, but who also require high-quality, reliable data to obtain valid quality studies and achieve their goals for improving care and promoting patient safety.

Vendor Engagement and Support in Reassessment and Design Enhancement

During the analysis of an existing electronic H&P at any stage, each practice should want and need the involvement and cooperation of its EHR vendor. The practice's ability to engage the vendor to participate in this process will vary for each practice, depending on the signed contract (as considered in Chapters 17-19) and, more important, on the existing relationship between the practice and the vendor. The willingness of the vendor to be an active participant in the reassessment and possible design enhancement process underscores the importance of including clauses that specify an evolutionary approach to vendor relationships and responsibilities, plus additional clauses that require the software to fulfill the practice's H&P design criteria and performance benchmarks, as presented in Chapter 19.

Including such clauses in the contract will determine whether additional costs, *if any*, will be incurred for such assistance and the extent of those costs.

continued

To achieve this and perhaps more, all practices' attorneys should include a binding clause that requires that vendors provide reassessment and design enhancements on an *as needed basis* to ensure compliant E/M documentation and coding, after using and pending further use of the EHR system by physicians. Under these conditions, identifying potentially noncompliant design features and/or coding programs that fail to consider medical necessity—before and after implementation—should provide required leverage, if necessary, for obtaining corrective enhancements.

Under less ideal circumstances, when an existing contract lacks such protective clauses, discussion with a vendor for design enhancements to correct identified H&P problems can lead to additional costs for the practice. The contract negotiations for these improvements also provide an opportunity to introduce new contract clauses about criteria, benchmarks, and evolutionary relationships. In addition, as previously emphasized, the time and money invested in HITr is rewarded many times over through improved EHR usability, enhanced quality of care, appropriate increases in productivity, assurance of compliant documentation and coding, and increased physician satisfaction.

STATUS OF GROUPS CURRENTLY USING EHRs

The practices that have purchased EHR systems fall into three general categories, and practices in each category should experience significant benefit from performing an assessment of the current status of the usability, clinical quality features, data integrity, and compliance of their electronic H&P record. Practices that have experienced a failed implementation may benefit from taking the opportunity to reexamine the problems with their software and identify training and/or design enhancements that could result in an effective clinical system and reenergize a successful HITr effort. Practices that are experiencing significant issues or challenges using their current EHRs will similarly benefit from a formal reassessment to identify the strengths and weaknesses of their systems and rectify the sources of the problems. Finally, medical practices whose physicians are satisfied with the performance of their electronic H&P record should be pleased to confirm their levels of success, and they and their vendors should welcome the opportunity to identify improvements that could further improve performance, ensure E/M coding compliance, and stimulate the development of features that will enhance the next generation of software.

THE EHR ASSESSMENT PROCESS FOR A PRACTICE

The process and tools for performing an *EHR status assessment* of a practice using an electronic H&P system can parallel the initial approach used for overall practice transformation incorporating modifications to accomodate each practice's particular experience and needs. The leadership should formally appoint an assessment team (if not already in place), which should include representatives of the physicians and clinical staff, the coding and compliance staff, and the practice administration. This team should compile formal sets of EHR design criteria and performance benchmarks, such as those considered in Chapter 18. The team should develop these measures as if the practice were starting a new EHR project from the inception to create optimal standards that can be used to fairly measure the features of the existing software system and physicians' ability to use them successfully. The team should then proceed with an overall assessment of the critical elements of the electronic H&P record.

E/M Audits for Compliance, Promoting Quality Care, and Data Integrity

The first step in evaluating an existing electronic H&P record should be to perform representative E/M audits of the documentation created by physicians using the current software system. The results will demonstrate the ability of the software to capture and present meaningful individualized clinical documentation, in addition to an in-depth analysis of how well it meets the standards of documentation and coding. These audits should be modeled on the type of "current status" audits described in Chapter 20, which include the following features:

- Comparison of the code levels selected with the level indicated by the NPP. This step is essential to determine whether E/M code designation fulfills Medicare and insurers' standard that "medical necessity of a service is the overarching criterion for payment."[5] It will also determine whether there is a pattern of overcoding or undercoding (or both) compared with the level of care warranted by the NPP.

- Determination of whether the software promotes and physicians regularly perform comprehensive medical histories during every visit, which is a necessary step for determining an accurate assessment of the severity of the NPP

- Determination of whether all elements of E/M documentation are recorded for every encounter. This particularly refers to all elements of medical decision making (MDM), including documentation of the three levels of risk (presenting problems, diagnostic procedures, and treatment options) and complexity of data.

- Determination of whether every record documents the severity of the NPP

- Determination of whether clinical documentation is sufficient to support submitted E/M codes in every case

- Identification of whether the electronic H&P record uses any intrinsically noncompliant design features, such as documentation by exception, copy forward, copy and paste pre-existing information, and/or preloaded generic macros to describe medical history or physical examination findings

The coding and compliance staff should perform these audits and review the results with the physicians on the assessment team. They should determine whether the current medical record documentation has shortcomings in meeting all of the reviewed criteria, particularly whether the software's E/M coding functionality is compatible with criteria for medical necessity (ie, the codes selected should be at levels appropriate for the NPP). Any compliance issues should be noted.

Physicians should review clinical records to ascertain whether the documentation consistently provides a cogent representation of patient-specific and visit-specific medical history, examination findings, and decision making.

They should be able to distinguish the clinical features of each encounter, and they should be able to clearly understand each physician's medical logic for determining diagnoses, further evaluations, and treatments. Any compromises related to quality care and data integrity issues should be noted.

Software Feature Assessment for Compliance

Following the diagnostic audit, coders and physicians should together perform an analytic review of each section of the electronic H&P record from a quality and compliance perspective. This review should identify any features that, when used as designed, lack the ability to permit compliant documentation or provide tools that may create noncompliant documentation. Figure 21.1 provides a sample audit checklist that includes many of the commonly encountered design issues that can create such E/M compliance problems.

FIGURE 21.1

Audit Checklist for Electronic H&P Design Features for Compliance. HPI indicates history of present illness; MDM, medical decision making; NPP, nature of the presenting problem; PFSH, past, family, and social history; and ROS, review of systems.

Section of Medical Record	Desired Design Feature for Compliance	Present	Not Present
PFSH	Ability to document sufficient information for quality and compliance	☐	☐
	Yes and *No* check-boxes for patient completion	☐	☐
	Space to enter free-text details for "yes" responses	☐	☐
ROS	Ability to document specific questions about signs and symptoms for at least 10 organ systems	☐	☐
	Yes and *No* check-boxes for patient completion	☐	☐
	Space to enter free-text details for "yes" responses	☐	☐
HPI	Ability to document true medical history in free text	☐	☐
	Documentation prompt describing "chronological description" and listing the 8 elements of HPI	☐	☐
	Absence of documentation tools that use copy-and-paste, pick-lists, and/or pre-entered generic macros	☐	☐
Physical Exam	Templates with check-boxes based on the 1997 Documentation Guidelines	☐	☐
	Normal and *Abnormal* check-boxes for rapid documentation of areas examined	☐	☐
	Space to enter free-text details for "abnormal" findings	☐	☐
	Documentation prompt associating extent of exam with level of care appropriate for NPP	☐	☐
MDM	Separation of "management options" from "data ordered" (optional enhancement)	☐	☐
	Documentation of complexity of data	☐	☐
	Documentation of risk of presenting problems	☐	☐
	Documentation of risk of diagnostic procedures	☐	☐
	Documentation of risk of management options	☐	☐
	Documentation prompts associating levels of MDM components with NPP	☐	☐
NPP	Documentation of severity of the NPP	☐	☐
	Documentation prompt associating severity of NPP with levels of care for each type of service	☐	☐

Software Feature Assessment for Usability and Efficiency

As noted in Part 1, a critical factor in achieving usability and efficiency in EHRs are designs and structures that can facilitate patient care that are compatible with physicians' diagnostic process. Another important factor is the use of graphic interface (eg, selection lists or templates with check-boxes) and narrative interface (ie, free-text) designs in the appropriate sections of the H&P. The audit checklist in Figure 21.1 helps the assessment team evaluate how each component of the electronic H&P contributes to the diagnostic process and whether each of the designs under consideration incorporates these optimal interfaces.

Another factor that contributes to the usability and efficiency of EHRs is the ability to provide physicians with a full range of data entry tools, which include the options for documentation by writing and dictation, in addition to keyboard and mouse. For most physicians, direct computer entry of individualized narrative descriptions using a keyboard at the point of care is slower than writing or dictation. Also, many physicians and patients have negative impressions of attempts at direct entry during a visit because such efforts require placement of the keyboard and computer screen between the physician and the patient, or that they force the physician to turn away from the patient to enter data. Either option tends to disrupt eye contact and can convey the impression that the physician is, at times, paying attention to the computer rather than to the patient.

The assessment team should review the data entry options of its existing software. Unless all physicians prefer direct keyboard entry for entering free-text narrative, the team should request design enhancements that provide one or more tools for data entry by writing and one or more tools for data entry by dictation.

Physician Interviews and Possible Time Trials

The assessment team should also obtain a measure of physicians' satisfaction with the usability, flexibility, efficiency, and quality of the documentation characteristics of the electronic H&P record. The team should design a questionnaire to obtain physicians' subjective impressions of their EHR experience, such as the example shown in Figure 21.2. Time trials may also be appropriate, with a member of the assessment team shadowing some physicians at the point of care and recording observations on a "time trials" form, such as the one illustrated in Chapter 20 in Figure 20.2.

Summary Report and Assessment

Following these assessments, the assessment team should compile a detailed summary report, including the audit checklist and the physician satisfaction survey, to document all facets of the electronic H&P record. This should include its findings regarding abilities of the current system to promote quality care; achieve consistently compliant documentation and coding; facilitate data integrity; and meet goals for usability, efficiency, and productivity. The team should be particularly sensitive to detection of designs that attempt to increase the speed of documentation at the expense of compliance and quality care factors.

F I G U R E 21.2

Sample Physician Satisfaction Survey for Evaluating Data Entry. Physicians can complete this type of form to share their personal level of satisfaction with use of their electronic history and physical examination (H&P) record during patient care. The top of the questionnaire may include shading to indicate data entry modalities that are not available on the existing software; in this situation, physicians should be asked whether they would prefer to have the missing option(s) available. EHR indicates electronic health record; E/M, evaluation and management; HPI, history of present illness; MDM, medical decision making; NPP, nature of the presenting problem; PFSH, past, family, and social history; and ROS, review of systems.

Physician's Name_____

Data entry tool(s) used: ☐ Typing on keyboard   ☐ Active mouse entry

☐ Writing for graphic sections (☐ digital pen   ☐ tablet PC   ☐ paper for indirect entry)

☐ Writing for narrative sections (☐ digital pen   ☐ tablet PC   ☐ paper for indirect entry)

☐ Dictation for narrative sections (☐ voice recognition software   ☐ transcription)

Please place a check in the column that best describes your impressions of EHR software capabilities.

Usability / Flexibility / Efficiency ?	Excellent	Satisfactory	Unsatisfactory
Medical History Section			
Patient completion of PFSH survey			
Patient completion of ROS survey			
Physician completion of PFSH/ROS details			
Staff completion of PFSH & ROS update for established patients			
Physician completion of individualized HPI			
Physical Examination Section			
Check boxes to document normal findings			
Entry of "pertinent normal findings"			
Entry of detailed/specific abnormal findings			
MDM Section			
Entry of data reviewed			
Entry of differential and rule-out diagnoses			
Ability to enter descriptions of probability			
Entry of treatment options			
Documentation of complexity of data			
Documentation of risk of presenting problems			
Documentation of risk of diagnostic procedures			
Documentation of risk of treatment options			
NPP Section			
Documentation of the NPP			
General Comments			
Ability to document patient-specific data			
Ability to understand patient's condition from documentation of prior visits			
Comfort with E/M compliance features			
Comfort with data entry options			

Improvement Programs

When sample audits indicate compliance and/or quality issues with the existing software, it is likely that corrective modifications will have to include enhanced design features for the software and additional physician training to properly use the improved programs. Ideally, EHR vendors should feel an imperative to provide design enhancements that address identified compliance deficiencies because physicians have a right to expect that their software will facilitate compliant documentation and coding and not subject them to the financial risk of failing an audit.

The assessment team can also implement a physician training program, as described in Chapter 20, so that physicians can address existing compliance concerns and be well prepared to use the requested software design modifications that will promote compliant documentation and coding.

TEMPORIZING MEASURES

It is hoped that EHR vendors will respond positively to requested improvements in software design and functionality that will benefit physicians, patients, and the health care system. However, if a medical practice encounters delays or resistance from its software vendor in modifying designs to improve compliance and/or efficiency, it has the option of temporarily entering compliant supplemental written and/or dictated information into the patient records to compensate for deficits. For example, the set of sample screens or paper forms provided in Appendix F includes all the H&P components required to ensure E/M compliance. From these forms the assessment team can create a template on paper that includes E/M elements that are missing from the electronic H&P form. Most often, this new form would at least include the features commonly absent from current software: the three elements of risk, data complexity, and NPP. Physicians would complete this additional form during patient care and have this scanned into the documents section of the patient's EHR file.

Sample Assessment and Response

The following is a hypothetical example. Following thorough review of the existing electronic H&P record, the assessment team identifies the following findings that the medical practice wants to improve:

- Inability to document details of positive responses in the ROS
- Inability to enter a free-text narrative to document the history of the present illness (HPI)
- Inability to document the MDM section's three levels of risk and complexity of data
- Inability to document the NPP
- Lack of documentation prompts to guide compliant levels of care and documentation
- Lack of capability for data entry by (legible) handwriting

The practice should request that the vendor's software designers develop screens that allow the compliant documentation required and that provide additional ability to enter hand-written information. While awaiting software

---

continued

modifications to address each of these issues, the assessment team could develop paper forms that include all the missing features and use them to train and prepare the practice's physicians for enhanced records that contain these features. The paper forms can also be used during patient care as a stop-gap measure to provide the required documentation components. In addition to including appropriate check-boxes in paper templates, adding narrative sections as necessary would also provide physicians the option of recording their findings by writing and/or dictation.

This additional information should be scanned into the electronic H&P record for permanent storage. Although the scanned information would not be available for search or data mining, its presence will fulfill the need for compliant and clinically complete documentation of the H&P.

SUMMARY

Health information technology is a rapidly evolving field, responding to a changing medical environment and pressures from multiple stakeholders. Currently, physicians and information management specialists have identified usability, compliance, information integrity, and quality care challenges inherent in some of the established electronic H&P designs. Medical practices presently using an EHR should establish a system of continuous reevaluation, while also working with their software vendors to ensure that their software designs meet their patient care goals, are compliant with *Current Procedural Terminology* (*CPT®*) standards for documentation and levels of care, and keep pace with the evolution of information technology. Similarly, EHR vendors should welcome guidance from their existing users to identify shortcomings and help refine their designs and improve them in future versions of their software.

Practices can establish an assessment team of physicians, coding and compliance staff, and administrators to perform audits of their current records; perform a critical analysis of software design and functionality; and survey their physicians' level of satisfaction with the usability, efficiency, and effectiveness of their electronic H&P record. If these assessments reveal significant problems, the team should analyze whether correcting the documentation problems requires further physician training, software design modifications, or a combination of both. These improvements can proceed according to the same HITr protocols similar to those presented for practices preparing for a new EHR system.

Creating a model for EHR reassessment and software design evolution should result in ongoing benefits for patient care that leads to improved reliability of clinical documentation and make a positive contribution toward the overall health system goals of increasing quality and patient safety.

References

1. Baertlein L. U.S. health info technology lags. Reuters, Washingtonpost.com, July 26, 2007. http://www.washingtonpost.com/wp-dyn/content/article/2007/07/26/AR2007072601510.html. Accessed July 30, 2007.

2. McClellan M. McClellan M. CMS Quality, Efficiency and Value-Based Purchasing Policies: The Role of Health Information Technology. Presented at: the Second Health Information Technology Summit; September 9, 2005; Washington, DC.

3. Vogenitz W. EMR and E/M: beware of software's potential to upcode. Part B News. May 1, 2006. http://www.eclinicalworks.com/2006-05-01-pr2.php. Accessed July 30, 2007.

4. Gustin G. What you don't know about electronic health record clinical progress notes and paper templates could be creating compliance risk, I: the compliance department needs to be involved in the selection and implementation process. J Health Care Compliance. January–February 2006:57-59.

5. Centers for Medicare & Medicaid Services. Selection of level of evaluation and management service. In: *Medicare Claims Processing Manual.* Chapter 12: section 30.6.1. http://new.cms.hhs.gov/manuals/downloads/clm104c12.pdf. Accessed July 30, 2007.

chapter 22

Conclusion: The Role of *Practical EHR* in Health Information Technology

"If you have built castles in the air, your work need not be lost; that is where they should be. Now put the foundations under them."[1]

Henry David Thoreau, *Walden*

Practical EHR has evolved in response to two fundamental observations:

- There is an unacceptably high rate of unsatisfactory EHR adoptions as a result of failed/unsuccessful implementation or physician dissatisfaction with their systems.

- Current electronic H&P designs do not adequately fulfill physicians' optimum requirements for a highly functional and comprehensively documented H&P record.

These problems are sufficiently pervasive to have created a barrier to successful integration of EHRs in many practices and a significant deterrent to purchase for others. These problems have, in essence, contributed to the "electronic chasm," a gulf that must be closed before all medical practices can have usable and effective EHR systems, allowing them to subsequently realize the other benefits of HIT, such as achieving the free flow of medical information and facilitating the development of tools and protocols to help ongoing improvement in patient safety and health care quality.

Until now, the energies of information technology experts and policy analysts have focused primarily on the patient care benefits to be gained by leveraging, correlating, and exchanging the clinical information that has previously been recorded in EHRs, without critical assessment of the quality, integrity, and/or reliability of that information or how it is recorded. In other words, far less attention has been directed to the design and functionality of the electronic H&P, despite the fact that this is the essential EHR component for capturing meaningful data and helping physicians provide quality care. In addition, on careful questioning, many physicians and practice administrators can identify problems with the electronic H&P as a primary cause of their current EHR challenges.

As emphasized throughout *Practical EHR*, the electronic H&P is the foundation physicians rely on during patient care, not only for recalling stored data and clinical descriptions and capturing meaningful new clinical information, but also for providing a roadmap that guides the quality care diagnostic process.

Practical EHR provides information to help physicians identify and understand the issues underlying effective design and functionality of the electronic H&P. It includes a variety of tools for distinguishing software designs that fulfill physicians' requirements from those that have the potential to interfere with or disrupt them. In addition, *Practical EHR*'s solutions for effective preparation, investigation, software modification, training, and verification provide physicians and their administrators with the knowledge and tools to succeed with the practice transformation process.

Finally, *Practical EHR* principles also provide a foundation to help physicians and EHR companies to work together to engineer solutions that can overcome current barriers and to create systems and processes that can fulfill the visions of increasing efficiency and quality that HIT can deliver to our health care system.*

Reference

1.   Thoreau HD. *Walden.* Boston, MA: Tickner and Fields; 1854.

---

*Appendix I summarizes the salient principles discussed throughout this book for creating effective electronic H&P designs and planning successful practice transformation.

Calculating Costs of Paper-Based Medical Records

Before evaluating the economic costs and benefits of investing in an electronic health record (EHR) system, it is helpful for medical practices to assess their starting point—the cost of using existing paper records. This assessment starts with identifying and compiling all factors contributing to the total cost. The accompanying forms provide a practical starting point for collecting these data and organizing them into a final figure that considers the cost per physician per month. This is a highly useful result because it can be compared with the projected costs per physician per month for purchase and upkeep of an EHR system. It is also very easy to multiply this result by the number of physicians in a practice to obtain the practice's total monthly cost.

The factors considered in this evaluation are as follows:

■ Labor cost for "chart pulls" (finding medical records and refiling them after use). This factor includes not only chart pulls during patient visits, but also chart pulls for filing laboratory and radiology reports, filing correspondence, answering patient phone calls, use during testing, etc.
■ Chart material costs
■ Filing and storage space costs
■ Transcription costs (may be added into this calculation or kept as a separate entity)

Figure A.1 illustrates a "chart-pull time sheet" that can be duplicated for individual staff members to document the time spent during each episode of pulling, filing, and searching for charts. Accurately tracking this information for 1 work week should provide a reasonable approximation of the amount of staff time invested in maintaining the existing paper record.

Figure A.2 can be used for a practice to compile all the data, beginning with the total time spent by the staff per week as recorded in the chart-pull time sheets. The remaining figures should be readily available from the practice manager. Following the instructions for the mathematical sequence allows calculation of a reasonable estimate of monthly costs for maintaining the practice's existing paper record system.

F I G U R E A.1

Chart-Pull Time Sheet

<u>**Chart-Pull Time Sheet**</u>   **Name:** _____   **Date** ____ / ____ / ____

Date	No. Physicians Present	Time Spent	Task (Optional)

Total Time Spent: _____ hours   Hours per Physician: _____

Directions: Record the time spent pulling charts for appointments; filing reports; answering phone calls from patients, physicians, or other health care providers; searching for charts; refiling charts; and any other activity related to pulling and refiling charts.

Cost of Paper Medical Records

Step I: Cost of chart pulls per month

    a)   Time per week for *all* chart pulls, including visits,

        phone calls, correspondence, testing, etc.   _____ hours

    b)   Multiply by 4 (to extrapolate to hours/month)   _____ hours

    c)   Multiply by average office staff salary

            {$_____ per hour}   = $_____

    d)   Multiply by 1.25 (to account for benefits)   = $_____

    e)   Divide by number of physicians {n = ____}

    Cost of chart pulls per physician per month: $_____

Step II: Cost of materials for new charts per month

    a)   Cost of each folder $_____

    b)   Cost of blank labels per folder $_____

    c)   Cost of date and letter labels per folder $_____

    d)   Add a + b + c for total cost per folder: $_____

    e)   Multiply "d" times number of new patients

            + consults per month {n = ____} for cost/month $_____

    f)   Divide by number of physicians {n = ____}

    Cost of chart materials per physician per month: $_____

Step III: Cost of space for active charts

            {chart storage = _____% of total space}

    a)   Monthly rental for office space for charts $_____

    b)   Monthly cost of real estate taxes for charts $_____

    c)   Add a + b for real estate monthly cost for charts: $_____

    d)   Divide by number of physicians   {n = ____}

    Cost of chart space per physician per/ month: $_____

Step IV (optional): Cost of transcription

    a)   Monthly transcription expenses (total) $_____

    b)   Divide by number of physicians   {n = ____}

    Cost of transcription per physician per month: $_____

Total cost per physician per month (add totals from steps I, II, III, and IV) $_____

Calculating Medical Practice Overhead Costs

Powerful insights are available to physicians and practice managers through the determination of hourly overhead costs and comparing these costs with the hourly overhead reimbursements provided by Medicare and private insurers through the resource-based relative value system (RBRVS) system. The RBRVS provides calculations for three components of each service identified in the *Current Procedural Terminology* (*CPT®*) manual:

- Physician work
- Practice expense
- Professional liability insurance

In theory, the physician work component should reimburse physicians for the time required to perform the service, technical skill and physical effort, mental effort and judgment, and psychological stress associated with the physician's concern about iatrogenic risk to patients.[1] The other two components address the costs physicians incur in providing these services. The relative value units (RVUs) assigned to each of the three components are added to calculate the total RVUs for a service. Medicare uses these values to determine reimbursements. It multiplies a service's total RVUs by a national Centers for Medicare & Medicaid Services conversion factor (and a geographic adjustment) to determine payment for each CPT-coded service. Most private insurers also use this system, commonly using a percentage of the Medicare conversion factor; in some cases, this percentage is greater than 100% and in some, it is less.

In theory, the RBRVS implies that its payment for overhead expenses and liability insurance expenses should be sufficient to compensate physicians for their true costs. In reality, there is usually a significant disparity between reimbursement for these two categories of expenses and practices' actual expenses. Practice management consultants use a variety of approaches, many based on RVUs to compare reimbursements with true costs. The three forms in this appendix present a practical approach to achieve this result in easily understood terms, with the final results presented in dollars and time rather than in RVUs.

Calculation 1 determines a straightforward total hourly overhead cost per physician. This initial expense assessment results from subtracting total physician benefits from the practice's total annual income to derive total annual overhead. It then divides this total by the number of physicians and the approximate hours worked per physician per year to calculate the hourly overhead cost per physician.

Calculation 2 adds an additional level of sophistication, focusing solely on income and expenses related to direct clinician care (including

Calculation 1: Overhead Cost per Hour per Physician

Step 1.1: List total practice income per year $_____

Step 1.2: List total physician income and benefits

        a) Total salaries $_____

        b) Retirement fund contributions $_____

        c) Vehicles $_____

        d) Insurance (eg, health, auto) $_____

        e) Conference expenses $_____

        f) Promotion and entertainment $_____

        g) Other physician expenses $_____

                Total $_____

Step 1.3: Calculate total annual practice expenses

        Subtract total for 1.2 from total for 1.1 $_____

Step 1.4: Calculate annual practice expense per physician

        Divide 1.3 by number of physicians {n = ____} $_____

Step 1.5: Calculate expense per physician per hour

        Divide 1.4 by annual hours worked per physician $_____

        (40 hours per week for 48 weeks = 1,920)

physicians, physicians' assistants, and nurse practitioners) that is reimbursed under the RBRVS system. It subtracts all income and expenses attributed to services and/or goods that are not directly the result of one-on-one patient care by clinicians. These supplemental income resources, which are found in many medical practices owing to the medical payment constrictions inherent in the current reimbursement system, include the following:

■ Medical services provided by ancillary personnel (eg, nurses, medical assistants, and technologists), such as laboratory testing, radiology studies, physiologic testing, physical therapy, and allergy treatments

■ Medical services not reimbursed under the RBRVS system, such as aesthetic procedures, vision corrective surgery, hair replacement procedures, and hair removal procedures

■ Sale of goods not reimbursed under the RBRVS system, such as eyeglasses, hearing aids, skin treatments, and medications

This calculation allows practices to remove consideration of all income and expenses related to nonclinician care, thereby identifying a more realistic cost per hour for the provision of actual medical services. This calculation provides another important and often insightful calculation. Step 2.2 compares the *net* income the practice receives from nonphysician services with the total amount of physician income and benefits. The difference between these two

Calculation 2: Overhead Cost per Hour, Medical Care Only
Refinement: subtracting nonphysician-related income and expenses

---

Step 2.1: Gross <u>medical-based</u> income for practice

      a) List total practice income per year (from step 1.1) $_____

      b) List gross income from ancillary (nonphysician) $_____
         sources (eg, audiometry, laboratory, X-ray, EKG,
         allergy tests and shots)

      c) Total: Subtract (b) from (a) $_____

Step 2.2: <u>Medical-based</u> total physician income and benefits

      a) List total physician income and benefits per year $_____
         (from step 1.2)

      b) List net income from ancillary (nonphysician) $_____
         sources (ancillary income less ancillary expenses)

      c) Total: Subtract (b) from (a) $_____

Step 2.3: Calculate <u>medical-based</u> annual practice expenses

      a) Net medical-based income (subtract 2.2c from 2.1c) $_____

      b) List expenses for ancillary (nonphysician) services $_____

      c) Total: Subtract (b) from (a) $_____

Step 2.4: Calculate annual <u>medical-based</u> practice expense per physician

      Divide 2.3c by number of physicians {n = _____} $_____

Step 2.5: Calculate <u>medical-based</u> expense per physician per hour

      Divide 2.4 by annual hours worked per physician $_____

      (40 hours per week for 48 weeks = 1,920 hours) {hours = _____}

---

values shows how much net income clinicians produce from direct patient care. In cases in which the profit from ancillary services equals or exceeds physicians' total income and benefits, the practice is actually losing money on the provision of patient care. In addition, when the result in 2.2c is a negative number, it demonstrates that profits from the ancillary services are subsidizing the medical care expenses. Substituting this number with zero allows the calculation of the actual medical practice expense and contributes to a true picture of practice costs.

Calculation 3 takes advantage of the fact that RVUs for evaluation and management (E/M) services incorporate a value for the amount of time that physicians "typically" spend for each type and level of service. For example, the *CPT* manual advises that the typical face-to-face physician time for code 99205 is 60 minutes, for code 99203 is 30 minutes, and for code 99213 is 15 minutes. The *CPT* manual provides these time values as "guidelines," and they are weighed in setting the RVU values for each of these codes. Calculation 3 applies these time values to reasonably convert payments for these services into the hourly reimbursement rate by Medicare for practice expenses and liability insurance

Calculation 3: Time Reimbursed for E/M Services
Comparing True Overhead Costs With Reimbursement for Overhead

---

Step 3.1: List <u>medical-based</u> expense per physician $_____
         per hour

         (from step 2.5)

Step 3.2: Medicare and insurer reimbursement for overhead expense

         a) RVUs per hour for {practice expense {PE} +
            liability insurance {LI}}   _____

            i)   PE RVU + LI RVU for 99213 $\times$ 4, or

            ii)   PE RVU + IE RVU for 99203 $\times$ 2

         b) Conversion factor for payment by Medicare $_____
            (or selected insurer)

         c) Overhead reimbursed per physician per hour $_____
            (multiply a $\times$ b)

Step 3.3: Percentage of overhead reimbursed   _____%
         for E/M care

         Divide 3.2c by 3.1

Step 3.4: Time per visit covered by Medicare (or insurer)
         reimbursement

         a) 99205 = 60 minutes $\times$ (% from 3.3)   _____ minutes

         b) 99204 = 45 minutes $\times$ (% from 3.3)   _____ minutes

         c) 99203 = 30 minutes $\times$ (% from 3.3)   _____ minutes

         d) 99214 = 25 minutes $\times$ (% from 3.3)   _____ minutes

         e) 99213 = 15 minutes $\times$ (% from 3.3)   _____ minutes

         f) 99244 = 60 minutes $\times$ (% from 3.3)   _____ minutes

         g) 99243 = 40 minutes $\times$ (% from 3.3)   _____ minutes

---

expenses. It then compares this hourly reimbursement with the actual practice overhead expense calculated in calculation 2, demonstrating the amount of time actually reimbursed by Medicare (or other insurers) for various E/M services. Practices can extend these calculations to other E/M services by accessing their typical times listed in the *CPT* manual. It is also helpful to realize that because the RBRVS system carefully equates the values for procedure services on the same scale as E/M cognitive services, this hourly reimbursement rate calculated for E/M is valid for procedure services as well.

References

1.   American Medical Association. *Medicare RBRVS 2007: The Physician's Guide.* Chicago, IL: American Medical Association; 2004:25.

TABLE OF RISK*

Level of Risk	Presenting Problem(s)	Diagnostic Procedure(s) Ordered	Management Options Selected
Minimal	• One self-limited or minor problem, eg, cold, insect bite, tinea corporis	• Laboratory tests requiring venipuncture • Chest x-rays • EKG/EEG • Urinalysis • Ultrasound, eg, echocardiography • KOH prep	• Rest • Gargles • Elastic bandages • Superficial dressings
Low	• Two or more self-limited or minor problems • One stable chronic illness, eg, well controlled hypertension, non-insulin dependent diabetes, cataract, BPH • Acute uncomplicated illness or injury, eg, cystitis, allergic rhinitis, simple sprain	• Physiologic tests not under stress, eg, pulmonary function tests • Non-cardiovascular imaging studies with contrast, eg, barium enema • Superficial needle biopsies • Clinical laboratory tests requiring arterial puncture • Skin biopsies	• Over-the-counter drugs • Minor surgery with no identified risk factors • Physical therapy • Occupational therapy • IV fluids without additives
Moderate	• One or more chronic illnesses with mild exacerbation, progression, or side effects of treatment • Two or more stable chronic illnesses • Undiagnosed new problem with uncertain prognosis, eg, lump in breast • Acute illness with systemic symptoms, eg, pyelonephritis, pneumonitis, colitis • Acute complicated injury, eg, head injury with brief loss of consciousness	• Physiologic tests under stress, eg, cardiac stress test, fetal contraction stress test • Diagnostic endoscopies with no identified risk factors • Deep needle or incisional biopsy • Cardiovascular imaging studies with contrast and no identified risk factors, eg, arteriogram, cardiac catheterization • Obtain fluid from body cavity, eg, lumbar puncture, thoracentesis, culdocentesis	• Minor surgery with identified risk factors • Elective major surgery (open, percutaneous or endoscopic) with no identified risk factors • Prescription drug management • Therapeutic nuclear medicine • IV fluids with additives • Closed treatment of fracture or dislocation without manipulation
High	• One or more chronic illnesses with severe exacerbation, progression, or side effects of treatment • Acute or chronic illnesses or injuries that pose a threat to life or bodily function, eg, multiple trauma, acute MI, pulmonary embolus, severe respiratory distress, progressive severe rheumatoid arthritis, psychiatric illness with potential threat to self or others, peritonitis, acute renal failure • An abrupt change in neurologic status, eg, seizure, TIA, weakness, sensory loss	• Cardiovascular imaging studies with contrast with identified risk factors • Cardiac electrophysiological tests • Diagnostic endoscopies with identified risk factors • Discography	• Elective major surgery (open, percutaneous or endoscopic) with identified risk factors • Emergency major surgery (open, percutaneous or endoscopic) • Parenteral controlled substances • Drug therapy requiring intensive monitoring for toxicity • Decision not to resuscitate or to de-escalate care because of poor prognosis

* From Health Care Financing Administration. *Documentation Guidelines for Evaluation and Management Services.* American Medical Association; 1997:31. BPH indicates benign prostatic hypertrophy; EEG, electroencephalogram; EKG, electrocardiogram; KOH, potassium hydroxide; IV, intravenous; MI, myocardial infarction and TIA, transient ischemic attack.

Relating NPP and E/M Levels of Care Compliance

Some electronic health records (EHRs) include software functionality for determining the level of evaluation and management (E/M) care documented during the patient encounter. In most current systems, this calculation is based solely on the medical history, examination, and decision making (ie, the three key components), without consideration of medical necessity. In contrast, the E/M descriptors incorporate medical necessity as the nature of the presenting problem (NPP), which is included in determining the appropriate levels of care for every type of service that also includes the three key components. Physicians' criteria for E/M documentation and coding compliance must include confirmation that the software takes into consideration the NPP. In addition, coders should confirm the compliance features of such software by ensuring that the levels of care warranted are compliant with *Current Procedural Terminology* (*CPT®*) descriptors. The following table lists, by type of service, the *maximum* level of care that the *CPT* manual indicates is medically appropriate for each level of severity of the NPP.

Type of Service	Severity of NPP	Maximum Indicated Level of Care
99201-99205	Self-limited or minor	1
outpatient initial visit	Low	1
	Low to moderate	2
	Moderate	3
	Moderate to high	4 or 5
	High	5

(*Continued*)

Type of Service	Severity of NPP	Maximum Indicated Level of Care
99211-99215	Minimal	1
outpatient established visit	Self-limited or minor	2
	Low	2
	Low to moderate	3
	Moderate	3
	Moderate to high	4 or 5
	High	5
99241-99245; outpatient consultation	Self-limited or minor	1
99251-99255; inpatient consultation	Low	2
	Low to moderate	2
	Moderate	3
	Moderate to high	4 or 5
	High	5
99218-99220	Low	99218
hospital observation	Low to moderate	99218
	Moderate	99219
	Moderate to high	99219
	High	99220
99221-99223; initial hospital care	Low*	1
	Low to moderate*	1
*Note: it is considered unlikely that a patient with "low" or "low to moderate" NPP would, in fact, warrant hospital admission	Moderate	2
	Moderate to high	2
	High	3
99231-99233; subsequent hospital care	Stable, recovering, or improving	1
(It is noteworthy that the NPP for this type of service uses atypical descriptors)	Responding inadequately or has minor complication	2
	Unstable, significant complication, or significant new problem	3

(*Continued*)

Type of Service	Severity of NPP	Maximum Indicated Level of Care
99281-99285	Self-limited or minor	1
emergency department services	Low	1
	Low to moderate	2
	Moderate	3
	Moderate to high	3
	High (no immediate threat)	4
	High (and immediate threat to life or physiologic function)	5
99304-99306	Low	99304
initial nursing facility care	Low to moderate	99304
	Moderate	99305
	Moderate to high	99305
	High	99306
99307-99310	Stable, recovering, or improving	99307
subsequent nursing facility care	Responding inadequately or has minor complication	99308
	Significant complication or a significant new problem	99309
	Unstable or significant new problem requiring immediate physician attention	99310
99324-99328	Low	99324
new patient, domiciliary, rest home,	Low to moderate	99324
or custodial care services	Moderate	99325
	Moderate to high	99326
	High	99327
	Unstable or significant new problem requiring immediate physician attention	99328

(*Continued*)

Type of Service	Severity of NPP	Maximum Indicated Level of Care
99334-99337	Self-limited or minor	99334
established patient, domiciliary,	Low	99334
rest home, or custodial care services	Low to moderate	99335
	Moderate	99335
	Moderate to high	99336 or 99337
	High	99337

Importance of Adhering to E/M Compliance With Electronic H&P

As discussed throughout this book, an effective electronic history and physical examination (H&P) record is a requirement for evaluation and management (E/M) compliance, productivity, confirming the extent of care performed if a physician is under review for potential professional liability, and, most important, assisting physicians in providing quality patient care.

Regardless of whether a physician is using a paper or electronic medical record, there is a potential for the design and functionality of the record to cause problems with the information documented (or not documented) by the physician. These problems can occur when the medical record lacks one or more features needed for optimal documentation or when a physician fails to correctly use the features that are available.

An "intelligent" medical record design should include all features essential to help physicians achieve maximal quality, efficiency, and compliance. To accomplish these goals, each physician must also use these tools correctly. The purpose of this Appendix is to examine the consequences of improper design and/or use, so that software designers can incorporate salient H&P record design features that facilitate compliance and optimal care and provide error-proofing designs that protect physicians against improper use of the electronic H&P record.

Table E.1 examines the possible ways that improper design or use of the H&P record could lead to less than ideal results for compliance, quality care, and medical liability protection. It is included to emphasize the importance of proper design and, most important, that physicians must understand the principles of E/M compliance and its relationship to quality care, regardless of how many benefits and protections are designed into an intelligent electronic H&P record.

Consequences of Improper Design and/or Use

Section of Medical Record	Category of Improper Design or Use	Issues and Possible Worst-Case Scenario
PFSH and ROS (1), initial visit	**Functionality:** Physician required to ask questions and document patient responses into EHR	a) **Efficiency:** Significant time expense compared with option of patient completing preprinted form
PFSH and ROS (2), initial visit	**Design:** Software lacks ability for physician to sign (or initial) to confirm review of all information in these sections (eg, information could have been entered by another member of the staff) **Functionality:** Software fails to require physician to add signature	a) **Compliance:** Audit of initial visit record concludes lack of documentation of PFSH and/or ROS; no credit given for PFSH/ROS (not documented, not done); causes downcode to level 2 or 1 b) **Compliance:** Audits showing repeated downcoding for lack of documentation of review of PFSH/ROS could lead to investigation for fraud, with severe financial penalties
PFSH and ROS (3), initial visit	**Design:** Software lacks ability for physician to document free-text details about positive responses **Functionality:** Software fails to require physician to document free-text details for each positive response	a) **Quality of care:** Physician fails to document and/or consider detailed information critical to patient care, eg, 1) Need to clarify details of positive personal history of cancer, diabetes, cardiovascular disease, or seizures 2) Need to clarify details of positive history of smoking, drinking, or drug use 3) Need to clarify details of positive family history of cancer, cardiovascular disease, or neurologic disorders 4) Need to clarify details of positive signs and symptoms in ROS; responses such as "chest pain," "headache," and "shortness of breath" need to be treated as a "mini" HPI b) **Medical liability:** Litigation owing to not finding and addressing medical issues such as those listed
PFSH and ROS (4), established patient visit	**Design:** Software copies and pastes identical medical history information from the patient's initial visit into record for subsequent visits **Functionality:** This process is automated. Although it permits physicians to modify the data entered automatically, doing this correctly would require physicians to review all positive and negative elements of the initial questionnaire.	a) **Compliance:** Although this automated process is fast, it creates cloned documentation. The software does not require the physician to review and update each item on the template, and physicians generally do not take the time to do so b) **Quality of care (and compliance):** The PFSH and ROS should report the patient's actual health status on the date of the visit, not the status from weeks or months ago. c) **Medical liability:** Litigation owing to failing to find significant new symptoms, because the record permitted "copy and paste" of old information instead of guiding the physician to obtain information about the patient's current health status
PFSH and ROS (5), established patient visit	**Design:** Software lacks ability for physician to document (including free-text) an update	a) **Efficiency and usability:** Physicians and patients object to repeating entire inventory of questions at every subsequent visit.

(Continued)

Section of Medical Record	Category of Improper Design or Use	Issues and Possible Worst-Case Scenario
	of PFSH and ROS since date of last visit (which should also be documented)	b) **Compliance:** Audit of established visit record concludes lack of documentation of PFSH and ROS; results in problem-focused history c) **Quality of care:** Physician fails to document and/or consider detailed recent information critical to patient care, such as examples in PFSH and ROS (3); results in problem-focused care d) **Medical liability:** Litigation owing to not identifying and addressing health issues such as those listed
HPI (1)	**Design:** a) Fails to provide for a narrative (free-text) entry, or b) Offers additional options along with narrative (eg, pick-lists, graphic section listing eight elements of HPI, or preloaded "macros")	a) **Efficiency:** Free-text narrative is more efficient than other options for entering a high-quality individualized medical history b) **Compliance:** Absence of narrative HPI precludes physicians from being able to document a chronological description of course of illness, which in an audit results in determination of a "brief" HPI (maximum level 2 initial visit or level 3 established visit) or determination that physician did not obtain a true HPI (potentially eliminating E/M service entirely on an initial visit) c) **Quality of care:** Quality narrative medical history is most effective diagnostic tool in the medical armamentarium. Failure of physicians to use this tool decreases probability of accurate diagnoses and increases reliance on costly laboratory and radiographic tests to make a diagnosis, rather than confirm one. d) **Medical liability:** Litigation owing to "failure to diagnose," based on inadequate medical history
HPI (2)	**Functionality:** Failure to provide documentation prompts indicating need for chronological description, providing a list of the eight elements of HPI, and guiding extent of information required for an "extended" HPI	a) **Compliance:** Use of a brief HPI supports maximum level of care at level 2 for initial visit, level 3 for established visit b) **Quality of care:** Use of a brief HPI limits physician's ability to obtain full insight into patient's illness and identify correct diagnoses
Physical examination (1)	**Design:** Software programmed to automatically insert normal comprehensive level examination for every visit **Functionality:** Physician instructed to "document by exception," entering abnormal findings to replace the pre-entered normal findings and theoretically deleting areas not examined	a) **Efficiency:** Documenting numerous abnormal findings by exception requires more time than dictating or writing the abnormal examination findings. b) **Efficiency:** When a physician performs less than a comprehensive examination, it requires more time to delete the portions not performed than it would to check off "normal" or "abnormal" boxes on a graphic interface. c) **Compliance:** Physicians rarely take the time to delete, from the pre-entered

(Continued)

Section of Medical Record	Category of Improper Design or Use	Issues and Possible Worst-Case Scenario
		documentation, the portions of the examination not performed. Therefore, nearly every visit documents a comprehensive examination and counts this level of care toward a high-level E/M code, without consideration of the lack of medical necessity for performing a comprehensive examination. d) **Medical liability:** Litigation owing to misleading documentation of normal examination findings for a body area not examined; could result in liability for "failure to diagnose" if the patient had an abnormality of the nonexamined area
Physical examination (2)	**Design:** Failure to provide a graphic interface for compliant documentation of all areas examined and whether findings are normal or abnormal	a) **Efficiency:** Graphic interface, based on 1997 Documentation Guidelines,* required to permit rapid documentation of examination elements b) **Compliance:** Documentation Guidelines require examination and documentation of "specific abnormal and relevant negative findings . . . of affected or symptomatic body area(s) or organ system(s)"
Physical examination (3)	**Design:** Failure of graphic interface to include a brief explanation of "normal" designation for each element of the examination	a) **Efficiency:** Failure of graphic interface to include description of normal findings requires additional time for physician to add such a description to the narrative (free-text) area during each encounter b) **Compliance:** Commonly, physicians fail to document normal findings in narrative section. Failure to describe normal findings does not fulfill Documentation Guidelines criteria.
Physical examination (4)	**Design:** Failure to provide a narrative interface for detailed and individualized documentation of all significant abnormal findings in affected and in asymptomatic body areas	a) **Efficiency:** Free-text narrative is more efficient than other options for describing individualized examination findings. b) **Compliance:** Documentation Guidelines require documentation of specific abnormal and relevant negative findings of affected areas. c) **Quality of care:** Lack of detailed description of abnormal examination findings can result in difficulty monitoring a patient's clinical progress, particularly assessing the extent to which problems are resolving or getting worse. d) **Medical liability:** Lack of individualized and detailed examination documentation reduces ability to defend medical decisions made and/or justify reasons for not making other decisions.

(Continued)

Section of Medical Record	Category of Improper Design or Use	Issues and Possible Worst-Case Scenario
Physical examination (5)	**Functionality:** Failure to provide documentation prompts that indicate levels of care appropriate for severity of NPP	a) **Compliance:** Lack of guidance fails to facilitate provision of appropriate level of examination. Level of examination lower that appropriate for the NPP (and/or for code submitted) can result in under coding by physician and/or downcoding in an audit. b) **Quality of care:** Lack of guidance can result in lower amount of care provided than warranted by the standard of care (as cited in the *CPT*® manual†).
MDM (1), diagnoses	**Design:** Use of pick lists (graphic interface; usually providing only ICD-9 codes and explanations) from which physician selects one or more diagnoses; systems that combine EHR and practice management software may also link selected diagnoses directly to charge entry	a) **Compliance:** Fails to provide a means of fulfilling Documentation Guidelines requirements for appropriate "number" of diagnoses, including inability to document differential diagnoses or "possible," "probable," or "rule out" diagnosis. This restriction becomes a requirement when numeric codes are automatically forwarded to practice management software for direct billing because claims submission guidelines prohibit use of rule out and possible diagnoses. b) **Compliance:** Documentation of only one diagnosis (when system incapable of documenting rule out diagnoses) commonly results in straightforward MDM, resulting in downcode to level 2 for initial visit; may result in downcode to level 2 for established visit c) **Compliance:** Use of a graphic interface without narrative capability eliminates ability to document, with an established diagnosis, the progress or lack of progress in problem resolution (as required by the Documentation Guidelines) d) **Quality of care:** Absence of narrative interface capability prevents physicians from including adjectives that indicate severity and/or probability of various diagnosis, information that is extremely helpful during subsequent visits and to other physicians who participate in the care of a patient e) **Medical liability:** Failure to include rule out diagnoses and adjectives that indicate severity and/or probability of various diagnoses may significantly compromise ability to present physician's consideration of all possible causes of a patient's illness.
MDM (2), diagnoses	**Functionality:** Failure to provide documentation prompts that indicate number of the diagnoses (or treatment options) appropriate for severity of the NPP	a) **Compliance:** Without guidance based on severity of the NPP, physicians commonly document only one "most probable" diagnosis. If matched with one "most appropriate" treatment option, this practice most

(Continued)

Section of Medical Record	Category of Improper Design or Use	Issues and Possible Worst-Case Scenario
		commonly results in a straightforward MDM and a downcode to level 2 for an initial visit; may result in downcode to level 2 for established visit b) **Compliance:** Audits that result in repeated downcoding because of documentation of only straightforward MDM could lead to investigation for fraud, with severe financial penalties c) **Quality of care:** Documentation of only one diagnosis may reflect active consideration of only one possible disease process at a time (rather than evaluation of several likely diagnoses), which could delay identifying correct diagnosis
MDM (3), plans	**Design:** Having one section that includes both data ordered and management options	a) **Compliance:** The *CPT* manual and Documentation Guidelines assign data ordered and management options as distinct and separate elements of MDM. Listing these separate elements together disrupts ability of physicians and/or integrated coding software to determine the correct level of complexity of MDM.
MDM (4), management options	**Design:** Use of pick-lists (graphic interface) from which physician selects one or more management options. Approach can be useful as a supplement to free-text, but not as a replacement	**Issues of pick-lists providing sole option for documenting treatment options:** a) **Efficiency:** Finding and selecting multiple treatment items from one or more pick-lists is commonly less efficient than free-text entry by writing, dictating, or typing. b) **Compliance:** Graphic interface fails to provide a means of fulfilling Documentation Guidelines requirements for appropriate "number" of management *options*, including inability to label (and, therefore, document) alternative treatments considered and not implemented and/or possible future treatments. c) **Quality of care:** List of management options may not include all potential treatments, particularly those related to environmental or dietary management. d) **Quality of care:** Physician tends to select solely from the preset list. *The list will often drive the care, rather than the care driving what is documented.* e) **Quality of care:** Use of a graphic interface without narrative capability eliminates ability to document a blueprint for future treatments that

(Continued)

Section of Medical Record	Category of Improper Design or Use	Issues and Possible Worst-Case Scenario
		may be appropriate based on results of pending tests and/or problems with initial treatment choice(s). f) **Medical liability:** Documentation of only the treatment option(s) actually ordered could significantly reduce ability to defend a claim based on lack of informed consent (which legally requires physicians to discuss all treatment options with the patient).
MDM (5), management options	**Functionality:** Failure to provide documentation prompts that indicate number of treatment options (or diagnoses) appropriate for severity of the NPP	a) **Compliance:** Without guidance based on severity of the NPP, physicians commonly document only one most appropriate treatment option. If matched with one most probable diagnosis, this most commonly results in a straightforward MDM and a downcode to level 2 for an initial visit; may result in downcode to level 2 for established visit b) **Compliance:** Audits that result in repeated downcoding because of documentation of straightforward MDM could lead to investigation for fraud, with severe financial penalties.
MDM (6), complexity of data to be reviewed	**Design:** Failure to provide interface for documentation of the *complexity* of data reviewed or ordered	a) **Compliance:** Failure to document the complexity of data leaves the interpretation of complexity to the discretion of a reviewer, which, in some cases, could result in inappropriate downcoding.
MDM (7), risks	**Design:** Failure to provide interface for documentation of the three types of risk described in the *CPT* manual and Documentation Guidelines	a) **Compliance:** Failure to document the elements of risk leaves the interpretation of the risk of the patient's illnesses, diagnostic evaluations, and treatments to the discretion of a reviewer, which, in some cases, could result in inappropriate downcoding. Under strict interpretation, an auditor could conclude that the lack of documentation of risks is equivalent to physician not considering the risks; this could lead to more stringent downcoding. b) **Compliance:** Audits that result in repeated downcoding because of documentation of a straightforward MDM could lead to investigation for fraud, with severe financial penalties.
NPP	**Design:** Failure to provide interface for documentation of the NPP	a) **Compliance:** Failure to document the NPP leaves the interpretation of the severity of the patient's illnesses (and, therefore, assessment of medical necessity) to the discretion of a reviewer, which, in some cases, could result in inappropriate downcoding. b) **Compliance:** Audits that result in repeated downcoding because of lack of medical necessity to support levels of care submitted could lead to investigation for fraud, with severe financial penalties.

(Continued)

Section of Medical Record	Category of Improper Design or Use	Issues and Possible Worst-Case Scenario
NPP (2)	**Functionality:** Failure to provide documentation prompts that indicate correlation among severity of illness, appropriate levels of care and documentation, and appropriate E/M code levels	a) **Compliance:** For CMS, the main criterion for payment is medical necessity. The clinical examples (which illustrate the NPP as the indicator for medical necessity) in the *CPT* manual assist in selecting correct codes. b) **Compliance:** Without the guidance of the NPP, physicians may document and submit codes at levels higher than medically necessary. c) **Quality of care:** Without the guidance of the NPP, physicians may provide care at levels lower than medically indicated and below the standard of care (as designated by medical specialty societies through the CPT clinical examples and E/M descriptors)

CMS indicates Centers for Medicare & Medicaid Services; CPT, *Current Procedural Terminology*; EHR, electronic health record; HPI, history of present illness; ICD-9, International Classification of Diseases, Ninth Revision, Clinical Modification; MDM, medical decision making; NPP, nature of the presenting problem; PFSH, past, family, and social history; and ROS, review of systems.

* Health Care Financing Administration. *Documentation Guidelines for Evaluation and Management Services.* American Medical Association. Chicago: IL. 1997

†American Medical Association. *Current Procedural Terminology (CPT®).* Chicago, IL: American Medical Association; 2007.

Sample Electronic H&P Screens and Forms

This appendix includes four sample designs for compliant history and physical examination (H&P) record screens (and corresponding paper forms) for reference in evaluating and enhancing electronic H&P record designs. The forms illustrate four of the most common types of service:

- Initial outpatient visit (and consultation) for the general multisystem examination defined by 1997 Documentation Guidelines. (The examination component of the template for the multisystem examination is more extensive than the template for single specialty examinations. Therefore, the examination section of the H&P record for this type of examination requires scrolling functionality on an electronic screen and a supplemental sheet in a paper form, as discussed in Chapter 14.)

- Follow-up outpatient visit (for a cardiology examination)

- Initial hospital admission (for an ear, nose, and throat examination)

- Subsequent hospital care visit (for an ear, nose, and throat examination)

These sample forms show the comprehensive H&P record structure that is the foundation for the diagnostic process and the basis for guiding evaluation and management documentation and coding compliance. Its design will be familiar to nearly all physicians from their training, with the exception of the small section near the end that guides documentation of the physician's assessment of the complexity of data, the three levels of risk, and the nature of the presenting problem(s). Although the basic structure of these forms is established by quality care and compliance parameters, the specific questions and descriptions can be modified to meet the preferences of each physician.

NOTE: In an EHR-screen with scrolling function, the physical examination form, *Initial Visit Form (Supplement)* on page 380 would follow directly after the *Initial Visit Form (p. 3)* on page 378.

Patient Name:_____   Account No._____   DOB:____/____/____

Outpatient Initial Visit Form (p. 1): Please provide the following medical information to the best of your ability:

Date:	Age:	List any ALLERGIES TO MEDICATIONS:
What problems are you here for today?		

Past Medical History:
1) Please check the "Yes" or "No" box to indicate if you have any of the following illnesses; for "Yes" answers, please explain.

	Yes	No			Yes	No	
Diabetes (Circle: type I / type II)	☐	☐	_____	Stomach or Intestinal problems	☐	☐	_____
Hypertension (high blood press)	☐	☐	_____	Allergy problems/therapy	☐	☐	_____
Thyroid problems	☐	☐	_____	Kidney problems	☐	☐	_____
Heart Disease/cholesterol probs	☐	☐	_____	Neurological problems	☐	☐	_____
Respiratory problems	☐	☐	_____	Cancer	☐	☐	_____
Bleeding disorder	☐	☐	_____	Other Medical Diagnosis	☐	☐	_____

2) Please list any operations (and dates) you have ever had *(including tonsils & adenoids)* :

3) Please list any current medications (and amounts, times per day):
(include aspirin, antacids, vitamins, hormone replacement, birth control, herbal supplements, OTC meds including sinus/allergy/weight loss meds):

Social History:

	Yes	No	Please list details below:
Do you use tobacco?	☐	☐	List type and how much: _____
If no, did you use it previously?	☐	☐	List type and how much: _____ When did you quit?
Do you drink alcohol?	☐	☐	List type and how much: _____
Do you use recreational drugs?	☐	☐	List type and how much: _____
What is your occupation?			_____

Family History:
Please check the "Yes" or "No" box to indicate whether any relatives have any of the following illnesses:
If yes, please indicate which relative(s) have the problem.

	Yes	No	
Heart problems/murmurs	☐	☐	_____
Allergy	☐	☐	_____
Diabetes	☐	☐	_____
Cancer	☐	☐	_____
Bleeding disorder	☐	☐	_____
Anesthesia problems	☐	☐	_____

☐ See attached dictation   Reviewed by:

page 1

376

Date____/____/____

Patient Name:_____ Account No._____ DOB:____/____/____

Outpatient Initial Visit Form (p. 2): Please provide the following medical information to the best of your ability:

Review of Systems:

1) Please check the "Yes" or "No" box to indicate whether you presently have any of the following symptoms:

2) For any "yes" responses, please check the "Current" box if this symptom relates to the reason for your visit today.

		Yes	No	Current		Yes	No	Current
GENERAL	chills	☐	☐	☐	weight loss or gain	☐	☐	☐
	fatigue	☐	☐	☐	daytime sleepiness	☐	☐	☐
ALLERGY	environmental allergy	☐	☐	☐	sneezing fits	☐	☐	☐
NEURO	headache	☐	☐	☐	weakness	☐	☐	☐
	passing out	☐	☐	☐	numbness, tingling	☐	☐	☐
EYES	eye pain/pressure	☐	☐	☐	vision changes	☐	☐	☐
	watery or itchy eyes	☐	☐	☐				
ENT	hearing loss	☐	☐	☐	ear noises	☐	☐	☐
	dizziness	☐	☐	☐	lightheadedness	☐	☐	☐
	nasal congestion	☐	☐	☐	sinus pressure or pain	☐	☐	☐
	hoarseness	☐	☐	☐	problem snoring, apnea	☐	☐	☐
	throat clearing	☐	☐	☐	throat pain	☐	☐	☐
RESPIR	cough	☐	☐	☐	coughing blood	☐	☐	☐
	wheezing	☐	☐	☐	shortness of breath	☐	☐	☐
CARDIAC	chest pain	☐	☐	☐	palpitations	☐	☐	☐
	wake short of breath	☐	☐	☐	ankle swelling	☐	☐	☐
GI	difficulty swallowing	☐	☐	☐	heartburn	☐	☐	☐
	abdominal pain	☐	☐	☐	nausea/vomiting	☐	☐	☐
	bowel irregularity	☐	☐	☐	rectal bleeding	☐	☐	☐
GU	frequent urination	☐	☐	☐	painful urination	☐	☐	☐
	blood in urine	☐	☐	☐	prostate problems	☐	☐	☐
HEME/LYM	swollen glands	☐	☐	☐	sweating at night	☐	☐	☐
	bleeding problems	☐	☐	☐	easy bruising	☐	☐	☐
ENDO	feel warmer than others	☐	☐	☐	feel cooler than others	☐	☐	☐
MSK	joint aches	☐	☐	☐	muscle aches	☐	☐	☐
SKIN	rash	☐	☐	☐	hives	☐	☐	☐
	itching	☐	☐	☐	skin or hair changes	☐	☐	☐
PSYCH	depression	☐	☐	☐	anxiety or panic	☐	☐	☐

PLEASE STOP HERE	☐ See attached dictation

Reviewed by:

Date ____/____/____

Patient States Consultation Requested By_____

Patient Name:_____

Account No._____   DOB:____/____/____

Outpatient Initial Visit Form (p. 3)

PRESENT ILLNESS	Chronology with: 1. one to three elements (level 2) 2. four to eight elements; OR status of 3 chronic or inactive conditions (level 3, 4 or 5)
	(1) duration (2) timing (3) severity (4) location (5) quality (6) context (7) modifying factors (8) assoc. signs & symptoms

☐ See attached dictation

PHYSICAL EXAMINATION: General Multisystem Exam

GENERAL   (at least 3 measurements of vital signs)   HT___ft___in   WT_____lbs

BP sitting-standing____/____mm Hg   BP supine____/____mm Hg

PULSE _____/min   regular - irregular   RESP ____/min   TEMP_____°(F-C)

			Normal/AB					Normal/AB	
	GENERAL APPEARANCE	Stature, nutrition	☐	☐	CHEST/	BREAST INSPECTION	Symmetry, color	☐	☐
EYES	CONJUNCTIVAE & LIDS	Appearance, color	☐	☐	BREASTS	BREAST/AXILLAE PALP	Nodules, masses	☐	☐
	PUPILS & IRISES	Size, reactivity	☐	☐	GI/ABD	MASSES/TENDERNESS	Palpation	☐	☐
	OPTIC DISCS	Fundi, vessels	☐	☐		LIVER/SPLEEN	Size, tenderness	☐	☐
ENT	EARS & NOSE, EXTERNAL	Appearance	☐	☐		HERNIA EVAL	Inspection, palpation	☐	☐
	OTOSCOPY	Canals, tymp membranes	☐	☐		ANUS/RECTUM/PERIN	Appearance, palpation	☐	☐
	HEARING	Response to sound	☐	☐		STOOL, HEMACULT	Eval for blood	☐	☐
	INTERNAL NOSE	Septum, mucosa, turbs	☐	☐	LYMPH	NECK/AXILLAE/GROIN/OTHER	Adenopathy	☐	☐
	LIPS,TEETH & GUMS	Mucosa, dentition	☐	☐		(circle areas examined; requires exam in 2 or more regions)			
	OROPHARYNX	Mucosa, tonsils, palate	☐	☐	MSKEL	GAIT & STATION	Stability & smoothness	☐	☐
NECK	MASSES & TRACHEA	Symmetry, masses	☐	☐	(partial)	DIGITS & NAILS	Color & appearance	☐	☐
	THYROID	Size, nodules	☐	☐	SKIN/	INSPECTION	Head, trunk, RUE	☐	☐
RESP	RESPIRATORY EFFORT	Inspiratory-expiratory	☐	☐	SUBCU		LUE,RLE, LLE	☐	☐
	CHEST PALPATION	Movement	☐	☐		PALPATION	Head, trunk, RUE	☐	☐
	CHEST PERCUSSION	Sound	☐	☐			LUE,RLE, LLE	☐	☐
	AUSCULTATION	Lung sounds	☐	☐	NEURO	CRANIAL NERVES	II - XII	☐	☐
CVS	HEART PALPATION	Rhythm	☐	☐		DEEP TENDON REFLEXES	Knee, ankle, Babinski	☐	☐
	HEART AUSCULTATION	Sounds	☐	☐		SENSATION	Light touch	☐	☐
	CAROTID ARTIERIES	Pulsation	☐	☐	PSYCH	JUDGEMENT & INSIGHT	Subjectively	☐	☐
	ABDOMINAL AORTA	Pulsation	☐	☐		ORIENTATION	Person, place, time	☐	☐
	FEMORAL ARTERIES	Pulsation	☐	☐		MEMORY	Recent & remote	☐	☐
	PEDAL PULSES	Pulsation	☐	☐		MOOD & AFFECT	Comments	☐	☐
	EDEMA,VARICES, LE	Appearance	☐	☐					

☐ Continued on supplemental page   ☐ See attached dictation

---

1. Problem focused = 1-5 elements (level 1)   2. Expanded = 6-11 elements (level 2)   3. Detailed = 12 or more elements [in 2 or more systems] (level 3)
4. Comprehensive = document two (or more) elements in each of nine (or more) systems (level 4 or 5)   *Optional

page 3

378

Patient Name:_____   Account No._____   DOB:____/____/____

Outpatient Initial Visit Form (p. 4)

MEDICAL DECISION MAKING	
DATA REVIEWED (c):	2 of the 3 sections (a vs a', b vs b' vs b'', c vs c' vs c'') must meet or exceed indicated level of care
	1. Minimal (level 2) 2. Limited (level 3) 3. Moderate (level 4) 4. Extensive (level 5)

☐ X-ray/CT scan   ☐ See attached dictation

☐ MRI

☐ Lab/blood work

IMPRESSIONS / DIFFERENTIAL DIAGNOSES (a):   **PLANS / MANAGEMENT OPTIONS (a')**

1. Minimal (level 2)   2. Limited (level 3)   3. Multiple (level 4)   4. Extensive (level 5)

1) _____   1) _____   ☐ See attached dictation

2) _____   2) _____

3) _____   3) _____

4) _____   4) _____

5) _____   5) _____

DATA ORDERED (c'):   1. Minimal or none (level 2)   2. Limited (level 3)   3. Moderate (level 4)   4. Extensive (level 5)

☐   ☐   ☐   ☐   ☐

                                                                                   ☐ See attached dictation

Information Sheets Given:	☐	☐	☐	☐
	☐	☐	☐	☐

COMPLEXITY OF DATA REVIEWED OR ORDERED (c'')

1. Minimal (level 2)	2. Limited (level 3)	3. Moderate (level 4)	4. Extensive (level 5)
1. min	2. limited	3. mod	4. extensive

RISK OF COMPLICATIONS &/OR MORBIDITY OR MORTALITY (see examples in Table of Risk)

	1. Minimal (level 2)	2. Low (level 3)	3. Moderate (level 4)	4. High (level 5)
risk of presenting problem(s) (b):	1. min	2. low	3. mod	4. high
risk of diagnostic procedure(s) ordered or reviewed (b'):	1. min	2. low	3. mod	4. high
risk of management option(s) selected (b''):	1. min	2. low	3. mod	4. high

NATURE OF PRESENTING PROBLEM(S)

1. minor	(level 1)	Problem runs definite and prescribed course, is transient in nature, and is not likely to permanently alter health status; OR, has a good prognosis with management and compliance.
2. low	(level 1)	Problem in which the risk of morbidity without treatment is low; there is little to no risk of mortality without treatment; full recovery without functional impairment is expected.
3. low - mod	(level 2)	Problem in which the risk of morbidity without treatment is low to moderate; there is low to moderate risk of mortality without treatment; full recovery without functional impairment is expected in most cases, with low probability of prolonged functional impairment
4. moderate	(level 3)	Problem in which the risk of morbidity without treatment is moderate; there is moderate risk of mortality without treatment; prognosis is uncertain, or there is an increased probability of prolonged functional impairment.
5. mod - high	(levels 4,5)	Problem in which the risk of morbidity without treatment is moderate to high; there is moderate risk of mortality without treatment; uncertain prognosis or increased probability of prolonged functional impairment
6. high	(levels 4,5)	Problem in which the risk of morbidity without treatment is high to extreme; there is moderate to high risk of mortality without treatment, or high probability of severe prolonged functional impairment.

Complete this section only if documented below > 50% of visit time involved counseling and/or coordinating care.

TIME: _____ minutes   ☐ > 50% of visit time involved counseling and/or coordination of care

Clinician's signature: _____

Date____/____/____

Patient Name:_____ Account No._____ DOB:____/____/____

Outpatient Initial Visit Form (Supplement)

| PHYSICAL EXAMINATION: | | | General Multisystem Exam (continued) | | | |

			Normal/AB							**Normal/AB**
GU/	SCROTAL CONTENTS	Appearance, palpation	☐ ☐	**MSKEL**	RT UPPER EXTREMITY	Inspec., palp., percussion	☐ ☐
MALE	PENIS	Appearance, palpation	☐ ☐			Range of motion	☐ ☐
	PROSTATE	Palpation	☐ ☐			Stability or laxity	☐ ☐
GU/	EXT GENITALIA	Appearance, palpation	☐ ☐			Muscle strength & tone	☐ ☐
FEMALE	URETHRA	Inspection	☐ ☐		LT UPPER EXTREMITY	Inspec., palp., percussion	☐ ☐
(PELVIC)	BLADDER	Palpation	☐ ☐			Range of motion	☐ ☐
	CERVIS	Palpation	☐ ☐			Stability or laxity	☐ ☐
	UTERUS	Palpation	☐ ☐			Muscle strength & tone	☐ ☐
	ADNEXA/PARAMET	Palpation	☐ ☐		RT LOWER EXTREMITY	Inspec., palp., percussion	☐ ☐
MSKEL	HEAD & NECK	Inspec., palp., percussion	☐ ☐			Range of motion	☐ ☐
		Range of motion	☐ ☐			Stability or laxity	☐ ☐
		Stability or laxity	☐ ☐			Muscle strength & tone	☐ ☐
		Muscle strength & tone	☐ ☐		LT LOWER EXTREMITY	Inspec., palp., percussion	☐ ☐
	SPINE, RIBS, PELVIS	Inspec., palp., percussion	☐ ☐			Range of motion	☐ ☐
		Range of motion	☐ ☐			Stability or laxity	☐ ☐
		Stability or laxity	☐ ☐			Muscle strength & tone	☐ ☐
		Muscle strength & tone	☐ ☐			☐ See attached dictation	

1. Problem focused = 1-5 elements (level 1)   2. Expanded = 6-11 elements (level 2)   3. Detailed = 12 or more elements [in 2 or more systems] (level 3)
4. Comprehensive = document two (or more) elements in each of nine (or more) systems (level 4 or 5)   *Optional

Patient Name:_____   Account No._____   DOB:____/____/____

Outpatient Established Patient Visit Form (p. 1)

Date: ____/____/____	**PMH/SH/FH**	no change since last visit date: _____

Except: _____

_____

New Allergies: _____   Existing allergies: _____

Current Medications: _____

Reviewed by: _____

ROS	no change since last visit date: _____

Except: _____

Reviewed by: _____

PRESENT ILLNESS   Chronology with: 1. one to three elements (level 2 or 3)   2. four to eight elements; OR status of 3 chronic or inactive conditions (level 4 or 5)
(1) duration   (2) timing   (3) severity   (4) location   (5) quality   (6) context   (7) modifying factors   (8) assoc. signs & symptoms

☐ See attached dictation

_____
_____
_____
_____
_____
_____
_____
_____

PHYSICAL EXAMINATION: Cardiology

GENERAL   (at least 3 measurements of vital signs)   HT___ft___in   WT____lbs

BP sitting-standing ____/____mm Hg   BP supine____/____mm Hg

PULSE _____/min   regular - irregular   RESP_____/min   TEMP _____° (F-C)

			Normal/AB				Normal/AB
	GENERAL APPEARANCE	Stature, nutrition	☐ ☐	RESPIR	EFFORT	Inspiratory-exp	☐ ☐
EYES	CONJUNCTIVAE & LIDS	Scleral color; vascularity	☐ ☐		AUSCULTATION	Breath sounds	☐ ☐
ENT	TEETH, GUMS, PALATE		☐ ☐	**GI/ABD**	EXAMINATION, PALPATION	Absence of masses/tenderness	☐ ☐
	ORAL MUCOSA	Absence of pallor, cyanosis	☐ ☐		LIVER, SPLEEN	Size, no tenderness	☐ ☐
NECK	JUGULAR VEINS	Size, absence of waves	☐ ☐		RECTAL	Prostate size/abs of masses	☐ ☐
	THYROID	Size, absence of masses	☐ ☐		STOOL, HEMACULT	IF on anticoagulant Rx	☐ ☐
CVS	HEART PALPATION	PMI	☐ ☐	**MSK**	BACK	Palpation, alignment	☐ ☐
	HEART AUSCULTATION	Sounds, murmurs, bruits	☐ ☐		GAIT & EXERCISE TOLERANCE	Ambulation	☐ ☐
	CAROTID ARTERIES	Upstroke, absence of bruits	☐ ☐		MUSCLE STRENGTH & TONE	Resting & moving	☐ ☐
	ABDOMINAL AORTA	Size, absence of bruits	☐ ☐	**EXTREMS**	DIGITS & NAILS	Absence of petecchiae	☐ ☐
	FEMORAL ARTERIES	Palpable, absence of bruits	☐ ☐	**SKIN**	INSPEC/PALPATION	Absence of rashes	☐ ☐
	PEDAL PULSES	Palpable	☐ ☐	**NEURO**	ORIENTATION		☐ ☐
	EXTRMITIES	No edema or varicosities	☐ ☐	**PSYCH**	MOOD & AFFECT		☐ ☐

☐ See attached dictation

_____
_____
_____
_____
_____
_____

---

1. Problem focused = 1-5 elements (level 2)	2. Expanded = 6-11 elements (level 3)	3. Detailed = 12 or more elements (level 4)
4. Comprehensive = document every element in basic areas AND at least 1 element in each optional area (level 5)		*Optional

page 1

Date____/____/____

Patient Name:_____ Account No._____ DOB:____/____/____

Outpatient Established Patient Visit Form (p. 2)

MEDICAL DECISION MAKING	2 of the 3 sections (a vs a', b vs b', c vs c") must meet or exceed indicated level of care
DATA REVIEWED (c):	1. Minimal (level 2) 2. Limited (level 3) 3. Moderate (level 4) 4. Extensive (level 5)

☐ X-ray/CT scan   ☐ See attached dictation

☐ MRI

☐ Lab/blood work

IMPRESSIONS / DIFFERENTIAL DIAGNOSES (a):   PLANS / MANAGEMENT OPTIONS (a')

1. Minimal (level 2)   2. Limited (level 3)   3. Multiple (level 4)   4. Extensive (level 5)

1) _____   1) _____   ☐ See attached dictation

2) _____   2) _____

3) _____   3) _____

4) _____   4) _____

5) _____   5) _____

DATA ORDERED (c'):   1. Minimal or none (level 2)   2. Limited (level 3)   3. Moderate (level 4)   4. Extensive (level 5)

☐   ☐   ☐   ☐

                                                                                          ☐ See attached dictation

Information Sheets Given:

COMPLEXITY OF DATA REVIEWED OR ORDERED (c")

	1. Minimal (level 2)	2. Limited (level 3)	3. Moderate (level 4)	4. Extensive (level 5)
	1. min	2. limited	3. mod	4. extensive

RISK OF COMPLICATIONS &/OR MORBIDITY OR MORTALITY (see examples in Table of Risk)

	1. Minimal (level 2)	2. Low (level 3)	3. Moderate (level 4)	4. High (level 5)
risk of presenting problem(s) (b):	1. min	2. low	3. mod	4. high
risk of diagnostic procedure(s) ordered or reviewed (b'):	1. min	2. low	3. mod	4. high
risk of management option(s) selected (b"):	1. min	2. low	3. mod	4. high

NATURE OF PRESENTING PROBLEM(S)

1. minor	(level 2)	Problem runs definite and prescribed course, is transient in nature, and is not likely to permanently alter health status; OR, has a good prognosis with management and compliance.
2. low	(level 2)	Problem in which the risk of morbidity without treatment is low; there is little to no risk of mortality without treatment; full recovery without functional impairment is expected.
3. low - mod	(level 3)	Problem in which the risk of morbidity without treatment is low to moderate; there is low to moderate risk of mortality without treatment; full recovery without functional impairment is expected in most cases, with low probability of prolonged functional impairment
4. moderate	(level 3)	Problem in which the risk of morbidity without treatment is moderate; there is moderate risk of mortality without treatment; prognosis is uncertain, or there is an increased probability of prolonged functional impairment.
5. mod - high	(levels 4,5)	Problem in which the risk of morbidity without treatment is moderate to high; there is moderate risk of mortality without treatment; uncertain prognosis or increased probability of prolonged functional impairment
6. high	(levels 4,5)	Problem in which the risk of morbidity without treatment is high to extreme; there is moderate to high risk of mortality without treatment, or high probability of severe prolonged functional impairment.

Complete this section only if documented below > 50% of visit time involved counseling and/or coordinating care.
TIME: _____ minutes   ☐ > 50% of visit time involved counseling and/or coordination of care

	Clinician's signature:

Patient Name:_____ Account No._____ DOB:___/___/___

Initial Hospital Care Form (p. 1): Please provide the following medical information to the best of your ability:

Date:	Age:	List any ALLERGIES TO MEDICATIONS:
What problems are you here for today?		

Past Medical History:
1) Please check the "Yes" or "No" box to indicate if you have any of the following illnesses; for "Yes" answers, please explain.

	Yes	No			Yes	No	
Diabetes	☐	☐	_____	**Stomach or Intestinal problems**	☐	☐	_____
Hypertension (high blood press)	☐	☐	_____	**Allergy problems/therapy**	☐	☐	_____
Thyroid problems	☐	☐	_____	**Kidney problems**	☐	☐	_____
Heart Disease/cholesterol probs	☐	☐	_____	**Neurological problems**	☐	☐	_____
Respiratory problems	☐	☐	_____	**Cancer**	☐	☐	_____
Bleeding disorder	☐	☐	_____	**Other Medical Diagnosis**	☐	☐	_____

2) Please list any operations (and dates) you have ever had *(including tonsils & adenoids)* :

3) **Please list any current medications (and amounts, times per day):**
(include aspirin, antacids, vitamins, hormone replacement, birth control, herbal supplements, OTC nasal sprays/cold/sinus/allergy meds):

Social History:	Yes	No	**Please list details below:**	
Do you use tobacco?	☐	☐	List type and how much: _____	
If no, did you use it previously?	☐	☐	List type and how much: _____	**When did you quit?**
Do you use recreational drugs?	☐	☐	List type and how much: _____	
Do you drink alcohol?	☐	☐	List type and how much: _____	
What is your occupation?			_____	

Family History:
  Please check the "Yes" or "No" box to indicate whether any relatives have any of the following illnesses:
  If yes, please indicate which relative(s) have the problem.

	Yes	No	
Heart problems/murmurs	☐	☐	_____
Allergy	☐	☐	_____
Diabetes	☐	☐	_____
Cancer	☐	☐	_____
Bleeding disorder	☐	☐	_____
Anesthesia problems	☐	☐	_____

☐ See attached dictation | Reviewed by: _____

page 1

383

Patient Name:_____   Account No._____   DOB:_____/_____/_____

Initial Hospital Care Form (p. 2): Please provide the following medical information to the best of your ability:

Review of Systems:

1) Please check the "Yes" or "No" box to indicate whether you presently have any of the following symptoms:

2) For any "yes" responses, please check the "Current" box if this symptom relates to the reason for your visit today.

		Yes	No	Current		Yes	No	Current
GENERAL	chills	☐	☐	☐	weight loss or gain	☐	☐	☐
	fatigue	☐	☐	☐	daytime sleepiness	☐	☐	☐
ALLERGY	environmental allergy	☐	☐	☐	sneezing fits	☐	☐	☐
NEURO	headache	☐	☐	☐	weakness	☐	☐	☐
	passing out	☐	☐	☐	numbness, tingling	☐	☐	☐
EYES	eye pain/pressure	☐	☐	☐	vision changes	☐	☐	☐
	watery or itchy eyes	☐	☐	☐				
ENT	hearing loss	☐	☐	☐	ear noises	☐	☐	☐
	dizziness	☐	☐	☐	lightheadedness	☐	☐	☐
	nasal congestion	☐	☐	☐	sinus pressure or pain	☐	☐	☐
	hoarseness	☐	☐	☐	problem snoring, apnea	☐	☐	☐
	throat clearing	☐	☐	☐	throat pain	☐	☐	☐
RESPIR	cough	☐	☐	☐	coughing blood	☐	☐	☐
	wheezing	☐	☐	☐	shortness of breath	☐	☐	☐
CARDIAC	chest pain	☐	☐	☐	palpitations	☐	☐	☐
	wake short of breath	☐	☐	☐	ankle swelling	☐	☐	☐
GI	difficulty swallowing	☐	☐	☐	heartburn	☐	☐	☐
	abdominal pain	☐	☐	☐	nausea/vomiting	☐	☐	☐
	bowel irregularity	☐	☐	☐	rectal bleeding	☐	☐	☐
GU	frequent urination	☐	☐	☐	painful urination	☐	☐	☐
	blood in urine	☐	☐	☐	prostate problems	☐	☐	☐
HEME/LYM	swollen glands	☐	☐	☐	sweating at night	☐	☐	☐
	bleeding problems	☐	☐	☐	easy bruising	☐	☐	☐
ENDO	feel warmer than others	☐	☐	☐	feel cooler than others	☐	☐	☐
MSK	joint aches	☐	☐	☐	muscle aches	☐	☐	☐
SKIN	rash	☐	☐	☐	hives	☐	☐	☐
	itching	☐	☐	☐	skin or hair changes	☐	☐	☐
PSYCH	depression	☐	☐	☐	anxiety or panic	☐	☐	☐

PLEASE STOP HERE   ☐ See attached dictation

Reviewed by:

Date ____/____/____

Patient Name:_____ Account No._____ DOB:____/____/____

Initial Hospital Care Form (p. 3)

PRESENT ILLNESS	Chronology with: four to eight elements REQUIRED (level 1, 2 or 3) *(NOTE: less than 4 elements documented is insufficient)*
	(1) duration (2) timing (3) severity (4) location (5) quality (6) context (7) modifying factors (8) assoc. signs & symptoms

☐ See attached dictation

PHYSICAL EXAMINATION: Ear, Nose & Throat

GENERAL   (at least 3 measurements of vital signs)

HT____ft____in   WT_____lbs

BP sitting-standing ____/____mm Hg   BP supine ____/____mm Hg

PULSE _____/min regular - irregular   RESP _____/min   TEMP _____° (F-C)

			Normal/AB					Normal/AB	
	GENERAL APPEARANCE	Stature, nutrition	☐	☐	NECK	MASSES & TRACHEA	Symmetry, masses	☐	☐
	COMMUNICATION & VOICE	Pitch, clarity	☐	☐		THYROID	Size, nodules	☐	☐
HEAD/	INSPECTION	Lesions, masses	☐	☐	EYES	OCULAR MOTILITY & GAZE	EOMs, nystagmus	☐	☐
FACE	PALPATION / PERCUSSION	Skeleton, sinuses	☐	☐	RESP	RESPIRATORY EFFORT	Inspiratory-expiratory	☐	☐
	SALIVARY GLANDS	Masses, tenderness	☐	☐		AUSCULTATION	Lung sounds	☐	☐
	FACIAL STRENGTH	Symmetry	☐	☐	CVS	HEART AUSCULTATION	Rhythm, heart sounds	☐	☐
ENT	PNEUMO-OTOSCOPY	EACs; TMs mobile	☐	☐		PERIPH VASC SYSTEM	Edema, color	☐	☐
	HEARING ASSESSMENT	Gross; Weber/Rinne	☐	☐	LYMPH	NECK/AXILLAE/GROIN/ETC.	Adenopathy	☐	☐
	EXTERNAL EAR & NOSE	Appearance	☐	☐	NEURO	CRANIAL NERVES	II - XII	☐	☐
	INTERNAL NOSE	Mucosa, turbinates	☐	☐	PSYCH	ORIENTATION	Person, place, time	☐	☐
	*AFTER DECONGESTANT	Septum, OMCs	☐	☐		MOOD & AFFECT	Comments	☐	☐
	LIPS,TEETH & GUMS	Mucosa, dentition	☐	☐		*ROMBERG		☐	☐
	ORAL CAVITY, OROPHARYNX	Mucosa, tonsils, palate	☐	☐		*TANDEM ROMBERG		☐	☐
	HYPOPHARYNX	Mucosa, pyriforms	☐	☐		*PAST POINTING		☐	☐
	LARYNX (mirror: adults)	Anatomy, vocal cord mobility	☐	☐					
	NASOPHAR (mirror: adults)	Mucosa, choanae	☐	☐					

☐ See attached dictation

---

3. Detailed = 12 or more elements (level 1)   *(NOTE: less than 12 elements documented is insufficient for initial hospital care)*

4. Comprehensive = document every element in basic areas AND at least 1 element in each optional area (level 2 or 3)   *Optional

Patient Name:_____   Account No._____   DOB:____/____/____

Initial Hospital Care Form (p. 4)

MEDICAL DECISION MAKING DATA REVIEWED (a):	2 of the 3 sections (a vs a' vs a", b vs b', c vs c' vs c") must meet or exceed indicated level of care
	1. Minimal (level 1) 2. Limited (level 1) 3. Moderate (level 2) 4. Extensive (level 3)

☐ See attached dictation

IMPRESSIONS / DIFFERENTIAL DIAGNOSES (b):   **PLANS / MANAGEMENT OPTIONS (b')**

1. Minimal (level 1)   2. Limited (level 1)   3. Multiple (level 2)   4. Extensive (level 3)

1)   1)   ☐ See attached dictation

2)   2)

3)   3)

4)   4)

5)   5)

DATA ORDERED (a'):   1. Minimal or none (level 1)   2. Limited (level 1)   3. Moderate (level 2)   4. Extensive (level 3)

☐   ☐   ☐   ☐   ☐

☐ See attached dictation

COMPLEXITY OF DATA REVIEWED OR ORDERED (a")

	1. Minimal (level 1)	2. Limited (level 1)	3. Moderate (level 2)	4. Extensive (level 3)
	1. min	2. limited	3. mod	4. extensive

RISK OF COMPLICATIONS &/OR MORBIDITY OR MORTALITY (see examples in Table of Risk)

	1. Minimal (level 1)	2. Low (level 1)	3. Moderate (level 2)	4. High (level 3)
risk of presenting problem(s) (c):	1. min	2. low	3. mod	4. high
risk of diagnostic procedure(s) ordered or reviewed (c'):	1. min	2. low	3. mod	4. high
risk of management option(s) selected (c"):	1. min	2. low	3. mod	4. high

NATURE OF PRESENTING PROBLEM(S)

1. minor	(level 1)	Problem runs definite and prescribed course, is transient in nature, and is not likely to permanently alter health status; OR, has a good prognosis with management and compliance.
2. low	(level 1)	Problem in which the risk of morbidity without treatment is low; there is little to no risk of mortality without treatment; full recovery without functional impairment is expected.
3. low - mod	(level 1)	Problem in which the risk of morbidity without treatment is low to moderate; there is low to moderate risk of mortality without treatment; full recovery without functional impairment is expected in most cases, with low probability of prolonged functional impairment
4. moderate	(level 2)	Problem in which the risk of morbidity without treatment is moderate; there is moderate risk of mortality without treatment; prognosis is uncertain, or there is an increased probability of prolonged functional impairment.
5. mod - high	(level 2)	Problem in which the risk of morbidity without treatment is moderate to high; there is moderate risk of mortality without treatment; uncertain prognosis or increased probability of prolonged functional impairment
6. high	(level 3)	Problem in which the risk of morbidity without treatment is high to extreme; there is moderate to high risk of mortality without treatment, or high probability of severe prolonged functional impairment.

Complete this section only if documented below > 50% of visit time involved counseling and/or coordinating care.

TIME: _____ minutes   ☐ > 50% of visit time involved counseling and/or coordination of care

Clinician's signature:

Patient Name:_____ Account No._____ DOB:____/____/____

Subsequent Inpatient Care Form (p. 1)

Date: ____/____/____ Time:_____AM / PM ROS: no change since last visit date: ____/____/____

☐ No chest pain ☐ No shortness of breath ☐ No calf pain or tenderness

Except: _____

PRESENT ILLNESS | Chronology with: 1. one to three elements (level 1 or 2) 2. four to eight elements; OR status of 3 chronic or inactive conditions (level 3)
(1) duration (2) timing (3) severity (4) location (5) quality (6) context (7) modifying factors (8) assoc signs & symptoms

☐ See attached dictation

PHYSICAL EXAMINATION: Ear, Nose & Throat

GENERAL (at least 3 measurements of vital signs)

HT___ft___in   WT_____lbs

BP sitting-standing____/____mm Hg   BP supine____/____mm Hg

PULSE _____/min regular - irregular   RESP _____/min   TEMP _____° (F-C)

			Normal/AB					Normal/AB	
	GENERAL APPEARANCE	Stature, nutrition	☐	☐	**NECK**	MASSES & TRACHEA	Symmetry, masses	☐	☐
	COMMUNICATION & VOICE	Pitch, clarity	☐	☐		THYROID	Size, nodules	☐	☐
HEAD/	INSPECTION	Lesions, masses	☐	☐	**EYES**	OCULAR MOTILITY & GAZE	EOMs, nystagmus	☐	☐
FACE	PALPATION/PERCUSSION	Skeleton, sinuses	☐	☐	**RESP**	RESPIRATORY EFFORT	Inspiratory-expiratory	☐	☐
	SALIVARY GLANDS	Masses, tenderness	☐	☐		AUSCULTATION	Lung sounds	☐	☐
	FACIAL STRENGTH	Symmetry	☐	☐	**CVS**	HEART AUSCULTATION	Rhythm, heart sounds	☐	☐
ENT	PNEUMO-OTOSCOPY	EACs; TMs mobile	☐	☐		PERIPH VASC SYSTEM	Edema, color	☐	☐
	HEARING ASSESSMENT	Gross; Weber/Rinne	☐	☐	**LYMPH**	NECK/AXILLAE/GROIN/ETC.	Adenopathy	☐	☐
	EXTERNAL EAR & NOSE	Appearance	☐	☐	**NEURO**	CRANIAL NERVES	II - XII	☐	☐
	INTERNAL NOSE	Mucosa, turbinates	☐	☐	**PSYCH**	ORIENTATION	Person, place, time	☐	☐
	*AFTER DECONGESTANT	Septum, OMCs	☐	☐		MOOD & AFFECT	Comments	☐	☐
	LIPS,TEETH & GUMS	Mucosa, dentition	☐	☐		*ROMBERG		☐	☐
	ORAL CAVITY, OROPHARYNX	Mucosa, tonsils, palate	☐	☐		*TANDEM ROMBERG		☐	☐
	HYPOPHARYNX	Mucosa, pyriforms	☐	☐		*PAST POINTING		☐	☐
	LARYNX (mirror: adults)	Anatomy, vocal cord mobility	☐	☐					
	NASOPHAR (mirror: adults)	Mucosa, choanae	☐	☐					

☐ See attached dictation

---

1. Problem focused = 1-5 elements (level 1)   2. Expanded = 6-11 elements (level 2)   3. Detailed = 12 or more elements (level 3)
*Optional

page 1

Date ____/____/____

Patient Name:_____ Account No._____ DOB:____/____/____

Subsequent Inpatient Care Form (p. 2)

MEDICAL DECISION MAKING	2 of the 3 sections (a vs a' vs a", b vs b', c vs c' vs c") must meet or exceed indicated level of care
DATA REVIEWED (c):	1. Minimal (level 1) 2. Limited (level 1) 3. Moderate (level 2) 4. Extensive (level 3)

☐ See attached dictation

_____
_____
_____
_____
_____
_____
_____

IMPRESSIONS / DIFFERENTIAL DIAGNOSES (a):   **PLANS / MANAGEMENT OPTIONS (a')**

1. Minimal (level 1)   2. Limited (level 1)   3. Multiple (level 2)   4. Extensive (level 3)

☐ See attached dictation

1)_____   1)_____

2)_____   2)_____

3)_____   3)_____

4)_____   4)_____

5)_____   5)_____

_____
_____

DATA ORDERED (c'):	1. Minimal or none (level 1) 2. Limited (level 1) 3. Moderate (level 2) 4. Extensive (level 3)
☐	☐ ☐ ☐ ☐

☐ See attached dictation

_____
_____
_____

COMPLEXITY OF DATA REVIEWED OR ORDERED (c")

	1. Minimal (level 1)	2. Limited (level 1)	3. Moderate (level 2)	4. Extensive (level 3)
	1. min	2. limited	3. mod	4. extensive

RISK OF COMPLICATIONS &/OR MORBIDITY OR MORTALITY (see examples in Table of Risk)

	1. Minimal (level 1)	2. Low (level 1)	3. Moderate (level 2)	4. High (level 3)
risk of presenting problem(s) (b):	1. min	2. low	3. mod	4. high
risk of diagnostic procedure(s) ordered or reviewed (b'):	1. min	2. low	3. mod	4. high
risk of management option(s) selected (b"):	1. min	2. low	3. mod	4. high

NATURE OF PRESENTING PROBLEM(S)

1   (level 1)   Usually, the patient is stable, recovering or improving.

2   (level 2)   Usually, the patient is responding inadequately to therapy or has developed a minor complication.

3   (level 3)   Usually, the patient is unstable or has developed a significant complication or a significant new problem.

Complete this section only if documented below > 50% of visit time involved counseling and/or coordinating care.
TIME: _____ minutes   ☐ > 50% of visit time involved counseling and/or coordination of care

	Clinician's signature:

Sample Forms for EHR Evaluation

This section contains two mock-up history and physical examination (H&P) forms that have been completed with sample information. They can be used for convenient evaluation of the usability and efficiency of entering data into the electronic H&P section of electronic health records (EHRs), as discussed in Chapter 19. By having a standard form, physicians can establish a baseline for comparison among different software systems.

These same forms can be copied and used during physician training and verification trials during the health information transformation process described in Chapter 20. Of course, practices are also invited to use their existing medical record documents or to copy forms from Appendix F and fill these with their own sample information.

NOTE: In an EHR-screen with scrolling function, the physical examination form, *Initial Visit Form (Supplement)* on page 394 would follow directly after the *Initial Visit Form (p. 3)* on page 392.

Patient Name: *Joan Jones*　　　　　　　　　　Account No. *123456*　　　　DOB: *1/1/1968*

Outpatient Initial Visit Form (p. 1): Please provide the following medical information to the best of your ability:

Date: *5/5/2007*	Age: *39*	List any ALLERGIES TO MEDICATIONS:
What problems are you here for today?		
Cough		*Penicillin*

Past Medical History:
1) Please check the "Yes" or "No" box to indicate if you have any of the following illnesses; for "Yes" answers, please explain.

	Yes	No			Yes	No	
Diabetes (Circle: type I / type II)	☐	☒	_____	Stomach or Intestinal problems	☐	☒	_____
Hypertension (high blood press)	☒	☐	_____	Allergy problems/therapy	☐	☒	_____
Thyroid problems	☐	☒	_____	Kidney problems	☐	☒	_____
Heart Disease/cholesterol probs	☒	☐	_____	Neurological problems	☐	☒	_____
Respiratory problems	☐	☒	_____	Cancer	☐	☒	_____
Bleeding disorder	☐	☒	_____	Other Medical Diagnosis	☒	☐	*Nasal polyps*

Hypertension diagnosed in 2004. With medication, BP runs 130/80

Elevated cholesterol, treated with Yyyyyyy; last lab - 210 total

2) Please list any operations (and dates) you have ever had *(including tonsils & adenoids)*:

Appendectomy 1980

3) Please list any current medications (and amounts, times per day);
(include aspirin, antacids, vitamins, hormone replacement, birth control, herbal supplements, OTC meds including sinus/allergy/weight loss meds):

Xxxxxxxx 50 mg. qd

Yyyyyyy 10 mg. qd

Zzzzzzz nasal inhaler, 2 puffs each nostril bid

Social History:

	Yes	No		Please list details below:
Do you use tobacco?	☒	☐	List type and how much:	*Cigarettes 1/2 ppd for 10 years*
If no, did you use it previously?	☐	☐	List type and how much:	When did you quit?
Do you use recreational drugs?	☐	☒	List type and how much:	_____
Do you drink alcohol?	☐	☒	List type and how much:	_____
What is your occupation?				*Electrician*

Family History:
Please check the "Yes" or "No" box to indicate whether any relatives have any of the following illnesses:
If yes, please indicate which relative(s) have the problem.

	Yes	No	
Heart problems/murmurs	☐	☒	_____
Allergy	☐	☒	_____
Diabetes	☐	☒	_____
Cancer	☐	☒	_____
Bleeding disorder	☐	☒	_____
Anesthesia problems	☐	☒	_____

☐ See attached dictation	Reviewed by:

page 1

Patient Name: **Joan Jones** Account No. *123456* DOB: *1/1/1968*

Outpatient Initial Visit Form (p. 2):   Please provide the following medical information to the best of your ability:

Review of Systems:

1) Please check the "Yes" or "No" box to indicate whether you presently have any of the following symptoms:

2) For any "yes" responses, please check the "Current" box if this symptom relates to the reason for your visit today.

		Yes	No	Current		Yes	No	Current
GENERAL	chills	☐	☒	☐	weight loss or gain	☐	☒	☐
	fatigue	☐	☒	☐	daytime sleepiness	☐	☒	☐
ALLERGY	environmental allergy	☐	☒	☐	sneezing fits	☐	☒	☐
NEURO	headache	☐	☒	☐	weakness	☐	☒	☐
	passing out	☐	☒	☐	numbness, tingling	☐	☒	☐
EYES	eye pain/pressure	☐	☒	☐	vision changes	☐	☒	☐
	watery or itchy eyes	☐	☒	☐				
ENT	hearing loss	☐	☒	☐	ear noises	☐	☒	☐
	dizziness	☐	☒	☐	lightheadedness	☐	☒	☐
	nasal congestion	☒	☐	☐	sinus pressure or pain	☒	☐	☐
	hoarseness	☐	☒	☐	problem snoring, apnea	☐	☒	☐
	throat clearing	☒	☐	☒	throat pain	☐	☒	☐
RESPIR	cough	☒	☐	☒	coughing blood	☐	☒	☐
	wheezing	☐	☒	☐	shortness of breath	☐	☒	☐
CARDIAC	chest pain	☐	☒	☐	palpitations	☐	☒	☐
	wake short of breath	☐	☒	☐	ankle swelling	☐	☒	☐
GI	difficulty swallowing	☐	☒	☐	heartburn	☒	☐	☐
	abdominal pain	☐	☒	☐	nausea/vomiting	☐	☒	☐
	bowel irregularity	☐	☒	☐	rectal bleeding	☐	☒	☐
GU	frequent urination	☐	☒	☐	painful urination	☐	☒	☐
	blood in urine	☐	☒	☐	prostate problems	☐	☒	☐
HEME/LYM	swollen glands	☐	☒	☐	sweating at night	☐	☒	☐
	bleeding problems	☐	☒	☐	easy bruising	☐	☒	☐
ENDO	feel warmer than others	☐	☒	☐	feel cooler than others	☐	☒	☐
MSK	joint aches	☐	☒	☐	muscle aches	☐	☒	☐
SKIN	rash	☐	☒	☐	hives	☐	☒	☐
	itching	☐	☒	☐	skin or hair changes	☐	☒	☐
PSYCH	depression	☐	☒	☐	anxiety or panic	☐	☒	☐

<u>PLEASE STOP HERE</u>   ☐ See attached dictation

Nose/sinus: Mild bilateral nasal congestion for many years. No recent change.

Occassional mild bi-frontal sinus pressure. No OTC nasal sprays.

No discharge or bleeding

Throat clearing: frequent throat clearing without productive phlegm

Heartburn: 4-5 months of intermittent mild heartburn,

mid-epigastric, worse in AM. Patient drinks 4-6 cups

of coffee per day. No dysphagia, nausea, or vomiting.

Enjoys spicy food. Eats Mexican or Chinese with

hot spices 2-3 times per week

Reviewed by:

Patient States Consultation Requested By_____

Patient Name: *Joan Jones*   Account No. *123456*   DOB: *1/1/1968*

Outpatient Initial Visit Form (p. 3)

PRESENT ILLNESS	Chronology with: 1. one to three elements (level 2) 2. four to eight elements; OR status of 3 chronic or in active conditions (level 3, 4 or 5)
	(1) duration (2) timing (3) severity (4) location (5) quality (6) context (7) modifying factors (8) assoc. signs & symptoms

Nurse Hx: *Three months of intermittent dry cough. Mild severity*

Clinician Hx: *3-4 episodes per day of dry, hacking cough. Episodes last 1-3 minutes.*   ☐ See attached dictation

No significant relief by drinking water. No associated phlegm, chest pain, wheezing,

or shortness of breath. Occasional problems waking at night with dry cough

PHYSICAL EXAMINATION: General Multisystem Exam

GENERAL (at least 3 measurements of vital signs)   HT _5_ ft _11_ in   WT _175_ lbs

BP sitting-standing _135_ / _84_ mm Hg   BP supine____/____mm Hg

PULSE ____/min   regular - irregular   RESP ____/min   TEMP _____ ° (F-C)

			Normal	AB				Normal	AB
	GENERAL APPEARANCE	Stature, nutrition	☒	☐	CHEST/	BREAST INSPECTION	Symmetry, color	☐	☐
EYES	CONJUNCTIVAE & LIDS	Appearance, color	☒	☐	BREASTS	BREAST/AXILLAE PALP	Nodules, masses	☐	☐
	PUPILS & IRISES	Size, reactivity	☒	☐	GI/ABD	MASSES/TENDERNESS	Palpation	☐	☐
	OPTIC DISCS	Fundi, vessels	☐	☐		LIVER/SPLEEN	Size, tenderness	☐	☐
ENT	EARS & NOSE, EXTERNAL	Appearance	☒	☐		HERNIA EVAL	Inspection, palpation	☐	☐
	OTOSCOPY	Canals, tymp membranes	☐	☐		ANUS/RECTUM/PERIN	Appearance, palpation	☐	☐
	HEARING	Response to sound	☒	☐		STOOL, HEMACULT	Eval for blood	☐	☐
	INTERNAL NOSE	Septum, mucosa, turbs	☐	☐	LYMPH	NECK/AXILLAE/GROIN/OTHER	Adenopathy	☒	☐
	LIPS,TEETH & GUMS	Mucosa, dentition	☒	☐		(circle areas examined; requires exam in 2 or more regions)			
	OROPHARYNX	Mucosa, tonsils, palate	☒	☐	MSKEL	GAIT & STATION	Stability & smoothness	☒	☐
NECK	MASSES & TRACHEA	Symmetry, masses	☒	☐	(partial)	DIGITS & NAILS	Color & appearance	☒	☐
	THYROID	Size, nodules	☒	☐	SKIN/	INSPECTION	Head, trunk, RUE	☐	☐
RESP	RESPIRATORY EFFORT	Inspiratory-expiratory	☒	☐	SUBCU		LUE, RLE, LLE	☐	☐
	CHEST PALPATION	Movement	☒	☐		PALPATION	Head, trunk, RUE	☐	☐
	CHEST PERCUSSION	Sound	☐	☐			LUE, RLE, LLE	☐	☐
	AUSCULTATION	Lung sounds	☐	☒	NEURO	CRANIAL NERVES	II - XII	☐	☐
CVS	HEART PALPATION	Rhythm	☐	☐		DEEP TENDON REFLEXES	Knee, ankle, Babinski	☐	☐
	HEART AUSCULTATION	Sounds	☒	☐		SENSATION	Light touch	☐	☐
	CAROTID ARTERIES	Pulsation	☐	☐	PSYCH	JUDGEMENT & INSIGHT	Subjectively	☒	☐
	ABDOMINAL AORTA	Pulsation	☐	☐		ORIENTATION	Person, place, time	☐	☐
	FEMORAL ARTERIES	Pulsation	☐	☐		MEMORY	Recent & remote	☐	☐
	PEDAL PULSES	Pulsation	☐	☐		MOOD & AFFECT	Comments	☒	☐
	EDEMA,VARICES, LE	Appearance	☒	☐	☒ Continued on supplemental page		☐ See attached dictation		

Lungs - mildly increased exp sounds throughout. Mild dry rales at both bases, R>L

1. Problem focused = 1-5 elements (level 1)	2. Expanded = 6-11 elements (level 2)	3. Detailed = 12 or more elements [in 2 or more systems] (level 3)
4. Comprehensive = document two (or more) elements in each of nine (or more) systems (level 4 or 5)		*Optional

Patient Name: **Joan Jones** Account No. *123456* DOB: *1/1/1968*

Outpatient Initial Visit Form (p. 4)

MEDICAL DECISION MAKING	
DATA REVIEWED (c):	2 of the 3 sections (a vs a', b vs b', c vs c' vs c") must meet or exceed indicated level of care **1.** Minimal (level 2) **2.** Limited (level 3) **3.** Moderate (level 4) **4.** Extensive (level 5)

☒ X-ray/CT scan *Chest X-ray, AP & lat, wnl.* ☐ See attached dictation

☐ MRI

☐ Lab/blood work

IMPRESSIONS / DIFFERENTIAL DIAGNOSES (a):

1. Minimal (level 2) **2.** Limited (level 3) **3.** Multiple (level 4) **4.** Extensive (level 5)

PLANS / MANAGEMENT OPTIONS (a')

1) *Chronic tracheobronchitis with cough*
2) *Likely secondary to smoking irritation &*
3) *Likely secondary to reflux (pharyngeal)*
4) *GERD with heartburn*
5) *Irritative rhinitis secondary to smoke*

1) *D/C all smoking* ☐ See attached dictation
2) *Discussed nicotine patch*
3) *Qqqqqq 20 mg. bid*
4) *Dietary modification, incl. D/C coffee*
5) *Elevate HOB*
6) *Return 3 weeks to monitor status*

DATA ORDERED (c'): **1.** Minimal or none (level 2) **2.** Limited (level 3) **3.** Moderate (level 4) **4.** Extensive (level 5)

☐ ☐ ☐ ☐ ☐

1) *If symptoms persist, consider PFTs &/or bronchoscopy* ☐ See attached dictation

Information Sheets Given: (Smoking Cessation) (Reflux)

COMPLEXITY OF DATA REVIEWED OR ORDERED (c")

1. Minimal (level 2) 2. Limited (level 3) 3. Moderate (level 4) 4. Extensive (level 5)

1. min (2. limited) 3. mod 4. extensive

RISK OF COMPLICATIONS &/OR MORBIDITY OR MORTALITY (see examples in Table of Risk)

1. Minimal (level 2) 2. Low (level 3) 3. Moderate (level 4) 4. High (level 5)

risk of presenting problem(s) (b): 1. min 2. low (3. mod) 4. high
risk of diagnostic procedure(s) ordered or reviewed (b'): 1. min 2. low 3. mod 4. high
risk of management option(s) selected (b"): 1. min 2. low (3. mod) 4. high

NATURE OF PRESENTING PROBLEM(S)

1. minor	(level 1)	Problem runs definite and prescribed course, is transient in nature, and is not likely to permanently alter health status; OR, has a good prognosis with management and compliance.
2. low	(level 1)	Problem in which the risk of morbidity without treatment is low; there is little to no risk of mortality without treatment; full recovery without functional impairment is expected.
3. low - mod	(level 2)	Problem in which the risk of morbidity without treatment is low to moderate; there is low to moderate risk of mortality without treatment; full recovery without functional impairment is expected in most cases, with low probability of prolonged functional impairment
4. moderate	(level 3)	Problem in which the risk of morbidity without treatment is moderate; there is moderate risk of mortality without treatment; prognosis is uncertain, or there is an increased probability of prolonged functional impairment.
(5. mod - high)	(levels 4,5)	Problem in which the risk of morbidity without treatment is moderate to high; there is moderate risk of mortality without treatment; uncertain prognosis or increased probability of prolonged functional impairment
6. high	(levels 4,5)	Problem in which the risk of morbidity without treatment is high to extreme; there is moderate to high risk of mortality without treatment, or high probability of severe prolonged functional impairment.

Complete this section only if documented below > 50% of visit time involved counseling and/or coordinating care.

TIME: _____ minutes ☐ > 50% of visit time involved counseling and/or coordination of care

Clinician's signature:

Date: ____/____/_____

Patient Name:._____ Account No._____ DOB:____/____/_____

Outpatient Initial Visit Form (Supplement)

PHYSICAL EXAMINATION:		General Multisystem Exam (continued)						

			Normal/AB					Normal/AB
GU/	SCROTAL CONTENTS	Appearance, palpation	☐	☐	MSKEL	RT UPPER EXTREMITY	Inspec., palp., percussion	☐ ☐
MALE	PENIS	Appearance, palpation	☐	☐			Range of motion	☐ ☐
	PROSTATE	Palpation	☐	☐			Stability or laxity	☐ ☐
GU/	EXT GENITALIA	Appearance, palpation	☐	☐			Muscle strength & tone	☐ ☐
FEMALE	URETHRA	Inspection	☐	☐		LT UPPER EXTREMITY	Inspec., palp., percussion	☐ ☐
(PELVIC)	BLADDER	Palpation	☐	☐			Range of motion	☐ ☐
	CERVIS	Palpation	☐	☐			Stability or laxity	☐ ☐
	UTERUS	Palpation	☐	☐			Muscle strength & tone	☐ ☐
	ADNEXA/PARAMET	Palpation	☐	☐		RT LOWER EXTREMITY	Inspec., palp., percussion	☐ ☐
MSKEL	HEAD & NECK	Inspec., palp., percussion	☐	☐			Range of motion	☐ ☐
		Range of motion	☐	☐			Stability or laxity	☐ ☐
		Stability or laxity	☐	☐			Muscle strength & tone	☐ ☐
		Muscle strength & tone	☐	☐		LT LOWER EXTREMITY	Inspec., palp., percussion	☐ ☐
	SPINE, RIBS, PELVIS	Inspec., palp., percussion	☐	☐			Range of motion	☐ ☐
		Range of motion	☐	☐			Stability or laxity	☐ ☐
		Stability or laxity	☐	☐			Muscle strength & tone	☐ ☐
		Muscle strength & tone	☐	☐			☐ See attached dictation	

1. Problem focused = 1-5 elements (level 1)   **2. Expanded = 6-11 elements (level 2)**   **3. Detailed = 12 or more elements [in 2 or more systems] (level 3)**
4. Comprehensive = document two (or more) elements in each of nine (or more) systems (level 4 or 5)   *Optional*

Patient Name: *Joan Jones* **Account No.** *123456* **DOB:** *1/1/1968*

Established Visit Form (p. 1)

Date: _5 / 26 / 2007_ PMH/SH/FH	no change since last visit date: _5 / 5 / 2007_

Except: *Mild sprain left ankle while jogging 10 days ago - recovered fully*

New Allergies: *None* **Existing allergies:** *Penicillin*

Current Medications: *Xxxxxxx 50 mg. qd, Yyyyyyy 10 mg. qd, Zzzzzzz nasal inhaler, 2 puffs each nostril bid,*
Qqqqqq 20 mg. bid **Reviewed by:**

ROS no change since last visit date: _5 / 5 / 2007_

Except: **Reviewed by:** *ABC*

PRESENT ILLNESS Chronology with: 1. one to three elements (level 2 or 3) 2. four to eight elements; OR status of 3 chronic or inactive conditions (level 4 or 5)
(1) duration (2) timing (3) severity (4) location (5) quality (6) context (7) modifying factors (8) assoc. signs & symptoms

Patient obtained patch and stopped smoking on 5/8. Notes gradual ☐ See attached dictation
decrease in frequency and intensity of cough since approx. 5/12. In last week, also notes significant
decrease in throat clearing and heartburn. Nasal congestion resolved - now breathing normally through nose.

PHYSICAL EXAMINATION: General Multisystem Exam

GENERAL (at least 3 measurements of vital signs) HT _5_ ft _11_ in   WT _175_ lbs

BP sitting-standing _130_ / _80_ mm Hg BP supine ___ / ___ mm Hg

PULSE ____/min regular - irregular RESP ____/min TEMP ____ °(F-C)

			Normal	AB				Normal	AB
	GENERAL APPEARANCE	Stature, nutrition	☒	☐	CVS	HEART PALPATION	Rhythm	☐	☐
EYES	CONJUNCTIVAE & LIDS	Appearance, color	☒	☐		HEART AUSCULTATION	Sounds	☐	☐
	PUPILS & IRISES	Size, reactivity	☒	☐		CAROTID ARTERIES	Pulsation	☐	☐
	OPTIC DISCS	Fundi, vessels	☐	☐		ABDOMINAL AORTA	Pulsation	☐	☐
ENT	EARS & NOSE, EXTERNAL	Appearance	☒	☐		FEMORAL ARTERIES	Pulsation	☐	☐
	OTOSCOPY	Canals, tymp membranes	☐	☐		PEDAL PULSES	Pulsation	☐	☐
	HEARING	Response to sound	☒	☐		EDEMA, VARICES, LE	Appearance, palpation	☐	☐
	INTERNAL NOSE	Septum, mucosa, turbs	☐	☐	CHEST/	BREAST INSPECTION	Symmetry, color	☐	☐
	LIPS, TEETH & GUMS	Mucosa, dentition	☒	☐	BREASTS	BREAST/AXILLAE PALP	Nodules, masses	☐	☐
	OROPHARYNX	Mucosa, tonsils, palate	☒	☐	GI/ABD	MASSES/TENDERNESS	Palpation	☐	☐
NECK	MASSES & TRACHEA	Symmetry, masses	☒	☐		LIVER/SPLEEN	Size, tenderness	☐	☐
	THYROID	Size, nodules	☒	☐		HERNIA EVAL	Inspection, palpation	☐	☐
RESP	RESPIRATORY EFFORT	Inspiratory-expiratory	☒	☐		ANUS/RECTUM/PERIN	Appearance, palpation	☐	☐
	CHEST PALPATION	Movement	☐	☐		STOOL, HEMACULT	Eval for blood	☐	☐
	CHEST PERCUSSION	Sound	☐	☐	LYMPH	NECK/AXILLAE/GROIN/OTHER	Adenopathy	☐	☐
	AUSCULTATION	Lung sounds	☐	☒		(circle areas examined; requires exam in 2 or more regions)			

☐ Continued on supplemental page ☐ See attached dictation

Lungs - mildly increased exp sounds throughout. Otherwise clear to ausc (rales resolved)

1. Problem focused = 1-5 elements (level 2) 2. Expanded = 6-11 elements (level 3) 3. Detailed = 12 or more elements (level 4)
4. Comprehensive = document two (or more) elements in each of nine (or more) systems (level 5) *Optional

page 1

Date ____/____/____

Patient Name: **Joan Jones**   Account No. **123456**   DOB: **1/1/1968**

Established Visit Form (p. 2)

MEDICAL DECISION MAKING	
DATA REVIEWED (c):	**2 of the 3 sections (a vs a', b vs b' vs b", c vs c' vs c") must meet or exceed indicated level of care**
	1. Minimal (level 2) 2. Limited (level 3) 3. Moderate (level 4) 4. Extensive (level 5)

☐ X-ray/CT scan   ☐ See attached dictation

☐ MRI

☐ Lab/blood work

IMPRESSIONS / DIFFERENTIAL DIAGNOSES (a):   **PLANS / MANAGEMENT OPTIONS (a')**

1. Minimal (level 2)   2. Limited (level 3)   3. Multiple (level 4)   4. Extensive (level 5)

☐ See attached dictation

1) *Irritative tracheitis & rhinitis, resolving*   1) *Continue nicotine patch & taper*

2) *GERD resolving with Rx*   2) *Xxxxxx bid for one more month, will then go to qd*

3)   3) *Return 1 month*

4)   4)

5)   5)

DATA ORDERED (c'):   **1. Minimal or none (level 2)   2. Limited (level 3)   3. Moderate (level 4)   4. Extensive (level 5)**

☐   ☐   ☐   ☐   ☐

☐ See attached dictation

Information Sheets Given:

COMPLEXITY OF DATA REVIEWED OR ORDERED (a")

1. Minimal (level 2)   2. Limited (level 3)   3. Moderate (level 4)   4. Extensive (level 5)

1. min   2. limited   3. mod   4. extensive

RISK OF COMPLICATIONS &/OR MORBIDITY OR MORTALITY (see examples in Table of Risk)

1. Minimal (level 2)   2. Low (level 3)   3. Moderate (level 4)   4. High (level 5)

risk of presenting problem(s) (c):   1. min   (2. low)   3. mod   4. high

risk of diagnostic procedure(s) ordered or reviewed (c'):   1. min   2. low   3. mod   4. high

risk of management option(s) selected (c"):   1. min   2. low   (3. mod)   4. high

NATURE OF PRESENTING PROBLEM(S)

1. minor	(level 2)	Problem runs definite and prescribed course, is transient in nature, and is not likely to permanently alter health status; OR, has a good prognosis with management and compliance.
2. low	(level 2)	Problem in which the risk of morbidity without treatment is low. There is little to no risk of mortality without treatment. Full recovery without functional impairment is expected.
(3. low - mod)	(level 3)	Problem in which the risk of morbidity without treatment is low to moderate; there is low to moderate risk of mortality without treatment; full recovery without functional impairment is expected in most cases, with low probability of prolonged functional impairment
4. moderate	(level 3)	Problem in which the risk of morbidity without treatment is moderate. There is moderate risk of mortality without treatment. Prognosis is uncertain, or there is an increased probability of prolonged functional impairment.
5. mod - high	(levels 4,5)	Problem in which the risk of morbidity without treatment is moderate to high; there is moderate risk of mortality without treatment; uncertain prognosis or increased probability of prolonged functional impairment
6. high	(levels 4,5)	Problem in which the risk of morbidity without treatment is high to extreme. There is moderate to high risk of mortality without treatment, or high probability of severe prolonged functional impairment.

Complete this section only if documented below > 50% of visit time involved counseling and/or coordinating care.

TIME: _____ minutes   ☐ > 50% of visit time involved counseling and/or coordination of care

Clinician's signature: *ABC*

page 2

Date ____/____/_____

Patient Name:_____   Account No._____ DOB:____/____/_____

Established Visit Form (Supplement)

PHYSICAL EXAMINATION:		General Multisystem Exam (continued)							

Normal/AB (left section) and **Normal/AB** (right section)

System	Item	Method	Normal	AB		System	Item	Method	Normal	AB
GU/	SCROTAL CONTENTS	Appearance, palpation	☐	☐	MSKEL	HEAD & NECK	Inspec., palp., percussion	☐	☐
MALE	PENIS	Appearance, palpation	☐	☐			Range of motion	☐	☐
	PROSTATE	Palpation	☐	☐			Stability or laxity	☐	☐
GU/	EXT GENITALIA	Appearance, palpation	☐	☐			Muscle strength & tone	☐	☐
FEMALE	URETHRA	Inspection	☐	☐		SPINE, RIBS, PELVIS	Inspec., palp., percussion	☐	☐
(PELVIC)	BLADDER	Palpation	☐	☐			Range of motion	☐	☐
	CERVIS	Palpation	☐	☐			Stability or laxity	☐	☐
	UTERUS	Palpation	☐	☐			Muscle strength & tone	☐	☐
	ADNEXA/PARAMET	Palpation	☐	☐		RT UPPER EXTREMITY	Inspec., palp., percussion	☐	☐
SKIN/	INSPECTION	Head, trunk, RUE	☐	☐			Range of motion	☐	☐
SUBCU		LUE, RLE, LLE	☐	☐			Stability or laxity	☐	☐
	PALPATION	Head, trunk, RUE	☐	☐			Muscle strength & tone	☐	☐
		LUE, RLE, LLE	☐	☐		LT UPPER EXTREMITY	Inspec., palp., percussion	☐	☐
NEURO	CRANIAL NERVES	II - XII	☐	☐			Range of motion	☐	☐
	DEEP TENDON REFLEXES	Knee, ankle, Babinski	☐	☐			Stability or laxity	☐	☐
	SENSATION	Light touch	☐	☐			Muscle strength & tone	☐	☐
PSYCH	JUDGEMENT & INSIGHT	Subjectively	☐	☐		RT LOWER EXTREMITY	Inspec., palp., percussion	☐	☐
	ORIENTATION	Person, place, time	☐	☐			Range of motion	☐	☐
	MEMORY	Recent & remote	☐	☐			Stability or laxity	☐	☐
	MOOD & AFFECT	Comments	☐	☐			Muscle strength & tone	☐	☐
MSKEL	GAIT & STATION	Stability & smoothness	☐	☐		LT LOWER EXTREMITY	Inspec., palp., percussion	☐	☐
	DIGITS & NAILS	Color & appearance	☐	☐			Range of motion	☐	☐
							Stability or laxity	☐	☐
	☐ See attached dictation						Muscle strength & tone	☐	☐

1. Problem focused = 1-5 elements (level 2)   2. Expanded = 6-11 elements (level 3)   3. Detailed = 12 or more elements (level 4)
4. Comprehensive = document two (or more) elements in each of nine (or more) systems (level 5)   *Optional

Exam Supplement

Benchmarks for EHR Design and Functionality

Physicians' primary goals and requirements for health information technology

1. Data storage and retrieval component
    a. Immediate access to medical charts from any location at any time
    b. Reduce or eliminate costs of operating a paper chart system

2. Data entry component
    a. Solve the problem of evaluation and management (E/M) compliance
    b. Improve the quality and efficiency of the medical history and physical examination (H&P) record
    c. Improve practice productivity

Benchmarks for electronic health record (EHR) software systems

1. Implementation success should be 100%

2. Training success: physician time for customization and full training in effective use of the H&P component should require less than 8 hours

3. Efficiency success: the electronic H&P record must facilitate completion of patient care and E/M compliant documentation for a comprehensive (ie, level 5) new patient visit, with appropriate medical necessity, in not more than ___ minutes of physician time
    a. Each specialty may have different time constraints, so each practice should enter its own benchmark for optimal efficiency. For example, experience in otolaryngology suggests than 15 minutes may be reasonable for many practitioners in that specialty

4. Productivity success: no decrease in practice productivity following EHR implementation
    a. Increased productivity for physicians not currently overcoding

5. Compliance success: design and functionality that, when used as designed, guide and ensure that every visit fulfills all requirements for E/M compliance, including consideration and documentation of medical necessity

6. Quality care success: requires entry of *individualized* narrative documentation, with absence of preloaded and/or generic clinical information for all appropriate sections of the H&P (ie, HPI, description of positive responses in the PFSH and ROS, description of abnormal and pertinent normal findings of physical examination, impressions section of the MDM, and the treatment options section of the MDM)

   a. Another physician, or an attorney, can read the clinical record and find it understandable and appropriate for the patient and that it makes medical sense.

Practical EHR Axioms

*P*ractical *EHR* has presented a number of fundamental principles related to physicians' goals and requirements. Many of them are compiled here for convenience.

1. Electronic Health Record (EHR) systems must be operable as well as interoperable (Chapter 1).

2. EHR systems must provide value to a practice as well as clinical capability (Chapter 1).

3. The data entry features *must* help physicians efficiently provide and document a high-quality (and compliant) history and physical examination (H&P) (Chapter 2).

4. Implementation success: 100% of EHR implementations should be successful (Chapter 2).

5. Efficiency Success: Design and functionality of EHR systems must facilitate completion of the care and compliant documentation for a medically indicated *comprehensive* new patient visit (ie, CPT code 99204 or 99205) in *not more than 15 minutes of a physician's time* (Chapter 2).

6. Productivity success: There should be no decrease in practice productivity on implementation of an effective EHR system (Chapter 2).

7. E/M compliance succcess: EHR must incorporate compliance-based design and functionality, thereby guiding physicians to provide and document an appropriate level of care during every medical encounter, based on consideration of medical necessity (Chapter 2).

8. Quality care success: EHRs must provide for documentation of free-text narrative descriptions in all sections of the H&P component that require input of *individualized* patient clinical information (Chapter 2).

9. Training success and efficiency: For physicians who are well trained in using an effective paper record, the training process for using the basic clinical information input features of a well-designed EHR should require no more than eight hours of a physician's time for software customization and learning (Chapter 2).

10. Although a major part of the *science* of medicine involves identifying the general disease category (ie, diagnosis) appropriate for each patient, a significant part of the *art* (and quality) of practicing medicine involves applying this diagnostic process, which helps to identify the distinctive aspects of each patient's medical issues and to determine when a patient's care warrants additional or atypical evaluation and/or management (Chapter 3).

11. A well-designed clinical record must support and record the physician's thought process, not supplant it (Chapter 3).

12. Although most physicians understand that documentation in the medical record should be a reflection of the quality of care provided, few appreciate the complementary insight that the depth and extent of the care they provide is very much influenced by the quality of the medical record they are using (Chapter 3).

13. While medical schools effectively train medical students to provide appropriate levels of comprehensive care using the medical diagnostic process, they also need to give them a set of tools that provides them with the ability to apply these principles under the demands of medical practice. It will be far easier to give students the tools that will keep them on the "right" road than it will be to try to rescue (and reeducate) them after they have detoured off of it (Chapter 3).

14. Data should supplement physicians' clinical impressions, not supplant them. The role of EHRs should be to help physicians implement the medical diagnostic process, not to replace physician expertise with automated responses based solely on laboratory findings and statistically based protocols (Chapter 4).

15. The foundation for quality care remains the identification of correct diagnoses in a timely manner, a goal that requires physicians to use the more sophisticated level of medical reasoning embodied in the diagnostic process (Chapter 4).

16. As with the external pressures for efficiency, the call for optimal productivity is the result of economic constriction created by reimbursement rates far lower than would be provided under a realistic resource-based system. A caution, which applies to physicians, administrators, and software developers, is that *overcoding is not an acceptable remedy to underpayment by insurers* (Chapter 5).

17. One of the cardinal rules of H&P design in EHRs must be that electronic systems cannot forgo quality care, compliance, and/or usability in an effort to increase speed (Chapter 5).

18. Physicians, insurers, and government agencies must all understand that there is a limit to how quickly physicians can see patients and continue to maintain *high-quality* evaluation and management (E/M) care, provide *appropriate* counseling to patients about their health issues, and complete *meaningful* documentation of those visits. It is important to note that physicians seem to have reached that limit. Any further decrease in the time that physicians have available for each patient visit owing to further reductions in reimbursement (and/or increases in practice expenses) may reasonably be expected to lead to decreases in quality care, patient safety, patient access, and cost-effectiveness (Chapter 7).

19. The electronic H&P component must avoid design or functionality that might promote, guide, or allow physician actions and documentation capable of interfering with optimal medical care and/or compliance (Chapter 7).

20. It is often even more important to find and address the differences among patients with similar clinical manifestations than it is to recognize their similarities (Chapter 7).

21. Although some currently available systems focus primarily on speed of documentation, *Practical EHR* mandates that usability, compliance, quality, and data integrity have the highest priority. Efficiency can be maximized only to the extent that it does not interfere with optimal results for these critical factors (Chapter 8).

22. Failure to recognize the necessity of maintaining and facilitating physicians' workflow and the entire diagnostic process is at the core of EHR issues that challenge usability, compliance, quality care standards, efficiency, and data integrity. As a fundamental principle, software design should not change or disrupt physicians' normal workflow for achieving optimal patient care; rather, designs should reinforce and facilitate this process (Chapter 8).

23. The EHR is a sophisticated tool whose design and functionality must be directed to helping physicians provide the best patient care possible. The EHR must supplement physicians' knowledge and judgment, not supplant them through automatic insertion of programmed clinical information and/or automated decisions regarding patient care (Chapter 10).

24. Physicians should anticipate achieving four major goals when employing compliant E/M methodology combined with intelligent medical record designs, even for records stored in a paper format:

    ■ Equal or increased quality of patient care.

    ■ Equal or improved efficiency (time spent).

    ■ E/M-compliant and "audit proof" documentation and coding.

    ■ Equal or increased levels of productivity, ie, compliant E/M code levels should increase [unless a physician is systematically overcoding] (Chapter 10).

25. *Practical EHR* recommends that in designing the various components of the electronic H&P, compliance should provide a starting platform on which each physician can build a quality-based superstructure that meets the highest standards of his or her specialty and personal values (Chapter 10).

26. Design elements intended to promote rapid entry of clinical information must also ensure compliant documentation and maintain the medical diagnostic process (Chapter 10).

27. The data input design should provide so much flexibility that physicians currently performing and recording a quality H&P will feel that the software is able to fit their personal documentation preferences and practice style, not require changing them (Chapter 11).

28. Physicians and their medical standards must dictate the direction and ultimate goals of a medical practice's transition to EHRs (Chapter 17).

29. The current approach to practice transformation (illustrated in Figure 17.1) has resulted in unsatisfactory outcomes and significant negative financial, professional, and emotional consequences for a large number of practices. Therefore, continuing to use the same approach to evaluating, purchasing, and implementing EHRs should not be an acceptable option (Chapter 19).

30. The stakes for success and failure are equally high for small and large practices; similarly the benefits of good preparation and laying a solid

foundation are just as great for both. Every hour invested in good preparation will be returned by the many hours saved during training, software verification, and implementation. Every dollar invested in obtaining expert guidance will generate a compounded return by preventing reductions in productivity, safely improving documentation and coding, and diminishing the risks of an unsatisfactory or failed implementation. From this perspective, no practice, large or small, can afford *not* to invest in a thorough and meticulous preparation (Chapter 19).

31. Speed is not efficiency. *Practical EHR* maintains a distinction between electronic H&P tools that promote efficiency and those that focus on speed. To be labeled as *efficient,* design tools that allow physicians to document faster must also continue to support the diagnostic process, ensure 100% E/M compliance, and permit only the recording of patient-specific and visit-specific clinical information. Designs that promote this type of efficiency are highly desirable. Designs that allow faster documentation but also introduce the potential for reducing the amount of care actually provided, impairing quality, failing to achieve compliance, and/or sacrificing data integrity are labeled as "speed tools," which are considered unacceptable (Chapter 20).

32. (On reassessing existing EHR systems): Physicians have every right to expect their software systems to facilitate compliant documentation and offer the high-quality H&P documentation required as a foundation for optimal care for their patients. Vendors who desire to have successful installations, with satisfied physicians and medical practices that endorse their software, will benefit (Chapter 21).